Pulmonary Manifestations of Rheumatic Disease

Paul F. Dellaripa · Aryeh Fischer
Kevin R. Flaherty
Editors

Pulmonary Manifestations of Rheumatic Disease

A Comprehensive Guide

With 64 Figures, 26 in Color

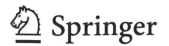

Editors
Paul F. Dellaripa
Division of Rheumatology
Department of Medicine
Brigham and Women's Hospital
Boston, MA, USA

Kevin R. Flaherty
Department of Internal Medicine
Division of Pulmonary/Critical Care
  Medicine
University of Michigan Medical School
Ann Arbor, MI, USA

Aryeh Fischer
Division of Rheumatology
Autoimmune and Interstitial Lung
  Disease Program
Department of Medicine
National Jewish Health
Denver, CO, USA

ISBN 978-1-4939-0769-4   ISBN 978-1-4939-0770-0 (eBook)
DOI 10.1007/978-1-4939-0770-0
Springer New York Heidelberg Dordrecht London

Library of Congress Control Number: 2014939120

Printed on acid-free paper

Springer is part of Springer Science+Business Media (www.springer.com)

We would like to dedicate this book to our wives, children, and parents.

P.D., A.F., K.F.

Preface

Our understanding and treatment of rheumatologic disease have undergone a revolution over the last 20 years that has resulted in markedly improved patient outcomes and quality of life. However, the area of pulmonary manifestations in the rheumatic diseases has historically been poorly understood and under-recognized, with the real potential for significant morbidity and mortality. Over the past 10 years, however, there has been a groundswell of clinical interest and inquiry through the formation of a consortium of diverse investigators from the fields of pulmonary medicine, rheumatology, pathology, and radiology, which has led to preliminary but important insights into these disorders. As such, we felt the time was right to dedicate a first-of-its-kind text to highlight and summarize our present knowledge, therapies, and potential future advances in the field of lung disease and the rheumatic diseases. This text focuses on clinical manifestations and management with a practical, case-based approach, and virtually all chapters are co-written by specialists from the fields of rheumatology and pulmonary medicine, as we try to address and appeal to a broad clinical audience that may be caring for such patients. We hope this text serves as a useful clinical resource for our readers as we move forward in this fascinating and clinically challenging intersection between autoimmunity and pulmonary disease.

We would like to thank all of the chapter authors of this text for their excellent contributions and, of course, we thank our patients. We also wish to thank our publisher, Springer Science + Business Media, and our editors (Kristopher Spring and Liz Corra) for their diligent efforts to complete this project.

Boston, MA, USA   Paul F. Dellaripa
Denver, CO, USA   Aryeh Fischer
Ann Arbor, MI, USA   Kevin R. Flaherty

Contents

Contributors

Kevin K. Brown, M.D. Department of Medicine, National Jewish Health, Denver, CO, USA

Kevin M. Chan, M.D. Division of Pulmonary and Critical Care Medicine, Department of Internal Medicine, University of Michigan Health System, Ann Arbor, MI, USA

Daniel A. Culver, D.O. Respiratory Institute, Cleveland Clinic, Cleveland, OH, USA

Sonye K. Danoff, M.D., Ph.D. Division of Pulmonary/Critical Care Medicine, Department of Medicine, Johns Hopkins University School of Medicine, Baltimore, MD, USA

Paul F. Dellaripa, M.D. Division of Rheumatology, Department of Medicine, Harvard Medical School, Brigham and Women's Hospital, Boston, MA, USA

Barri J. Fessler, M.D., M.S.P.H. Division of Clinical Immunology and Rheumatology, University of Alabama at Birmingham, Birmingham, AL, USA

Aryeh Fischer, M.D. Division of Rheumatology, Department of Medicine, Autoimmune Lung Center, National Jewish Health, Denver, CO, USA

Kevin R. Flaherty, M.D., M.S. Department of Internal Medicine, Division of Pulmonary/Critical Care Medicine, University of Michigan Medical School, Ann Arbor, MI, USA

Ritu R. Gill, M.D., M.P.H. Department of Radiology, Brigham and Women's Hospital, Boston, MA, USA

Ryan Hadley, M.D. Division of Pulmonary and Critical Care Medicine, Department of Internal Medicine, University of Michigan Health System, Ann Arbor, MI, USA

Kristin B. Highland, M.D., M.S.C.R. Respiratory Institute, Cleveland Clinic, Cleveland, OH, USA

Laura K. Hummers, M.D., Sc.M. Department of Medicine/Rheumatology, Johns Hopkins University School of Medicine, Baltimore, MD, USA

Cheilonda Johnson, M.D., M.H.S. Division of Pulmonary/Critical Care Medicine, Department of Medicine, Johns Hopkins University Hospital, School of Medicine, Baltimore, MD, USA

Joel T. Katz, M.D., M.A. Department of Medicine, Brigham and Women's Hospital, Boston, MA, USA

Tracy R. Luckhardt, M.D., M.S. Department of Pulmonary, Allergy and Critical Care Medicine, University of Alabama Birmingham, Birmingham, AL, USA

Toby M. Maher, M.B., M.Sc., Ph.D., F.R.C.P. Interstitial Lung Disease Unit, Royal Brompton & Harefield Foundation NHS Trust, London, UK

Stephen C. Mathai, M.D., M.H.S. Division of Pulmonary and Critical Care Medicine, Johns Hopkins University School of Medicine, Baltimore, MD, USA

Eric L. Matteson, M.D., M.P.H. Division of Rheumatology, Department of Medicine, Mayo Clinic College of Medicine, Rochester, MN, USA

Division of Epidemiology, Department of Health Science Research, Mayo Clinic College of Medicine, Rochester, MN, USA

Shikha Mittoo, M.D., M.H.S., F.R.C.P.C. Department of Medicine/Rheumatology, Mount Sinai Hospital, Toronto, ON, Canada

Chester V. Oddis, M.D. Division of Rheumatology, Department of Medicine, University of Pittsburgh Medical Center, Pittsburgh, PA, USA

Jonathan B. Parr, M.D., M.P.H. Department of Medicine, Brigham and Women's Hospital, Boston, MA, USA

Jay H. Ryu, M.D. Division of Pulmonary and Critical Care Medicine, Mayo Clinic College of Medicine, Rochester, MN, USA

Richard M. Silver, M.D. Division of Rheumatology and Immunology, Medical University of South Carolina, Charleston, SC, USA

Ulrich Specks, M.D. Division of Pulmonary and Critical Care Medicine, Mayo Clinic Rochester, Rochester, MN, USA

Virginia Steen, M.D. Department of Medicine, Georgetown University Medical Center, Washington, DC, USA

Jeffrey J. Swigris, D.O., M.S. Autoimmune Lung Center and Interstitial Lung Disease Program, National Jewish Health, Denver, CO, USA

Nargues Weir, M.D. Department of Medicine, NIH-Inova Advanced Lung Disease Program, Falls Church, VA, USA

The Lung in Rheumatic Diseases

Paul F. Dellaripa and Kevin R. Flaherty

Introduction

Pulmonary manifestations of rheumatic disease are among the least understood but potentially life-threatening complications among rheumatic diseases. It has only been within recent years that a concerted effort has been made to understand lung diseases in connective tissue disease (CTD) in terms of classification, appropriate diagnostic testing, and treatment strategies especially with regard to interstitial lung diseases (ILDs). Part of the challenge associated with CTD ILD has been the fact that these conditions are rare, clinical presentations can be heterogeneous, and the natural history is unpredictable and still not well understood. Furthermore, while much of our understanding regarding CTD ILD is based on our experiences in scleroderma, it is unclear how well these findings carry over into other CTDs in terms of natural history, mechanisms of disease, and potential response to treatment. In this chapter and text, we will provide an overview of our current knowledge of this fascinating intersection of rheumatology, autoimmunity, and pulmonary medicine by illustrating important emerging concepts and providing cases that reflect the complexity and challenges associated with lung disease in patients with CTDs, with a particular focus on parenchymal lung disease.

Disease Classification

One of the most difficult aspects in classifying patients with ILD is that the symptoms, physiologic abnormalities, radiographic findings, and even histopathology can be identical for patients with idiopathic disease (idiopathic interstitial pneumonia, IIP), ILD in the setting of CTD, or ILD due to other infectious, environmental, or even medication exposures. Thus, it is critical during the evaluation of a patient with ILD to determine if the patient has idiopathic ILD, connective tissue-associated ILD, or other possible causes of parenchymal lung disease. This evaluation should be ongoing as in some patients the pulmonary manifestations of a CTD precede involvement in other systems. This distinction appears to be important from a survival perspective [1, 2], whereby patients with CTD/ILD overall have a better prognosis, with the exception of RA-associated UIP [3]. Recent data also suggest that immunosuppressive therapy for IPF may be harmful while it remains a cornerstone of treatment for CTD ILD [4]. ILD associated with undifferentiated connective disease and the so-called

P.F. Dellaripa, M.D. (✉)
Division of Rheumatology, Department of Medicine, Harvard Medical School, Brigham and Women's Hospital, 75 Francis Street, Boston, MA 02115, USA
e-mail: pdellaripa@partners.org

K.R. Flaherty, M.D., M.S.
Department of Internal Medicine, Division of Pulmonary/Critical Care Medicine, University of Michigan Medical School, 1500 East Medical Center Drive, 3916 Taubman Center, Ann Arbor, MI 48109, USA

P.F. Dellaripa et al. (eds.), *Pulmonary Manifestations of Rheumatic Disease: A Comprehensive Guide*,
DOI 10.1007/978-1-4939-0770-0_1, © Springer Science+Business Media New York 2014

"lung-dominant" CTD where ILD is the principal manifestation of an underlying autoimmune disease is a challenging but important area of investigation, since such patients may benefit from anti-inflammatory therapy. A classification scheme that incorporates clinical manifestations (pulmonary and extrapulmonary), radiographic features, physiology, antibody profiles, and tissue type (when available) is at this time not well constructed but could be useful to help guide the clinician in deciding if CTD/ILD is present as well as aiding in monitoring response to treatment.

Similar to IPF, decline in lung function for CTD ILD patients is often unpredictable as in many patients, disease progression will be slow or will remain subclinical. Thus, aggressive treatment intervention without a clear sense of prognosis or disease course runs the risk of overtreatment or inappropriate treatment. For example, in the treatment of scleroderma, selection of patients that are at most risk for decline in forced vital capacity (FVC) and extent of lung involvement represents patients with the highest risk of progression and most appropriate for treatment and inclusion into clinical trials [5]. Biomarkers in the serum or bronchoalveolar lavage (BAL) such as KL-6 and surfactant protein D offer another potential approach to define those at highest risk for progression or gauge response to therapy and represent an area of active investigation [6]. In addition, there is not yet an agreement on which parameters—clinical (such as patient-reported outcomes), physiologic (pulmonary function testing, oxygen use, etc.), or radiographic (ground glass, fibrosis)—should be used to monitor for disease progression, although FVC remains the most utilized marker to date.

Scleroderma

Pulmonary complications are common in scleroderma, specifically ILD, and are clinically significant in at least 50 % of patients with diffuse disease and in up to 30 % of patients with limited disease. ILD tends to be more severe in African Americans [7]. Typical pathologic patterns include NSIP most commonly with UIP, COP,

and DAD less common. ILD is a leading cause of mortality and morbidity in this disease, yet the clinical progression and natural history can be variable, making it difficult to identify which patients are at highest risk for decline in pulmonary function and thus warrant treatment. The pathogenesis of lung disease involves the innate and adaptive immune systems, fibroblastic proliferation, and endothelial dysfunction. Activated macrophages and T cells induce growth factors such as TGF-beta, which appears to be a central player in the development of fibrosis. Other growth factors, such as platelet-derived growth factor, chitinases, and metalloproteinases such as MMP 12 may play a role in the inflammatory process and serve as potential targets therapeutically [8, 9]. Esophageal dysfunction and dysmotility leading to overt or microaspiration occur with significant frequency in scleroderma and may play an important role in either initiation or propagation of parenchymal lung disease in scleroderma and other CTDs and is an area of active clinical investigation [10].

Treatment of Scleroderma Lung Disease

As noted, decisions regarding treatment in scleroderma lung disease are complicated by a lack of clear clinical end points or biomarkers that predict which patients will develop aggressive or progressive disease. However, prospective data is emerging that may begin to clarify and predict prognosis and thus guide treatment decisions, including extent of fibrosis on HRCT, decline of FVC, level of skin involvement, genetic variants identified in GWAS studies, and specific characteristics of alveolar fluid [5, 11–14].

Data from two studies utilizing cyclophosphamide showed a modest improvement in FVC, most notably in patients with greater degrees of fibrosis, though the benefits of this medication are limited by side effects and limitations to duration of therapy. Again, inclusion in these studies did not discriminate for those that might be most responsive to therapy [15, 16]. The use of mycophenolate mofetil in scleroderma ILD has shown promise and is under clinical investigation [17]. The B cell-deleting agent rituximab is also under active investigation as a therapeutic agent in scleroderma though its role in ILD is uncertain and controlled trials are not yet available [18].

Other agents such as tyrosine kinase inhibitors, histone deacetylase inhibitors, and inhibition of morphogenic pathways offer novel approaches to attenuate fibrosis in scleroderma and other fibrosing disorders [19].

The role of steroids in the treatment of ILD is uncertain and has not been studied in a prospective trial. As there are concerns for inducing renal crisis in susceptible patients who are given high-dose steroids, many clinicians will consider using moderate or low doses of corticosteroids in combination with other immunosuppressive agents.

At this time, in those patients with active or progressive parenchymal lung diseases, immunomodulation with agents such as cyclophosphamide either intravenously or orally or mycophenolate or azathioprine are reasonable options in patients with suspected progressive or aggressive lung disease. Patients with concomitant ILD and pulmonary hypertension represent additional clinical challenges. Treatment with both immunomodulating therapies and therapy for PAH can be difficult and mortality is likely higher in these patients.

Case Vignette 1 that follows illustrates how aggressive treatment in a patient with limited scleroderma can result in substantial improvement in radiographic appearance of ILD though concomitant development of pulmonary hypertension can develop and require therapy.

Case Vignette 1

A 50-year-old male with limited scleroderma developed painful hands, sclerodactyly, and progressive dyspnea, with declining lung function (DLCO 50 %). Figure 1.1a shows bilateral ground-glass opacities and reticular changes. He was treated with 30 mg prednisone and IV cyclophosphamide monthly for 9 months, and in Fig. 1.1b there is substantial clearing of these findings post 9 months of treatment. He was transitioned to mycophenolate, but due to a continued decline in DLCO (39 %), a right heart catheterization was performed and indicated the development of early pulmonary hypertension which was treated with sildenafil.

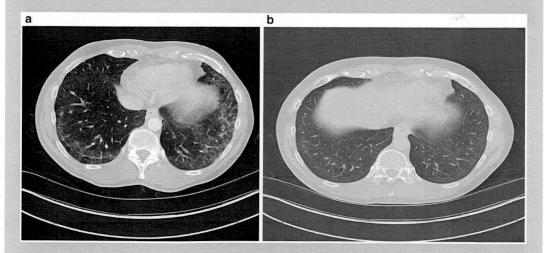

Fig. 1.1 (a) Bilateral ground-glass opacities and reticular changes in the subpleural regions of both lungs. (b) Substantial clearing of these findings post 9 months of treatment with cyclophosphamide

Rheumatoid Arthritis

In RA, all aspects of the respiratory system can be involved, but the lung parenchyma and airways present specific challenges that can impact morbidity and mortality and may often be involved together. Population data suggests the presence of ILD in RA results in a higher mortality among RA patients and that ILD can present prior to, concomitant with, or after the development of articular symptoms. Based on national population data, ILD occurs in approximately 10 % of patients with RA, and the predominant pathologic phenotype is UIP, with mortality in some studies approaching that seen with IPF [20–22]. The role of smoking and RA and the development of ILD are an area of active research as well as the increasing recognition of the presence of ILD and emphysema concomitantly in

RA patients [23]. Interesting research in the role of the shared epitope suggests a higher risk of ILD in RA patients expressing HLA DR2, potentially identifying a subgroup of RA patients at risk for ILD [24].

Airway involvement in the lung in RA presents unique challenges. Airway involvement includes BOOP/COP, follicular bronchiolitis, and obliterative bronchiolitis (OB), which may present with predominately obstructive disease that has variable response to anti-inflammatory and immunomodulatory therapy [25]. In some instances, such as in OB, there is no effective therapy and lung transplant becomes the only viable option. As Case Vignette 2 that follows illustrates, recognition of distinct clues to diagnosis, such as the presence of mosaicism on CT scan and obstruction on spirometry, can correlate with inflammatory bronchiolar disease on pathology and can influence treatment decisions.

Case Vignette 2

Pt x is a 56-year-old female with longstanding RA who developed slowly progressive dyspnea on exertion, and obstruction on pulmonary functions testing, thought to be related to asthma. Short courses of steroids resulted in temporary improvement in respiratory symptoms. In Fig. 1.2a, a CT scan shows air trapping or mosaicism. Lung biopsy (Fig. 1.2b) confirms the presence of dense lymphoid follicles

surrounding bronchioles. The patient was treated with Rituxan with stabilization in symptoms and improvement in obstruction in PFTs.

Rheumatoid nodulosis is a common finding on lung imaging of patients with RA and can sometimes be problematic. Though unusual, select cases can result in rupture of nodules which can lead to pneumothorax and these lesions can occasionally become infected, which can be difficult to treat.

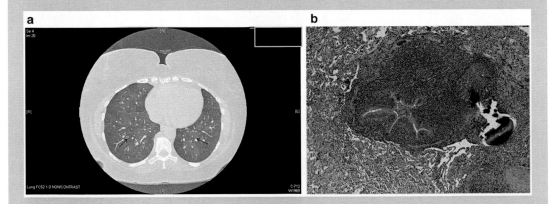

Fig. 1.2 (**a**) Chest CT shows air trapping or mosaicism. (**b**) Lung biopsy confirms the presence of dense lymphoid follicles surrounding bronchioles

(continued)

Inflammatory Myositis

Lung involvement in inflammatory myositis (IIM) is relatively common, variable in its severity and potentially life threatening. Parenchymal lung disease can be complicated by concomitant muscle weakness due to myositis and aspiration related to esophageal dysmotility. While overall morbidity and mortality may be more favorable than RA ILD and scleroderma ILD, recent reports suggest rapidly progressive disease can occur, especially in patients with amyopathic disease and those with the MDA 5 antibody [29]. The pathology seen most frequently in IIM/ILD is NSIP, while UIP, COP, and DAD are seen less commonly. In patients with inflammatory myositis with rapidly progressive ILD, aggressive immunosuppressive therapy is indicated and may be potentially lifesaving but may not be sufficient to prevent decline, and so transplant evaluation must sometimes be considered in concert with medical therapy. ILD is particularly common among myositis patients with the antisynthetase syndrome, as in patient with Jo-1 antibody, and in some series lung disease is the primary manifestation and myositis is less common [30–32].

Spontaneous pneumomediastinum is an unusual complication seen in IIM and often seen in concert with ILD and often associated with amyopathic cases of DM. The etiology of this phenomenon is unknown though it may represent the presence of either vasculopathic lesions in the airways or be related to architectural distortion due to interstitial disease. Treatment typically focuses on treatment of the underlying parenchymal lung disorder as Case Vignette 3 that follows illustrates [33].

(continued)

Case Vignette 3 (continued)

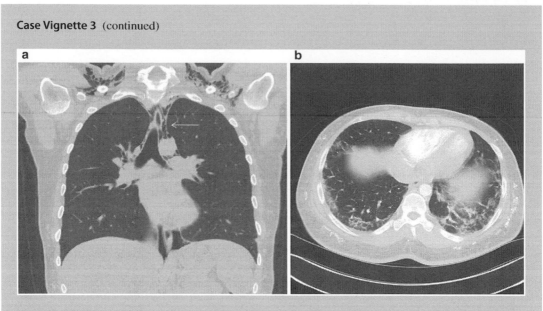

Fig. 1.3 (a) CT of the chest shows evidence of air in the mediastinum. (b) Reticular infiltrates in the subpleural regions

Systemic Lupus Erythematosus

Systemic lupus can present with many manifestations, including pleurisy, acute pneumonitis, and very rarely chronic progressive ILD. In rare patients, diffuse alveolar hemorrhage may present as part of the initial disease manifestation, requiring aggressive therapeutic intervention though large case series and prospective data are lacking. Given the role of immune complexes in such patients, this may be one of the few circumstances in addition to vasculitic syndromes where plasmapheresis may play a role in initial therapy for severe respiratory failure in the face of alveolar hemorrhage.

In the shrinking lung syndrome, recent evidence suggests that lung compliance and the relationship of pain associated with pleurisy may play an important role in this poorly understood syndrome though the role of immunomodulatory therapy in this condition is uncertain [34]. In addition, the presence of antiphospholipid antibodies can be associated with PE, DAH, and pulmonary hypertension. Finally, as in scleroderma, pulmonary hypertension may develop with or without other lung manifestations and must be considered in all systemic lupus erythematosus (SLE) patients with worsening dyspnea.

Sjogren's Syndrome

Sjogren's Syndrome (SS) can present with a variety of lung manifestations ranging from xerotrachea; bronchial disease such as follicular bronchiolitis; parenchymal lung disease including UIP, NSIP, and LIP; amyloidosis; and nodular and cystic lung disease [35]. Distinguishing between benign lymphoid aggregates and underlying lymphoma can be difficult and in some cases lung biopsy may be necessary. Given the central role of B cell proliferation in SS, B cell deletion therapy may play an important role in selected cases where lung biopsy suggests that lymphocytic infiltration is a significant pathological feature [36].

Vasculitis

Pulmonary manifestations in vasculitis include nodular lung disease, pleuritis, and parenchymal disease. Diffuse alveolar hemorrhage is an important and life-threatening feature of vasculitic syndromes seen in ANCA-associated disease such as granulomatosis with polyangiitis (GPA) and microscopic polyangiitis (MPA), Goodpasture's disease, and rarely cryoglobulinemia and SLE. Pulmonary vasculitis and pulmonary aneurysms can be seen in Behcet's and is a significant source of morbidity in that disorder. Capillaritis may manifest with frank hemop-tysis or may be notable only on CT scan, evidenced by ground-glass opacities, and may at times not be evident on bronchoscopy. In some patients, a falling hematocrit or elevated diffusion capacity may be a clinical clue to ongoing hemorrhage. The presence of concomitant interstitial fibrosis (UIP) and airway obstruction with vasculitis has been noted in some cases of ANCA-associated disease, and the risk of VTE in ANCA-associated disease has been well established [37]. Ongoing research focusing on the role of plasmapheresis in patients with pulmonary hemorrhage and vasculitis and emerging therapies with biologic therapies will hopefully improve outcomes and limit drug toxicity.

Case Vignette 4

In this case, a 55-year-old male presented for evaluation for what was thought to be IPF. He was noted to have concomitant epistaxis, and his ANCA was markedly pos ANCA myeloperoxidase. HRCT (Fig. 1.4a) showed honeycombing (arrows), and a lung biopsy showed evidence of both fibrosis inflammation (Fig. 1.4b) and numerous lymphocytic aggregates. He was treated with a combination of rituximab and steroids and transitioned to mycophenolate with stabilization in lung function.

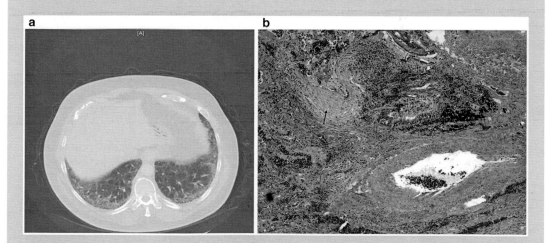

Fig. 1.4 (**a**) HRCT shows honeycombing (*arrows*) with reticular changes at the bases of both lung fields. (**b**) Evidence of fibrosis and lymphocytic aggregates on lung biopsy with *arrows* noting a fibroblastic foci

Drug-Induced Interstitial Lung Disease

While drug-induced ILD in rheumatic disease patients is rare, virtually every medication used in such patients has been implicated in causing ILD [38]. In many cases of drug-induced ILD, the initiation of a specific DMARD or biologic agent will lead to a noninfectious pulmonary process in a temporally identifiable period of time that clearly defines a drug-induced parenchymal reaction. However, identification of a drug-induced ILD may be difficult in those patients with preexisting ILD or where infection is suspected but no infectious agent is clearly identified. Drug reactions may range from localized infiltrates with fever and cough to diffuse infiltrates suggestive of acute lung injury (DAD), resulting in hypoxemic respiratory failure and death. Mechanisms of injury may be related to drug-induced direct cytotoxic injury to pneumocytes and respiratory endothelium such as with methotrexate or in some cases may be related to immune-mediated injury [39, 40].

While clearly identifiable cases of drug toxicity have been identified, such as with methotrexate or TNF inhibitors, gold, and other agents, there is considerable controversy as to whether these agents can exacerbate preexisting parenchymal lung disease. In particular, there has been concern with the use of TNF inhibitors in patients with underlying ILD, especially in RA. However, separating out confounding factors such as concomitant use of other drugs that may increase risk of ILD (such as MTX) or severity of underlying rheumatic disease make drawing such conclusions regarding worsening or initiation of ILD by the suspected drug extremely challenging. In the future, biomarkers may be available that help identify those populations that are at higher risk for drug-induced ILD [41]. Suffice to say that in patients with rheumatic disease where even mild ILD exists who require DMARD or biologic therapy, close surveillance and collaboration between the rheumatologist and pulmonologist is appropriate and necessary.

Undifferentiated and Lung-Dominant CTD

In some cases, patients present with poorly differentiated features of CTD with emerging ILD. In such cases, ILD may present with features of autoimmune disease that are subtle (e.g., periungual erythema and photosensitive rash in the absence of muscle weakness) or they may present with ILD with serologic markers that suggest specific rheumatic diseases without clinical features of a specific CTD (e.g., ILD in a patient who is CCP antibody positive but who has not developed arthritis as in Case Vignette 5 that follows). The recently introduced concept of *lung-dominant CTD* has been proposed, whereby certain pathological findings noted on lung biopsy in the absence of typical clinical features of CTD and concomitant antibody profiles suggest autoimmune disease that is essentially limited to the lung [42].

Case Vignette 5

In this case, an 85-year-old male presented with incidental findings of multiple lung nodules (Fig. 1.5a) but no respiratory symptoms and normal pulmonary function testing. He subsequently developed a cough and a VATS was performed which showed organizing pneumonia, fibrosis, and bronchiolar infiltration (Fig. 1.5b, arrow). Serologic evaluation revealed a high-titer CCP antibody but no other clinical features for RA to date.

(continued)

Case Vignette 5 (continued)

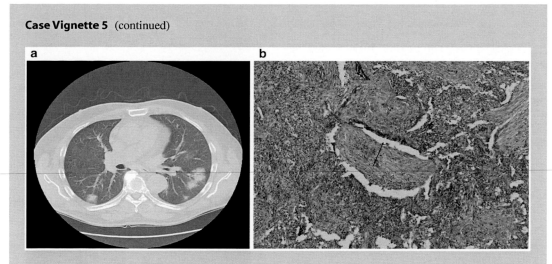

Fig. 1.5 (**a**) CT shows asymptomatic pulmonary nodules. (**b**) Lung biopsy shows organizing pneumonia, fibrosis, and bronchiolar infiltration

Conclusion

In summary, it is imperative for the pulmonologist to keep an open mind to the possibility that a patient with ILD may have an underlying systemic autoimmune disorder and that clinical features of those systemic disorders may be either subtle or initially absent and rheumatologists must be keenly aware and vigilant for the development of these complications in patients with rheumatic diseases. As such, close cooperation in a multidisciplinary fashion between specialties such as rheumatology and pulmonary medicine is imperative both for clinical care and research to improve the clinical outcomes and quality of life for these truly challenging patients [43].

References

1. Bouros D, Wells AU, Nicholson AG, et al. Histologic subsets of fibrosing alveolitis in patients with systemic sclerosis and their relationship to outcome. Am J Respir Med. 2002;165:1581–6.
2. Park JH, Kim DS, Park IN, et al. Prognosis of fibrotic interstitial pneumonia: idiopathic versus collagen vascular disease related subtypes. Am J Respir Crit Care Med. 2007;175:705–11.
3. Kim EJ, Elicker BM, Maldonado F, et al. Usual interstitial pneumonia in rheumatoid arthritis associated interstitial lung disease. Eur Respir J. 2010;35: 1322–8.
4. Raghu G, Anstrom KJ, King Jr TE, Lasky JA, Martinez FJ. Prednisone, azathioprine, and N-acetylcysteine for pulmonary fibrosis. Idiopathic Pulmonary Fibrosis Clinical Research Network. N Engl J Med. 2012;366(21):1968–77.
5. Goh NS, Desai SR, Veeraraghaven S, et al. Interstitial lung disease in systemic sclerosis: a simple staging system. Am J Respir Crit Care Med. 2008;177: 1248–54.
6. Bonella F, Volpe A, Caranachi P, et al. Surfactant protein D and KL-6 serum levels in systemic sclerosis: correlation with lung and systemic involvement. Sarcoidosis Vasc Diffuse Lung Dis. 2011;28:27–33.
7. Steen V, Domsic RT, Lucas M, Fertig N, Medsger Jr TA. A clinical and serologic comparison of African American and Caucasian patients with systemic sclerosis. Arthritis Rheum. 2012;64(9):2986–94.
8. Manetti M, Guiducci S, Romano E, et al. Increased serum levels and tissue expression of matrix metalloproteinase-12 n patients with systemic sclerosis: correlation with severity of skin and pulmonary fibrosis and vascular damage. Ann Rheum Dis. 2012;71(6): 1064–72.
9. Lee CG, Herzog EL, Ahangari F, et al. Chitinase I is a biomarker for and therapeutic target in scleroderma associated interstitial lung disease that augments TGF-B1 signaling. J Immunol. 2012;189(5): 2635–44.
10. Christmans RB, Wells AU, Capelozzi VL, Silver RM. GE reflux incites interstitial lung disease in systemic

sclerosis: clinical, radiologic, histopathologic and treatment evidence. Semin Arthritis Rheum. 2010; 40(3):241–9.

11. Roth MD, Tseng CH, Clements PJ, et al. Predicting treatment outcomes and responder subsets in scleroderma-related ILD. Arthritis Rheum. 2011; 63(9):2797–808.

12. Sharif R, Mayes MD, Tan FK, et al. IRF5 polymorphisms predicts prognosis in pts with SS. Ann Rheum Dis. 2012;71(7):1197–202.

13. Sfriso P, Cozzi F, Oliviero F, et al. CXCL11 in BAL and PFT decline in SS. Clin Exp Rheumatol. 2012;30(2 suppl 71):S71–5.

14. Tiev KP, Hua-Huy T, Kettaneh A, et al. Alveolar concentration of nitric oxide predicts in PFT deterioration in scleroderma. Thorax. 2012;67(2):157–63.

15. Tashkin DP, Elashof R, Clement P, et al. Cyclophosphamide versus placebo in scleroderma lung disease. N Engl J Med. 2006;354:2655–66.

16. Hoyles RK, Ellis RW, Wellsbury J, et al. A multicenter prospective randomized double blind placebo controlled trial of corticosteroids and intravenous cyclophosphamide followed by azathioprine for the treatment of pulmonary fibrosis in scleroderma. Arthritis Rheum. 2006;54:1962–70.

17. Mendoza FA, Nagle SJ, Lee JB, Jimenez SA. A prospective observational study of mycophenolate mofetil treatment in progressive diffuse cutaneous systemic sclerosis of recent onset. J Rheumatol. 2012;39(6):1241–7.

18. Daoussis D, Liossis SN, Tsamandas AC, Kalogeropoulou C, Paliogianni F, Sirinian C, Yiannopoulos G, Andonopoulos AP. Effect of long-term treatment with rituximab on pulmonary function and skin fibrosis in patients with diffuse systemic sclerosis. Clin Exp Rheumatol. 2012;30(2 Suppl 71): S17–22.

19. Beyer C, Distler O, Distler JH. Innovative antifibrotic therapies in SS. Curr Opin Rheumatol. 2012;24(3): 274–80.

20. Tsuchiya Y, Takayanagi N, Sugiura H, et al. Lung disease directly associated with rheumatoid arthritis and their relationship to outcome. Eur Respir J. 2011; 37(6):1411–7.

21. Olson AL, Swigris JJ, Springer DB, et al. rheumatoid arthritis—interstitial lung disease-associated mortality. Am J Respir Crit Care Med. 2011;183(3): 372–6.

22. Kim EJ, Collard HR, King Jr TE. Rheumatoid arthritis-associated interstitial lung disease: the relevance of histopathologic and radiographic pattern. Chest. 2009;136(5):1397–405.

23. Cottin V, Nunes H, Brillet PY, et al. Combined pulmonary fibrosis and emphysema: a distinct underrecognised entity. Eur Respir J. 2005;26(4):586–93.

24. Furukawa H, Oka S, Shimada K, et al. Associate of human leukocyte antigen with interstitial lung disease in rheumatoid arthritis: a protective role of shared epitopes. PLoS One. 2012;7(5):e33133.

25. Lynch 3rd JP, Weigt SS, DerHovanessian A, Fishbein MC, Gutierrez A, Belperio JA. Obliterative (constrictive) bronchiolitis. Semin Respir Crit Care Med. 2012;33(5):509–32.

26. Perez-Alvarez R, Perez-de-Lis M, Diaz-Lagares C, et al. Interstitial lung disease induced or exacerbated by TNF-targeted therapies: analysis of 122 cases. Semin Arthritis Rheum. 2011;41(2):256–64.

27. Dixon WG, Hyrich KL, Watson KD, et al. Influence of anti-TNF therapy on mortality in patients with rheumatoid arthritis associated interstitial lung disease: results from the British Society for Rheumatology Biologics Register. Ann Rheum Dis. 2010;69(6):1086–91.

28. Hadjinicoaou AV, Nisar MK, Bhagat S, et al. Non infectious pulmonary complications of newer biologic agents for rheumatic diseases; a systemic review of the literature. Rheumatology (Oxford). 2011; 50(12):2297–305.

29. Cao H, Pan M, Kang Y, et al. Clinical manifestations of dermatomyositis and clinical amyopathic dermatomyositis patient with positive expression of anti-MDA5 antibody. Arthritis Care Res. 2012;64(10): 1602–10.

30. Marie I, Hatron PY, Dominiqye S, et al. Short term and long term outcomes of interstitial lung disease in polymyositis and dermatomyositis :a series of 107 patients. Arthritis Rheum. 2011;63(11):3439–47.

31. Stanciu R, Guiguet M, Musset DT, et al. Antisynthetase syndrome with anti-Jo-1 antibodies in 48 patients: pulmonary involvement predicts disease-modifying antirheumatic drug use. J Rheumatol. 2012;39: 1835–9.

32. Kalluri M, Sahn SA, Oddis CV, et al. Clinical profile of anti-PL-12 autoantibody. Cohort study and review of the literature. Chest. 2009;135(6):1550–6.

33. Le Goff B, Chérin P, Cantagrel A, et al. Pneumomediastinum in interstitial lung disease associated with dermatomyositis and polymyositis. Arthritis Rheum. 2009;61(1):108.

34. Henderson LA, Loring SH, Gill RR, et al. Shrinking lung syndrome as a manifestation of pleuritis: a new model based on pulmonary physiological studies. J Rheumatol. 2013;40(3):273–81.

35. Watanabe M, Naniwa T, Hara M, Arakawa T, Maeda TSO. Pulmonary manifestations in Sjogren's syndrome: correlation analysis between chest computed tomographic findings and clinical subsets with poor prognosis in 80 patients. J Rheumatol. 2010;37(2): 365–73.

36. Swartz MA, Vivino FB. Dramatic reversal of lymphocytic interstitial pneumonitis in Sjögren's syndrome with rituximab. J Clin Rheumatol. 2011 Dec;17(8):454. J Rheumatol. 2010;37(2):365.

37. Seo P, Yuan IM, Holbrook JT, et al. For the WGET Research Group. Damage caused by Wegener's granulomatosis and its treatment: prospective data Form the Wegener's Granulomatosis Etanercept Trial (WGET). Arthritis Rheum. 2005;52:2168–78.

38. Roubille C, Haraui B. Interstitial lung diseases induced or exacerbated by DMARDS and biologic agents in rheumatoid arthritis: a systemic literature review. Semin Arthritis Rheum. 2013 Oct 5. pii: S0049-0172(13)00201-1. doi: 10.1016/j.semarthrit.2013. 09.005. [Epub ahead of print].

39. Kim YJ, Song M, Ryu JC. Mechanisms underlying methotrexate-induced pulmonary toxicity. Expert Opin Drug Saf. 2009;8:451–8.

40. Guillon JM, Joly P, Autran B, et al. Minocycline-induced cell mediated hypersensitivity pneumonitis. Ann Intern Med. 1992;117:476–81.

41. Furukama H, Oka S, Shimada K. HLA-A *31:01 and methotrexate-induced interstitial lung disease in Japanese rheumatoid arthritis patients: a multidrug hypersensitivity marker? Ann Rheum Dis. 2013;72: 153–5.

42. Fischer A, West SG, Swigris JJ, et al. CTD associated ILD: a call for clarification. Chest. 2010;138(2): 251–6.

43. Castellino F, Goldberg H, Dellaripa PF. The impact of rheumatologic evaluation in the management of patients with interstitial lung disease. Rheumatology. 2011;50:483–93.

Evaluation of Lung Disease in Patients with Connective Tissue Disease

Aryeh Fischer and Kevin K. Brown

Introduction

The connective tissue diseases (CTDs) refer to the spectrum of systemic rheumatologic illnesses characterized by immune dysregulation with autoimmune phenomena (e.g., circulating auto-antibodies) and immune-mediated organ dysfunction. In general, they include rheumatoid arthritis (RA), systemic lupus erythematosus (SLE), systemic sclerosis (SSc), polymyositis/dermatomyositis (including anti-synthetase syndrome), primary Sjögren's syndrome, mixed CTD (MCTD), and undifferentiated CTD. While these disorders are often considered as a group, there is significant clinical heterogeneity among them. Each can potentially impact all organ systems, with the lungs as a common target; and all patients with CTD are at risk for developing associated clinically significant lung disease [1, 2].

As reviewed in Chap. 7, there are a wide variety of pulmonary manifestations associated with the CTDs, with essentially every anatomic compartment of the respiratory tract at risk of injury [1–3]. Certain characterized diseases are more commonly associated with specific patterns of lung involvement (Table 2.1) [1]. As examples, in patients with SSc, pulmonary involvement is the leading cause of mortality and is typically manifested by interstitial lung disease (ILD) or pulmonary hypertension (PH). In contrast, in SLE, ILD and PH occur much less frequently—while pleural disease occurs quite commonly. Patients with rheumatoid arthritis (RA) and Sjögren's syndrome often develop airways disease (bronchiolitis and bronchiectasis) and ILD, whereas patients with poly-/dermatomyositis frequently develop ILD and yet rarely develop airway complications [1].

Depending upon the clinical context, CTD-associated lung disease varies by time of onset, pattern of lung involvement, and disease severity. Indeed, ILD may be the initial manifestation of a CTD (with extrathoracic features of the CTD developing months or even years later) [4–7] or may be identified in well-established, long-standing CTD [2]. Furthermore, abnormalities found on chest imaging or pulmonary physiology may be subclinical, asymptomatic and stable, or chronically progressive or may present in a fulminant, life-threatening manner.

In this chapter we discuss our approach to the evaluation of lung disease in the CTD patient. We focus specifically on the ILD evaluation because this lung manifestation occurs across the entire spectrum of CTD, is an area in which the importance of a multidisciplinary approach has been demonstrated, is potentially the most clinically

A. Fischer, M.D. (✉)
Division of Rheumatology, Department of Medicine, Autoimmune Lung Center, National Jewish Health, 1400 Jackson Street G07, Denver, CO 80206, USA
e-mail: fischera@njhealth.org

K.K. Brown, M.D.
Department of Medicine, National Jewish Health, 1400 Jackson Street, Denver, CO 80401, USA

P.F. Dellaripa et al. (eds.), *Pulmonary Manifestations of Rheumatic Disease: A Comprehensive Guide*, DOI 10.1007/978-1-4939-0770-0_2, © Springer Science+Business Media New York 2014

Table 2.1 Most common CTD-associated pulmonary manifestations

	SSc	RA	Primary Sjögren's	MCTD	PM/DM	SLE
Airways	–	++	++	+	–	+
ILD	+++	++	++	++	+++	+
Pleural	–	++	+	+	–	+++
Vascular	+++	–	+	++	+	+
DAH	–	–	–	–	–	++

The number of + signs indicates relative prevalence of each manifestation
SSc systemic sclerosis, *RA* rheumatoid arthritis, *CTD* connective tissue disease, *MCTD* mixed connective tissue disease, *PM/DM* polymyositis/dermatomyositis, *SLE* systemic lupus erythematosus, *ILD* interstitial lung disease, *DAH* diffuse alveolar hemorrhage
Used with permission from Fischer A, du Bois RM. A Practical Approach to Connective Tissue Disease-Associated Lung Disease. In Baughman RP, duBois RM (eds): Diffuse Lung Disease: A Practical Approach. 2nd ed. New York: Springer; 2012

meaningful pulmonary manifestation, and often poses a significant diagnostic and management challenge for the practicing clinician.

The Pulmonary Evaluation by Clinical Context

Case Vignette 1
A 55-year-old man with well-established seropositive RA presents with recent-onset cough and dyspnea. He is a former smoker. The articular aspects of his RA are well controlled on chronic methotrexate, inflix-imab, and low-dose corticosteroids. His examination does not reveal synovitis. He has audible crackles in his lower lung zones bilaterally. He has a normal complete blood count and normal comprehensive metabolic panel. His erythrocyte sedimentation rate (ESR) is normal. He has a mild restrictive defect on pulmonary function testing and resting room-air pulse oximeter reading of 91 %. His high-resolution computed tomographic imaging shows evidence of a fibrotic interstitial pneumonia (Fig. 2.1).

Does this patient have CTD-ILD? How should we approach his evaluation?

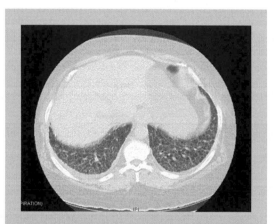

Fig. 2.1 High-resolution computed tomographic image in a patient with rheumatoid arthritis demonstrating evidence of a lower lobe-predominant fibrosing interstitial pneumonia

ILD in Established CTD

Chest imaging evidence of ILD is commonly identified in patients with an established, preexisting CTD. In fact, recent studies have shown radiographic prevalence rates of subclinical ILD of 33–57 % in various CTD cohorts [8]. ILD is particularly common in patients with SSc, PM/DM, RA, primary Sjögren's syndrome, and MCTD. However, just because a patient with CTD is identified to have parenchymal lung disease does not mean the two are necessarily related. For example, the presence of preexisting SSc may be associated with the development of lung injury due to other causes (e.g., aspiration-associated pneumonitis). Furthermore, because CTD patients are often on immunosuppressive medications, the finding of new pulmonary infiltrates in these patients should raise suspicion of respiratory infection—with either typical or atypical pathogens—and medication-induced lung toxicity. As with any patient that presents with interstitial infiltrates, a comprehensive evaluation is needed to explore all potential etiologies (e.g., infection, medication toxicity, environmental and occupational exposures, familial disease, smoking-related lung disease, malignancy, etc.). The determination that the ILD is truly *associated* with the preexisting CTD requires a thorough process of elimination, and this evaluation is enhanced by a multidisciplinary approach [5, 9].

In general, when considering the evaluation of ILD in patients with CTD, we consider the steps discussed next.

Confirm the Presence of a CTD

This may be simple, especially when the background CTD is well characterized and established, such as with small joint synovitis and RF and CCP positive RA. Yet, quite often, the precise rheumatologic diagnosis is uncertain and the development of ILD may impact its classification. Take for instance the patient with an isolated positive SS-A autoantibody that may have been considered to have primary Sjögren's syndrome. If the patient evolves to a presentation of fulminant acute respiratory distress syndrome with lung injury patterns of nonspecific interstitial pneumonia (NSIP), diffuse alveolar damage, and overlapping organizing pneumonia (OP), along with radiographic features of esophageal dysmotility and the peripheral digital fissuring of "mechanic's hands," one might consider an anti-synthetase syndrome, rather than what was initially suspected—in the absence of lung disease—to be more likely a case of primary Sjögren's syndrome.

Determine Whether the ILD Pattern "Fits"

All of the well-characterized lung injury patterns as defined by high-resolution computerized tomographic (HRCT) scanning are known to occur across the spectrum of CTD [10], with some patterns occurring more commonly with specific CTD. For example, a NSIP pattern is the most frequent ILD pattern seen in the setting of SSc [11, 12], while the usual interstitial pneumonia (UIP) pattern appears to be more common in RA [13–15]. Overlapping patterns such as UIP and NSIP or NSIP and organizing pneumonia (OP) are not unusual and can be considered almost routine in disorders such as PM/DM. More unusual patterns such as lymphocytic interstitial pneumonia (LIP) with cystic lung disease (e.g., especially with Sjögren's) and primary airways disease (e.g., bronchiolitis) may also occur in specific settings.

Exclude Infection and Medication-Induced Pneumonitis

As emphasized, just because the patient has a CTD does not preclude the possibility of alternative etiologies for ILD. A comprehensive and multidisciplinary evaluation is needed in patients with CTD and ILD and rendering a diagnosis of CTD-*associated* ILD requires exclusion of other etiologies for the ILD. In particular pulmonary infection and drug-induced lung disease are almost always in the differential.

Perform Bronchoalveolar Lavage When Clinically Indicated to Exclude Infection

In CTD-ILD patients, bronchoalveolar lavage (BAL) can be useful in sorting through the initial differential diagnosis, especially to exclude infection. Its usefulness as a baseline predictor of disease progression however is unclear. Silver and colleagues have shown that BAL neutrophilia or eosinophilia in patients with SSc-ILD is useful as a predictor of progressive ILD [16, 17]. However, two recent well-designed prospective studies failed to demonstrate any prognostic significance obtained from BAL in patients with SSc-ILD [18, 19], and hence, the routine use of BAL to solely predict the likelihood of disease progression in CTD-ILD is not recommended.

Transbronchial biopsy is of limited value in the evaluation of parenchymal lung disease in CTD, but may be diagnostic in more airway-centric complications such as bronchiolitis or assessing for malignancy.

Biopsy the Atypical Scenario

Because data have yet to show that determining a specific histopathologic pattern of lung injury impacts prognosis in CTD-ILD, the role of surgical lung biopsy in patients with preexisting CTD remains controversial. The distinction between the specific ILD subtypes (e.g., UIP vs. NSIP) is known to have baseline prognostic significance among patients with idiopathic interstitial pneumonia (IIP)—but does not appear to be as prognostically significant in patients with CTD. In the largest series of biopsied SSc-ILD subjects ($n=80$), Bouros and colleagues showed that changes in diffusing capacity over time—but not baseline histopathologic pattern—predicted prognosis [11]. Similarly, in their cohort of 93 patients with a variety of CTD-ILD, Park and colleagues demonstrated that age, pulmonary function, and degree of dyspnea were of prognostic importance—but differences in pattern of lung injury did not impact survival [20]. The relatively small study cohort sizes and the impact of selection and referral bias cannot be discounted and therefore the predictive power of different patterns of lung histopathology remains uncertain in CTD-ILD. Furthermore, CTD-ILD patients tend to be treated with immunosuppressive therapies—targeting both progressive ILD and the extrathoracic inflammatory features—irrespective of specific ILD pattern. In this context, because the biopsy finding may not impact on treatment decisions, including immunosuppression, when the chest imaging pattern provides a strongly suggestive but not definitive pattern diagnosis that is consistent with what would be expected under the clinical conditions, clinicians often elect not to proceed with a surgical biopsy.

In general, we believe a surgical lung biopsy may be appropriate in patients with preexisting CTD in cases when there are clinically significant concerns for an alternative explanation for the underlying lung disease (e.g., hypersensitivity pneumonitis), when the chest imaging pattern on HRCT is atypical for underlying CTD, when the HRCT features suggest malignancy or infection (e.g., progressive nodules, cavitation, consolidation, pleural thickening, or effusion), or when a specific pattern cannot be identified by HRCT.

Ultimately, the decision of whether to proceed with surgical lung biopsy is individualized, with due consideration for its associated risks, and whether its findings will impact on management and prognosis.

Case Vignette 2

A 40-year-old woman presents with acute onset of exertional fatigue, dyspnea, and cough. She has no relevant past medical history, takes no medications, and is a never smoker. Her review of systems is notable for recent development of arthralgias, digital edema, and Raynaud's phenomenon. On examination she has puffy hands without synovitis or sclerodactyly, a few scattered palmar telangiectasia, mild periungual erythema, and audible lower zone crackles bilaterally. Her laboratory studies note a positive antinuclear antibody (ANA) with a titer of 1:1,280 and nucleolar-staining pattern. She also has a positive anti-Scl-70 antibody. She has a normal set of pulmonary function tests. Her HRCT demonstrates suggestive features of the NSIP pattern of lung injury (Fig. 2.2).

Does this patient have CTD-ILD? How should we approach her evaluation?

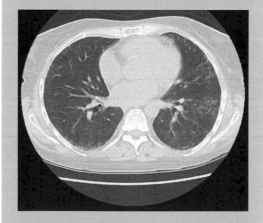

Fig. 2.2 High-resolution computed tomographic image in a patient presenting with an idiopathic interstitial pneumonia in a pattern suggestive of nonspecific interstitial pneumonia

ILD as the First Manifestation of a CTD

Considering the possibility of underlying CTD is an important aspect of the evaluation of patients presenting with an IIP. Within this scenario, the identification of occult CTD is common. A recent study reported that of 114 consecutive ILD patients evaluated at a tertiary referral center, 17 (15 %) were confirmed to have a new CTD diagnosis [21]. There is no standardized approach to the assessment of underlying CTD. Current practice includes performing a thorough history and physical examination and testing for circulating autoantibodies. Many centers have found that a multidisciplinary approach that includes rheumatologic consultation may also be useful. In practice, it is both unrealistic and impractical to have rheumatologic evaluation for all new cases of ILD, but certain proposed guidelines for deciding when to get rheumatologic consultation may be more realistic (Table 2.2) [5].

Because the extrathoracic features of occult CTD can be subtle, confirming the presence of underlying CTD can be challenging. One such study evaluated whether ILD as the sole presentation of CTD can be differentiated from an IIP [22]. Sixty-eight patients that presented with an ILD were followed prospectively over 11 years. Thirteen (19 %) eventually developed a characterizable CTD. The prevalence of a positive rheumatoid factor (RF) or ANA was no different in the group that developed CTD compared with those that did not. The authors concluded that patients defined as having an IIP could not be distinguished from those that develop CTD-ILD before the systematic manifestations appear [22].

As the following select studies demonstrate, a thorough—and multidisciplinary—evaluation with heightened surveillance for subtle extrathoracic features of CTD, assessing a broader array of autoantibodies, and consideration of radiographic and histopathologic features make the detection of occult CTD more likely.

One small series from a multidisciplinary ILD program that incorporated rheumatologic evaluation described six patients evaluated within a

Table 2.2 Suggested categories of ILD patients that require further rheumatologic evaluation

1. Women, particularly those younger than 50
2. Any patient with extrathoracic manifestations highly suggestive of CTD
a. That is, Raynaud's phenomenon, esophageal hypomotility, inflammatory arthritis of the metacarpal-phalangeal joints or wrists, digital edema, or symptomatic keratoconjunctivitis sicca
3. All cases of NSIP, LIP, or any ILD pattern with secondary histopathology features that might suggest CTD
a. That is, extensive pleuritis, dense perivascular collagen, lymphoid aggregates with germinal center formation, prominent plasmacytic infiltration
4. Patients with a positive ANA or RF in high titer (generally considered to be ANA > 1:320 or RF > 60 IU/mL), a nucleolar-staining ANA at any titer, or any positive autoantibody specific as to a particular CTD
a. That is, anti-CCP, anti-Scl-70, anti-Ro, anti-La, anti-dsDNA, anti-Smith, anti-RNP, anti-tRNA synthetase

Used with permission from Fischer A, du Bois RM. A Practical Approach to Connective Tissue Disease-Associated Lung Disease. In Baughman RP, duBois RM (eds): Diffuse Lung Disease: A Practical Approach. 2nd ed. New York: Springer; 2012

12-month span for presumed IIP [23]. All were found to have a positive nucleolar-pattern ANA, along with either an anti-Th/To or anti-Scl-70 antibody, and all had subtle extrathoracic features of SSc that included telangiectasia, Raynaud's phenomenon, digital edema, or esophageal hypomotility. This small series reinforced the concept that ILD may be the presenting manifestation of SSc, that engaging rheumatology for ILD evaluation can be helpful, and that suspicions for SSc are warranted in patients with a nucleolar-pattern ANA and NSIP or UIP [23, 24]. Another study from a multidisciplinary ILD program described a retrospectively evaluated cohort of 114 consecutive patients [21]. Thirty-four subjects (30 %) were found to have CTD-ILD and of these, only half had presented with a preexisting CTD. These authors argued that when confronted with an IIP, the presence of younger age, high-titer ANA, and elevated muscle enzymes were associated with underlying CTD. In another study, a cohort of 50 ILD patients referred to a tertiary referral center were retrospectively assessed and described [25]. Of the 25 patients confirmed to have a diagnosis of CTD-ILD—only after multidisciplinary evaluation—28 % had been initially referred with a diagnosis of IPF!

Another recent study highlights the importance of maintaining a heightened suspicion for underlying CTD in cases of NSIP—even when the ANA and RF are negative [6]. Nine patients evaluated over a 2-year period with idiopathic NSIP were ANA and RF negative but found to have the anti-synthetase syndrome based on the presence of a tRNA synthetase antibody (PL-7 or PL-12), NSIP, and subtle extrathoracic features that included "mechanic's hands," Raynaud's phenomenon, inflammatory arthritis, myositis, or esophageal hypomotility [6]. In another study, 198 consecutive cases of IIP were screened with a panel of anti-tRNA synthetase antibodies and identified positive anti-synthetase antibodies in 13 cases (7 %) [26]. They reported that those with positive antibodies were younger and more likely to have NSIP or UIP with lymphoid follicules. Furthermore, among the 13 with a positive tRNA synthetase antibody, extrathoracic manifestations of anti-synthetase syndrome were retrospectively identified in 7 cases [26].

Taken together, there are many variables to consider when evaluating a patient with presumed IIP for the presence of occult CTD. We have found that careful attention to the following items is often helpful.

Clinical Features

Demographic features can help distinguish the patient with an underlying CTD. In comparison to IPF, patients with CTD-ILD are more likely to be younger and female. A detailed review of systems and thorough physical examination is useful. Certain specific clinical features lend more support for underlying CTD than others. Of the CTD symptoms encountered in patients with IIP, perhaps none is as important as Raynaud's phenomenon. The presence of Raynaud's phenomenon is associated with a pattern of NSIP and when identified in a patient with ILD should raise strong suspicions for underlying CTD in general

Fig. 2.3 A nailfold capillary microscopic image from a patient with systemic sclerosis. Note the presence of marked capillary loop tortuosity, dilation, and areas of vascular dropout. (Used with permission from Fischer A, du Bois RM. A Practical Approach to Connective Tissue Disease-Associated Lung Disease. In Baughman RP, duBois RM (eds): Diffuse Lung Disease: A Practical Approach. 2nd ed. New York: Springer; 2012)

and SSc (with or without overt skin thickening) in particular. Indeed, Raynaud's phenomenon is encountered in nearly all patients with SSc and is a common finding in patients with PM/DM, anti-synthetase syndrome, primary Sjögren's syndrome, MCTD, SLE, and UCTD. Performing nailfold capillary microscopy is useful when assessing a patient with Raynaud's phenomenon. In particular, the presence of dilated or tortuous capillary loops or significant areas lacking capillary loops (i.e., capillary dropout) may be suggestive of SSc or PM/DM (Fig. 2.3).

The reporting of symmetric joint swelling or stiffness, or identifying synovitis on physical examination, is very useful. Because inflammatory arthritis is encountered in all of the CTDs, autoantibody profiles may be needed to clarify which specific CTD is present. In contrast, symptoms such as gastroesophageal reflux, pain, fatigue, dry eyes, dry mouth, alopecia, and weight loss are not nearly as helpful because they are ubiquitous and not nearly as specific for CTD.

The cutaneous manifestations of SSc and anti-synthetase syndrome are worthy of special mention because these two disorders are so commonly associated with ILD and their extrathoracic features are very specific and yet often quite subtle. It is important to recognize that the "mechanic's hands" sign of anti-synthetase syndrome can be

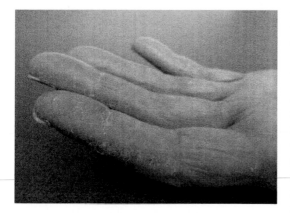

Fig. 2.4 A photograph of the distal digital fissuring characteristic of "mechanic's hands" in a patient with the anti-synthetase syndrome

Table 2.3 Useful antibodies for CTD-ILD assessment

Autoantibody	Commonly associated CTD
High-titer ANA (≥1:320 titer)	Many
High-titer RF (≥60 IU/mL)	RA, Sjögren's syndrome, SLE
Anti-CCP	RA
Anti-centromere	Systemic sclerosis
Anti-nucleolar-ANA	Systemic sclerosis
Anti-Ro (SS-A)	Many
Anti-La (SS-B)	SLE, Sjögren's syndrome
Anti-Smith	SLE
Anti-ribonucleoprotein	SLE, MCTD
Anti-dsDNA	SLE
Anti-topoisomerase (Scl-70)	Systemic sclerosis
Anti-tRNA synthetase antibodies	Poly-/dermatomyositis (anti-synthetase syndrome)
Anti-PM-Scl	Systemic sclerosis/myositis overlap
Anti-Th/To	Systemic sclerosis
Anti-U3 ribonucleoprotein	Systemic sclerosis
Anti-MDA-5 (CADM)	Clinical amyopathic dermatomyositis

Used with permission from Fischer A, du Bois RM. A Practical Approach to Connective Tissue Disease-Associated Lung Disease. In Baughman RP, duBois RM (eds): Diffuse Lung Disease: A Practical Approach. 2nd ed. New York: Springer; 2012

as subtle as only mild distal digital fissuring (Fig. 2.4) and that palmar telangiectasia may be limited to the finding of only few scattered dilated capillaries. Nonetheless, when such findings are present in a patient with an IIP, they are highly suggestive of underlying CTD.

Circulating Autoantibodies

Autoantibody assessment is an important part of the evaluation of patients with IIP. For patients with ILD in whom there is clinical suspicion of an underlying CTD, we recommend a broad panel of autoantibodies as a screening test (Table 2.3). It is also important to take note of the pattern of immunofluorescence when the ANA is positive, as the nucleolar-staining ANA pattern in patients with ILD may suggest SSc spectrum of disease [23, 24, 27].

Importantly, we highlight that the ANA and RF are relatively poor screening tests: they have low specificity—particularly when present at low titer—and can be seen in healthy individuals. In addition, given that a negative ANA and RF may dissuade some clinicians from pursuing further evaluation, cases of occult CTD that may be ANA and RF negative (e.g., anti-synthetase syndrome) are missed.

Chest Imaging Features

Thoracic HRCT imaging plays a central role in the evaluation of ILD by providing detailed infor-

mation on the pattern, distribution and extent of the ILD, and the presence of extraparenchymal abnormalities including pleural disease and pericardial and esophageal features. In contrast to IIP, patients with CTD-ILD are more likely to have pleural effusions, pericardial effusions, pericardial thickening, and esophageal dilatation [28]. Patients with CTD are also more likely to have an HRCT pattern suggestive of NSIP when compared to patients without CTD [28]. HRCT has varying degrees of correlation with histopathologic pattern. Among CTD-ILD patients with a typical HRCT pattern for UIP, the histopathology almost always correlates [28–30]. Interestingly, the converse does not hold true; CTD patients with histopathologic patterns of UIP may have HRCT patterns suggestive of NSIP [28–30]. As discussed previously, noting atypical patterns of lung injury may impact decisions to perform surgical lung biopsy.

Histopathologic Features

Several histopathologic features may be useful when trying to distinguish an IIP from CTD-ILD. An initial clue to an underlying CTD is the presence of multi-compartment involvement on the biopsy; in addition to parenchymal lung injury, there may be components of airways, vascular, or pleural disease [31, 32]. When compared to IPF, CTD-UIP is characterized by fewer fibroblastic foci, less overall fibrosis, and less honeycombing [33, 34]. Flaherty and colleagues compared the histopathologic features of 9 patients with CTD-UIP to that of 99 patients with IPF [34]. Those with CTD-UIP were younger, had better lung function, and shorter duration of symptoms. They found that those with IPF had significantly higher fibroblast focus scores than CTD-UIP and that the fibroblast focus score was the most discriminative feature between these groups [34]. Song and colleagues compared histopathologic features in 39 patients with CTD-UIP to 61 patients with IPF [33]. They found that the biopsies in those with CTD-UIP had fewer fibroblast foci and less honeycombing but had more germinal center formation and more evidence of inflammation than seen with IPF.

Additional histopathologic features that lend support for the presence of underlying CTD include the presence of lymphoid aggregates, germinal centers, increased perivascular collagen, follicular bronchiolitis, lymphoplasmacytic inflammation, eosinophil infiltration, or pleuritis [31, 32].

Determining Severity of Impairment

A standardized assessment for disease progression is important for the longitudinal monitoring of patients with CTD-ILD and helps guide therapeutic decision-making regarding the initiation, modification, or cessation of therapy. A number of objective modalities commonly employed for disease monitoring are detailed in this section.

Dyspnea and Quality of Life Measures

The use of a reproducible, subjective indicator of a patient's level of breathlessness, exercise capacity, and quality of life can provide clinically important data. By using a standardized and validated clinical tool to evaluate dyspnea, the clinician may assess respiratory disease progression and functionality over time. A number of dyspnea indices have been validated in respiratory disease and the choice of which index to use is less important than their consistent implementation by practitioners to reliably quantify subjective dyspnea. In one study, the self-reported measures of the Multi-Dimensional Health Assessment Questionnaire, University of California San Diego Dyspnea Questionnaire, and Dyspnea-12 Questionnaire were found to be useful in the assessment of patients with a wide spectrum of CTD-ILD [35]. These measures yielded meaningful information beyond that provided by pulmonary physiology and confirmed that dyspnea is strongly associated with perceived day-to-day functioning and global well-being in CTD-ILD.

Pulmonary Function Testing

Serial assessment of the forced vital capacity (FVC) and diffusing capacity for carbon monoxide (DLCO) allows for objective quantification of ventilatory capacity and gas exchange, respectively. These parameters are useful in assessing the degree of respiratory impairment due to ILD and may provide clues about the presence of coexistent PH as well. They are especially helpful when trying to assess for disease progression and response to therapy. Changes in FVC, and to a lesser degree of confidence in DLCO, over time predict survival in IPF and, therefore, are commonly used as surrogate markers for response to therapy in ILD in general [36]. Patients who decline ≥ 10 % of predicted FVC or ≥ 15 % of DLCO are considered to have clear and clinically significant evidence of progressive disease. In patients with CTD-ILD, pulmonary physiology appears to be a stronger predictor of survival than underlying histopathologic pattern seen at the time of diagnosis [11, 20].

Six-Minute Walk Test

The 6-minute walk test (6MWT) objectively assesses for ILD severity, disease progression, and response to therapy [37–39]. In a multicenter treatment trial in which the 6MWT was specifically evaluated in SSc-ILD, the investigators found that although the distance walked was reproducible, it correlated only weakly with FVC and Borg dyspnea index, suggesting that these tests measure different facets of disease progression [39]. Furthermore, because of significant extrathoracic variables—and musculoskeletal impairment in particular—the use of 6MWT as an end point for clinical trials in CTD-ILD has been disputed. In clinical practice, however, we find the 6MWT to be a generally useful test to perform longitudinally. It is relatively inexpensive, easy to perform, and provides an additional objective measure of exercise capacity for which to help plot the longitudinal clinical course of a patient.

Thoracic High-Resolution Computed Tomography

As discussed previously, HRCT imaging yields valuable information about ILD including the pattern and extent of disease, an assessment of disease progression, and the evaluation of extraparenchymal abnormalities. In many cases of CTD-ILD, a specific radiologic pattern (e.g., UIP or NSIP) can be determined with a high degree of confidence. This pattern recognition within specific clinical scenarios may obviate the need for surgical lung biopsy and provide prognostic information. The presence of a fibrotic radiographic pattern as evidenced by reticular opacities, traction bronchiectasis, and honeycombing is predictive of poor outcomes in both IIP and RA-ILD [13, 29, 40, 41]. A recent study of 215 subjects with SSc-ILD demonstrated that the HRCT extent of fibrosis and degree of FVC reduction provide discriminatory prognostic information [42]. The authors proposed a subclassification of SSc-ILD as "limited" or "extensive" based upon the estimation of extent of fibrosis on HRCT and impairment in FVC. This simple staging system provided a more accurate

prognostic separation than has been achieved with any single index in isolation [42].

Management Considerations

It is important to recognize that not all patients with CTD-ILD require pharmacologic treatment (see Chap. 14). Radiographic findings of ILD on HRCT are common, but only a subset of patients will show clinically significant, progressive disease. The decision to treat CTD-ILD often rests upon whether the patient is clinically impaired by their lung disease, whether it is progressive, and what comorbid conditions or mitigating factors exist [43]. Therapy for CTD-ILD is generally reserved for those patients with clinically significant, progressive disease, and this determination is based upon a constellation of clinical assessment tools that include both subjective and objective measures of respiratory impairment [43].

The evaluation and management of patients with CTD-ILD is optimized by effective multidisciplinary interactions among pulmonologists and rheumatologists. In particular, when considering immunomodulatory therapy options for CTD-ILD, both intrathoracic and extrathoracic disease manifestations and degrees of activity need to be assessed and taken into consideration when designing a therapeutic regimen. Given the heterogeneity in disease presentation, the multiple systems that may be affected, and the broad range of disease severity, coordinated care is essential. In all cases of CTD-ILD, disease monitoring, choice of therapy, and ongoing longitudinal assessment and reassessment of a treatment response are complex and are optimized by effective collaborative care among pulmonologists, rheumatologists, and other health-care providers.

Summary

Lung disease is a common manifestation of CTD and is associated with significant morbidity and mortality. The evaluation of lung disease, and ILD in particular, in patients with CTD is complex because of the heterogeneity of the CTDs and the varied types and degrees of severity of ILD encountered and because ILD can be identified at any point in time in these patients. A thorough— and multidisciplinary—evaluation is needed when CTD patients develop ILD or when evaluating ILD patients for the presence of occult CTD. Determining that ILD is associated with an established CTD requires the exclusion of alternative etiologies and thorough assessments of the clinical features of both the CTD and ILD. The detection of occult CTD in patients with so-called "idiopathic" ILD requires careful attention to the demographic profile, historical clues, subtle physical examination findings, specific autoantibody positivity, and radiologic and histopathologic features and can be optimized by a multidisciplinary approach that includes rheumatologic collaboration. A standardized assessment with the serial implementation of objective tests to determine disease severity and evidence of progression is important for the longitudinal monitoring of patients with CTD-ILD and helps guide management considerations.

References

1. Fischer A, du Bois R. Interstitial lung disease in connective tissue disorders. Lancet. 2012;380:689–98.
2. Frankel SK, Brown KK. Collagen vascular diseases of the lung. Clin Pulm Med. 2006;13:25–36.
3. Olson AL, Brown KK. Connective tissue disease-associated lung disorders. Eur Respir Mon. 2009; 46:225–50.
4. Cottin V. Interstitial lung disease: are we missing formes frustes of connective tissue disease? Eur Respir J. 2006;28:893–6.
5. Fischer A, du Bois RM. A practical approach to connective tissue disease-associated lung disease. In: Baughman RP, du Bois RM, editors. Diffuse lung disease: a practical approach. 2nd ed. New York: Springer; 2012.
6. Fischer A, Swigris JJ, du Bois RM, et al. Antisynthetase syndrome in ANA and anti-Jo-1 negative patients presenting with idiopathic interstitial pneumonia. Respir Med. 2009;103:1719–24.
7. Fischer A, West SG, Swigris JJ, Brown KK, du Bois RM. Connective tissue disease-associated interstitial lung disease: a call for clarification. Chest. 2010; 138:251–6.
8. Doyle TJ, Hunninghake GM, Rosas IO. Subclinical interstitial lung disease: why you should care. Am J Respir Crit Care Med. 2012;185:1147–53.
9. Fischer A. Interstitial lung disease: a rheumatologist's perspective. J Clin Rheumatol. 2009;15:95–9.
10. ATS/ERS. American Thoracic Society/European Respiratory Society International Multidisciplinary Consensus Classification of the Idiopathic Interstitial Pneumonias. This joint statement of the American Thoracic Society (ATS), and the European Respiratory Society (ERS) was adopted by the ATS board of directors, June 2001 and by the ERS Executive Committee, June 2001. Am J Respir Crit Care Med. 2002;165:277–304.
11. Bouros D, Wells AU, Nicholson AG, et al. Histopathologic subsets of fibrosing alveolitis in patients with systemic sclerosis and their relationship to outcome. Am J Respir Crit Care Med. 2002; 165:1581–6.
12. Kim DS, Yoo B, Lee JS, et al. The major histopathologic pattern of pulmonary fibrosis in scleroderma is nonspecific interstitial pneumonia. Sarcoidosis Vasc Diffuse Lung Dis. 2002;19:121–7.
13. Kim EJ, Collard HR, King Jr TE. Rheumatoid arthritis-associated interstitial lung disease: the relevance of histopathologic and radiographic pattern. Chest. 2009;136:1397–405.
14. Kim EJ, Elicker BM, Maldonado F, et al. Usual interstitial pneumonia in rheumatoid arthritis-associated interstitial lung disease. Eur Respir J. 2010; 35: 1322–8.
15. Lee HK, Kim DS, Yoo B, et al. Histopathologic pattern and clinical features of rheumatoid arthritis-associated interstitial lung disease. Chest. 2005; 127: 2019–27.
16. Kowal-Bielecka O, Kowal K, Highland KB, Silver RM. Bronchoalveolar lavage fluid in scleroderma interstitial lung disease: technical aspects and clinical correlations: review of the literature. Semin Arthritis Rheum. 2012;40:73–88.
17. Silver RM, Miller KS, Kinsella MB, Smith EA, Schabel SI. Evaluation and management of scleroderma lung disease using bronchoalveolar lavage. Am J Med. 1990;88:470–6.
18. Goh NS, Veeraraghavan S, Desai SR, et al. Bronchoalveolar lavage cellular profiles in patients with systemic sclerosis-associated interstitial lung disease are not predictive of disease progression. Arthritis Rheum. 2007;56:2005–12.
19. Strange C, Bolster MB, Roth MD, et al. Bronchoalveolar lavage and response to cyclophosphamide in scleroderma interstitial lung disease. Am J Respir Crit Care Med. 2008;177:91–8.
20. Park JH, Kim DS, Park IN, et al. Prognosis of fibrotic interstitial pneumonia: idiopathic versus collagen vascular disease-related subtypes. Am J Respir Crit Care Med. 2007;175:705–11.
21. Mittoo S, Gelber AC, Christopher-Stine L, Horton MR, Lechtzin N, Danoff SK. Ascertainment of

collagen vascular disease in patients presenting with interstitial lung disease. Respir Med. 2009;103:1152–8.

22. Homma Y, Ohtsuka Y, Tanimura K, et al. Can interstitial pneumonia as the sole presentation of collagen vascular diseases be differentiated from idiopathic interstitial pneumonia? Respiration. 1995;62:248–51.

23. Fischer A, Meehan RT, Feghali-Bostwick CA, West SG, Brown KK. Unique characteristics of systemic sclerosis sine scleroderma-associated interstitial lung disease. Chest. 2006;130:976–81.

24. Fischer A, Pfalzgraf FJ, Feghali-Bostwick CA, et al. Anti-th/to-positivity in a cohort of patients with idiopathic pulmonary fibrosis. J Rheumatol. 2006;33: 1600–5.

25. Castelino FV, Goldberg H, Dellaripa PF. The impact of rheumatological evaluation in the management of patients with interstitial lung disease. Rheumatology (Oxford). 2011;50:489–93.

26. Watanabe K, Handa T, Tanizawa K, et al. Detection of antisynthetase syndrome in patients with idiopathic interstitial pneumonias. Respir Med. 2011;105:1238–47.

27. Steen VD. Autoantibodies in systemic sclerosis. Semin Arthritis Rheum. 2005;35:35–42.

28. Hwang JH, Misumi S, Sahin H, Brown KK, Newell JD, Lynch DA. Computed tomographic features of idiopathic fibrosing interstitial pneumonia: comparison with pulmonary fibrosis related to collagen vascular disease. J Comput Assist Tomogr. 2009;33: 410–5.

29. Lynch DA. Quantitative CT of fibrotic interstitial lung disease. Chest. 2007;131:643–4.

30. Lynch DA, Travis WD, Muller NL, et al. Idiopathic interstitial pneumonias: CT features. Radiology. 2005;236:10–21.

31. Fukuoka JLK. Practical pulmonary pathology. A diagnostic approach. 1st ed. Philadelphia: Churchill-Livingstone; 2005.

32. Leslie KO, Trahan S, Gruden J. Pulmonary pathology of the rheumatic diseases. Semin Respir Crit Care Med. 2007;28:369–78.

33. Song JW, Do KH, Kim MY, Jang SJ, Colby TV, Kim DS. Pathologic and radiologic differences between idiopathic and collagen vascular disease-related usual interstitial pneumonia. Chest. 2009; 136:23–30.

34. Flaherty KR, Colby TV, Travis WD, et al. Fibroblastic foci in usual interstitial pneumonia: idiopathic versus collagen vascular disease. Am J Respir Crit Care Med. 2003;167:1410–5.

35. Swigris JJ, Yorke J, Sprunger DB, et al. Assessing dyspnea and its impact on patients with connective tissue disease-related interstitial lung disease. Respir Med. 2010;104:1350–5.

36. du Bois RM, Weycker D, Albera C, et al. Forced vital capacity in patients with idiopathic pulmonary fibrosis: test properties and minimal clinically important difference. Am J Respir Crit Care Med. 2011; 184:1382–9.

37. Buch MH, Denton CP, Furst DE, et al. Submaximal exercise testing in the assessment of interstitial lung disease secondary to systemic sclerosis: reproducibility and correlations of the 6-min walk test. Ann Rheum Dis. 2007;66:169–73.

38. Eaton T, Young P, Milne D, Wells AU. Six-minute walk, maximal exercise tests: reproducibility in fibrotic interstitial pneumonia. Am J Respir Crit Care Med. 2005;171:1150–7.

39. Hallstrand TS, Boitano LJ, Johnson WC, Spada CA, Hayes JG, Raghu G. The timed walk test as a measure of severity and survival in idiopathic pulmonary fibrosis. Eur Respir J. 2005;25:96–103.

40. Flaherty KR, Mumford JA, Murray S, et al. Prognostic implications of physiologic and radiographic changes in idiopathic interstitial pneumonia. Am J Respir Crit Care Med. 2003;168:543–8.

41. Kocheril SV, Appleton BE, Somers EC, et al. Comparison of disease progression and mortality of connective tissue disease-related interstitial lung disease and idiopathic interstitial pneumonia. Arthritis Rheum. 2005;53:549–57.

42. Goh NS, Desai SR, Veeraraghavan S, et al. Interstitial lung disease in systemic sclerosis: a simple staging system. Am J Respir Crit Care Med. 2008;177: 1248–54.

43. Fischer A, Brown KK, Frankel SK. Treatment of connective tissue disease related interstitial lung disease. Clin Pulm Med. 2009;16:74–80.

Rheumatoid Arthritis

3

Jay H. Ryu and Eric L. Matteson

Rheumatoid Arthritis

Introduction

Rheumatoid arthritis (RA) is the most common autoimmune-mediated joint disease affecting especially small and medium size joints leading to inflammation of the synovium with destruction of cartilage and bone [1]. It is also a systemic disorder, and the effects of systemic inflammation, and patients who have severe extraarticular rheumatoid arthritis disease manifestations have increased morbidity and are at higher risk of premature death [2, 3].

J.H. Ryu, M.D. (✉)
Division of Pulmonary and Critical Care Medicine,
Mayo Clinic College of Medicine,
Gonda 18 South, Mayo Clinic, 200 1st Street, SW,
Rochester, MN 55905, USA
e-mail: Ryu.jay@mayo.edu

E.L. Matteson, M.D., M.P.H.
Division of Rheumatology, Department of Medicine,
Mayo Clinic College of Medicine,
Rochester, MN 55905, USA

Division of Epidemiology, Department of Health
Science Research, Mayo Clinic College of Medicine,
200 1st Street, SW, Rochester, MN 55905, USA
e-mail: Matteson.eric@mayo.edu

Epidemiology

Rheumatoid arthritis affects approximately 1 % of the US population and is more common in persons of European and Asian ancestry. Approximately 75 % of patients with RA are women. Rheumatoid arthritis can affect persons at any age, with the mean age of onset of about 55 years of age [1, 4]. Extraarticular disease manifestations occur in more than 40 % of patients during the disease course and include keratoconjunctivitis sicca and rheumatoid nodules [4, 5]. Severe extraarticular manifestations such as vasculitis, Felty's syndrome, glomerulonephritis, pericarditis, pleuritis, scleritis, and interstitial lung disease (ILD) develop in approximately 15 % of patients during the course of the disease [4, 5].

Etiology and Pathogenesis

Rheumatoid arthritis is an autoimmune disease, which is due fundamentally to a loss of self-immunological tolerance [6]. The causes of the loss of immunological tolerance are not known; however, several factors are important in the disease pathogenesis. Genetic predisposition, including the presence of HLA-DR4, CTLA5, PTPN22, and environmental factors, the best studied of which is smoking, increase the risk of development of RA [1, 6]. The immune response is characterized by the development of specific autoantibodies including rheumatoid factor and anti-citrullinated protein antibodies (ACPA) [7, 8].

P.F. Dellaripa et al. (eds.), *Pulmonary Manifestations of Rheumatic Disease: A Comprehensive Guide*,
DOI 10.1007/978-1-4939-0770-0_3, © Springer Science+Business Media New York 2014

The immune dysfunction in RA is mediated by antigen-specific T-cell activation as well as B-cell and TH17-cell co-stimulation. The result is joint inflammation and ultimately osteoclastogenesis with bone and cartilage degradation, and pannus formation leading to the typical pattern of joint destruction and erosive disease seen on joint radiographs [1].

Patients who smoke are at higher risk of developing extraarticular manifestations including lung disease [5, 9–11]. In particular, patients who have HLA-DR4, HLA-B40, HLA-DQB1, and HLA-B54 and possibly alpha-1 proteinase inhibitor appear to have an increased likelihood of lung disease, particularly in the setting of smoking [6, 9, 12]. ACPAs, which are thought to be pathogenetic in RA, may be found in the lung in patients with RA, and there is evidence of increased levels of CD4, CD8, and CD54 T-cells as well as macrophages and CD20-positive B-cells in the lung tissue from patients with RA as well [13–15]. Low levels of interferon gamma and TGF-beta 2 are associated with the presence of fibrosis [16]. It has been speculated that TNF-alpha and interleukin-6 production by macrophages is increased in patients with RA-related ILD, and the presence of high proliferative potential colony forming cells in the peripheral blood has been associated with RA-related ILD [17, 18].

Clinical and Radiologic Features

Joint involvement in patients with RA is characterized by symmetrical swelling of appendicular joints, especially the interphalangeal joints, the metacarpophalangeal joints, the metatarsophalangeal joints, and often medium and large joints. In approximately one-quarter of patients, however, the disease onset is oligoarticular, often beginning in the knee.

Extraarticular disease manifestations can occur at any point during the disease and even occasionally may precede the development of joint disease [1, 4]. Signs of systemic inflammation include constitutional symptoms of fatigue, low-grade fever, weight loss, and elevated levels of inflammatory biomarkers including the C-reactive protein

and erythrocyte sedimentation rate. Rheumatoid nodules develop in approximately 30 % of all patients with RA sometime during the disease course, typically over pressure areas such as the elbow [5]. Active RA is associated with anemia of chronic disease. Chronic neutropenia with splenomegaly in the absence of lymphoma occurs in patients with Felty's syndrome, typically occurring in patients with longstanding, seropositive, nodular, deforming RA. Systemic vasculitis may present with involvement of small- and medium-sized vessels of the skin and progressive sensorimotor neuropathy with mononeuritis multiplex and vasculitis of the lower extremities, nailfold infarcts, leg ulcers, purpura, and digital gangrene [1, 4, 5].

Pulmonary involvement in RA is frequent, although not always clinically recognized, and is one of the leading causes of death in patients with RA [19, 20]. The most common forms of lung disease include ILD, constrictive (obliterative) bronchiolitis, and pleuritis. Pericarditis is the most frequent cardiac manifestation of rheumatoid arthritis, which can present as acute chest pain and dyspnea with tamponade, and lead to chronic constrictive pericarditis. Scleritis and peripheral ulcerative scleritis are severe complications of RA and typically occur with longstanding joint disease, which may or may not be active when the scleritis occurs. Patients with RA may also develop milder eye manifestations such as episcleritis, often in the setting of active disease, or keratoconjunctivitis sicca in the setting of secondary Sjögren's syndrome associated with xerostomia. As well, patients with RA, and especially those with severe extraarticular RA are at approximately a twofold increased risk of developing cardiovascular disease and severe infections as well as osteoporosis [21–24].

Rheumatoid factor is present in approximately 80 % of patients with RA, although the specificity is low. ACPA occur in approximately 40–50 % of patients with RA and have a specificity of 90–95 % for the disease [8]. Conventional radiographic examination reveals erosions in patients with established disease. Erosions and findings of synovitis may also be detected on magnetic resonance imaging and ultrasonography.

Diagnosis

The diagnosis of RA is based on the presence of characteristic joint swelling and presence of autoantibodies such as rheumatoid factor and ACPA. The key diagnostic features of RA include morning stiffness of greater than 1 h, arthritis of three or more joint areas, arthritis of the hands, symmetric arthritis, presence of rheumatoid nodules, presence of autoantibodies, and typical radiographic changes in the small joints of the hands and feet [1].

In an effort to facilitate the early diagnosis of RA, a new classification system has been developed, which focuses on features at earlier stages of the disease that are associated with persistent and erosive disease rather than defining the disease by its late-stage features such as erosive disease on radiographs. In the absence of other competing diagnoses, patients can be classified as having definite RA based on the confirmed presence of synovitis in at least one joint, absence of an alternative diagnosis that better explains the synovitis, and achievement of a total score of 6 or greater (of a possible 10) from individual scores in four domains: number and site of involved joints (score range, 0–5), serologic abnormality (score range, 0–3), elevated acute-phase response (score range, 0–1), and symptom duration (2 levels; 0 = symptom duration of less than 6 weeks; 1 = duration of symptom of greater than 6 weeks) [25].

Treatment

The treatment of RA is directed toward the underlying autoimmune disease pathology and guided by the severity of symptoms and signs [26]. Several quantitative measures of disease activity which are based on patient and physician global assessment, presence of joint pain, joint swelling, a patient reported measure of physical disability, and acute-phase reactants are used in the formal assessment of patients with RA. These measures are summarized as the disease activity score 28 (DAS-28), which includes 28 joint count, as well as other measures, such as the simplified disease activity index (SDAI), the clinical disease activity index (CDAI), and others. These summary measures are useful in assessment of disease severity and in management in practice [26].

In the past decade, important advances in the understanding of RA and its management and treatment, including the new classification criteria and better definitions of disease outcome and remission and the introduction of biologic response modifying drugs to inhibit the inflammatory process have greatly altered the approach to managing RA [26, 27]. Early diagnosis and more aggressive management of disease early and throughout the course of disease using standard disease assessment tools have resulted in improvement in function, quality of life, reduction in co-morbidities, and improved survival.

The goals of therapy for RA are to control the underlying inflammatory disease, to alleviate pain, restore quality of life, and preserve independence and the ability of patients to function in their activities of daily living. Prevention of joint destruction and co-morbidities of disease, including heart and lung disease are essential to these treatment goals.

The primary target of therapy in RA is remission, which is defined as the absence of signs or symptoms of inflammatory disease activity. The initial treatment approach in patients with RA is directed toward reduction of inflammatory symptoms and signs and includes the use of disease modifying anti-rheumatic drugs (DMARDs), usually methotrexate, with or without glucocorticosteroids, supplemented by nonsteroidal anti-inflammatory agents where helpful. Combinations of conventional DMARDs including hydroxychloroquine, sulfasalazine, and methotrexate are often used, with early assessment of response and intensification of therapy in the first 12 weeks following initiation of therapy as needed.

Treatment is intensified in patients who have high disease activity scores by the DAS-28 or CDAI or other. For patients on monotherapy, treatment can be escalated to triple DMARD therapy with the addition of sulfasalazine and hydroxychloroquine or the addition of biologic response modifiers including TNF inhibition, anti-cytokine therapy, T-cell co-stimulatory blockade, or kinase inhibition. For patients already taking combined methotrexate and a TNF inhibitor, an alternative biologic response modifier can be used for persistent active disease [1, 27, 28]. Currently approved biologic response modifiers for RA include anti TNF agents (infliximab, adalimumab, etanercept, certolizumab, golimumab), T-cell costimulatory factor inhibitor (abatacept), anti-IL1 blocker (anakinra), anti-IL6 receptor monoclonal antibody (tocilizumab), Janus kinase inhibitor (tofacitinib) and anti-CD20-directed therapy (rituximab).

Modern treatment of RA also includes attention to physical therapy, occupational therapy, and disease education for both the patient and their families. It is important to address the prevention of disease and treatment-related side effects including osteoporosis and cardiovascular disease, and pursue age-appropriate immunizations to reduce the likelihood of infections [26]. Treatment of extraarticular disease is directed at the specific extraarticular disease manifestations and can include, for example, topical therapies for dry eyes and dry mouth, and systemic immunosuppression with azathioprine, mycophenolate mofetil, and/or cyclophosphamide for more severe disease manifestations including vasculitis, scleritis, and lung disease.

Prognosis

Rheumatoid arthritis is associated with significant disability [1]. More than 75 % of patients with RA are partially disabled, and about 15 % of patients are completely disabled after a decade of disease. The disability begins early, with up to 20–30 % of patients disabled within the first 2–3 years of disease. Life expectancy is shortened by up to 3–7 years, especially in patients with extraarticular disease; infections and serious treatment-related side effects including tumors and gastrointestinal toxic effects from drugs used to treat RA further contribute disease morbidity and premature mortality [2, 4].

Patients who have RA are at 50 % higher risk of heart attack and more than twofold risk for heart failure with attendant decreased survivorship. Patients with RA-related ILD are at more than twofold increased risk of premature death [1, 2, 4].

Pulmonary Manifestations of Rheumatoid Arthritis

Introduction

A broad spectrum of pulmonary manifestations may be encountered in patients with RA and can involve any of the intrathoracic compartments including the lung parenchyma, pleura, airways, and the pulmonary vasculature (Table 3.1). Parenchymal lung disease consists of ILD and rheumatoid lung nodules. Rheumatoid lung nodules can be confused for malignancy. Airway diseases include cricoarytenoiditis, bronchiectasis, and small airways disease including constrictive bronchiolitis which can cause progressive airflow obstruction. Other forms of intrathoracic involvement include pleuritis, pleural effusion, and pulmonary vasculitis. In addition, drug-induced

Table 3.1 Spectrum of pulmonary manifestations in rheumatoid arthritis

Parenchymal
Usual interstitial pneumonia (UIP)
Nonspecific interstitial pneumonia (NSIP)
Organizing pneumonia (OP)
Lymphoid interstitial pneumonia (LIP)
Diffuse alveolar damage (DAD)
Desquamative interstitial pneumonia (DIP)
Eosinophilic pneumonia (EP)
Overlapping patterns of interstitial pneumonias
Rheumatoid lung nodule
Caplan's syndrome
Airways
Bronchiectasis
Constrictive bronchiolitis
Follicular bronchiolitis
Cricoarytenoiditis (upper airway obstruction)
Pleural
Pleuritis
Pleural effusion
Empyema
Pulmonary vascular
Vasculitis
Pulmonary hypertension
Others
Drug-induced lung disease
Infections

lung disease and pulmonary infections are relatively common in this patient population.

Pulmonary manifestation can be the presenting feature of RA, preceding articular manifestations in 10–20 % of RA patients [16, 29]. Clinical presentation of pulmonary disease may range from subclinical abnormalities identified by radiologic imaging or pulmonary function testing in the absence of accompanying symptoms to acute respiratory failure.

Interstitial Lung Disease

ILD is likely the most common pulmonary manifestations in RA and has been detected in 7–58 % of patients using chest imaging and pulmonary function testing [20, 30–34]. The wide range of this estimate is, in part, due to differing survey methods, e.g., chest radiography versus high-resolution computed tomography (HRCT) scan, but also on the criteria used to define the disease and the study population (e.g., stage of RA). Rheumatoid arthritis-related ILD is more commonly encountered in men who are middle-aged [34, 35]. High rheumatoid factor level, active joint disease, and smoking are risk factors for RA-related LD [5, 30, 36–38].

Various underlying histopathologic patterns may be seen in patients with RA-related ILD. Most common patterns are usual interstitial pneumonia (UIP) and nonspecific interstitial pneumonia (NSIP) but other patterns including diffuse alveolar damage (DAD), organizing pneumonia (OP), lymphocytic interstitial pneumonia (LIP), desquamative interstitial pneumonia (DIP), and eosinophilic pneumonia may also be encountered [29, 38–41]. Distinguishing these histopathologic patterns generally requires larger lung specimens as obtained via surgical lung biopsy rather than bronchoscopic biopsy. Underlying histopathologic patterns appear to have prognostic implications. For example, patients with UIP or DAD have shorter survival compared to those with NSIP or OP pattern [29, 39]. However, overlapping histopathologic patterns may be seen on lung biopsy, e.g., UIP with OP, in patients with RA-related ILD.

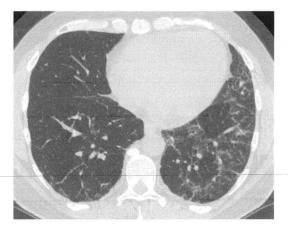

Fig. 3.1 High-resolution computed tomography (HRCT) scan of a 51-year-old man, ex-smoker, with rheumatoid arthritis and exertional dyspnea. Asymmetric parenchymal infiltrates are seen characterized by ground-glass opacities located peripherally, mainly in the left lung. Bronchoscopic biopsy showed organizing pneumonia

In some patients HRCT findings may suggest the dominant histologic pattern obviating the need for a lung biopsy [42].

Clinical features associated with ILD are non-specific and usually include progressive exertional dyspnea and non-productive cough [16, 43]. In the early stages of ILD, patients may not experience any respiratory symptoms [16, 30, 43]. Sometimes, RA-related ILD may present in an acute manner, resembling acute respiratory distress syndrome. In such situations, lung biopsy, if performed, usually reveals DAD [44–46].

Lung auscultation usually reveals inspiratory crackles over the lung bases [16, 33, 43]. Digital clubbing is uncommon. With advanced ILD, signs of respiratory distress and pulmonary hypertension may be present.

Chest radiography typically reveals bilateral interstitial infiltrates (reticular or reticulonodular opacities), more prominent in the lower lobes [16, 33, 43]. Sometimes the infiltrates may be patchy and homogeneous (ground-glass or consolidative opacities), especially when the underlying histopathologic pattern is OP (Fig. 3.1). High-resolution CT of the chest will provide a more detailed depiction of parenchymal opacities which will mostly consist of reticular and ground-glass opacities, with or without subpleural

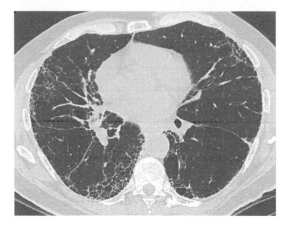

Fig. 3.2 HRCT scan of a 67-year-old man, nonsmoker, with a 6-year history of rheumatoid arthritis and slowly progressive exertional dyspnea over the preceding 2 years. Subpleural honeycombing is seen in both lungs, characteristic of usual interstitial pneumonia (UIP) pattern

honeycombing (seen in UIP pattern) (Fig. 3.2) [39, 47–49]. Radiologic findings on HRCT may suggest the predominant histopathologic pattern of underlying ILD but at other times present nonspecific results.

Pulmonary function testing will yield restrictive abnormalities similar to other ILDs with reduced lung volumes and diffusing capacity [16, 33, 43]. A mixed pattern of abnormalities, e.g., combined pattern of obstructive and restrictive changes, may be seen in patients with preexisting obstructive lung diseases such as chronic obstructive pulmonary disease or coexisting bronchiolar disease related to RA [50, 51]. Oxygen desaturation with exercise may be seen but hypoxemia at rest suggests advanced ILD.

In the majority of patients with RA and evidence of ILD, lung biopsy is not needed for diagnosis and management [16, 43, 52]. Bronchoscopy or surgical lung biopsy may be needed if there are atypical clinical or radiologic features that suggest a disorder other than that directly related to RA, e.g., infection, lymphoproliferative disease, etc.

The decision of whether treat RA-related ILD or not hinges on multiple factors including the severity of lung disease and symptoms, evidence of progression, comorbidities, likelihood of treatment response, potential side effects, and patient preferences [16, 43]. Most of the treatment data

in RA-related ILD consists of case series and other uncontrolled studies [16, 43, 52, 53].

For patients with progressive RA-related ILD, pharmacologic therapy usually involves corticosteroids which produce variable subjective and objective improvement [16, 33, 43, 54]. Typically, oral prednisone is used at a dose of 0.5–1.0 mg/kg/day. Other immunosuppressive agents that have been reported to be useful include azathioprine, cyclophosphamide, hydroxychloroquine, cyclosporine, mycophenolate mofetil, and tumor necrosis factor-α (TNF-α) inhibitors [16, 43, 54–56]. However, TNF-α inhibitors have also been reported to cause acute progression of RA-related ILD [57–60]. Rituximab has also been used in the management of RA-related ILD, with uncertain benefits; like TNF-inhibitors, it has also been reported to cause pulmonary decompensation in patients treated with it for cancer [61, 62]. It cannot be assumed that effective treatment for articular disease in RA will necessarily be effective in treating extraarticular manifestations including RA-related ILD. Methodical studies investigating the use of pharmacologic therapy in the treatment of RA-related ILD is needed including the use of novel biologic response modifiers. Lung transplantation is an option for patients with advanced RA-related ILD in the absence of contraindications.

In most patients with RA-related ILD, the lung disease slowly progresses over a number of years. The risk of death approximately three times higher in patients with RA-related ILD compared to RA patients without ILD [20]. Additionally, acute worsening ("acute exacerbation") of RA-related ILD has been reported and is commonly fatal (Fig. 3.3) [44–46].

Rheumatoid Lung Nodules and Caplan's Syndrome

Rheumatoid lung nodules are detected by chest radiography in 1 % of patients with RA whereas HRCT can detect lung nodules in up to 22 % [31, 63, 64]. The nodules are usually multiple and well-circumscribed, ranging in size from few millimeters to several centimeters (Fig. 3.4).

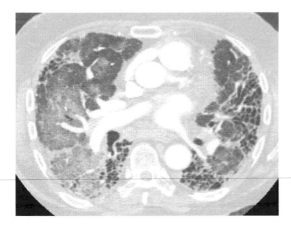

Fig. 3.3 HRCT scan of a 72-year-old man, ex-smoker, with a long history of rheumatoid arthritis and interstitial lung disease (ILD) presenting with acutely worsening dyspnea over the preceding few days. New ground-glass opacities are seen superimposed on preexisting ILD characterized by subpleural honeycombing bilaterally likely representing diffuse alveolar damage superimposed on UIP pattern. Two weeks later, the patient died of progressive respiratory failure

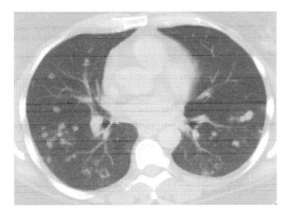

Fig. 3.4 HRCT scan of a 51-year-old woman, non-smoker, with a long history of rheumatoid arthritis and bilateral lung nodules. Numerous nodules, some cavitated, are seen in both lungs. Transthoracic needle aspiration biopsy confirmed the diagnosis of rheumatoid lung nodules

Pathologically, rheumatoid lung nodules appear granulomatous with collections of macrophages, lymphocytes, plasma cells, and palisading epithelioid cells around a necrotic core [38, 40, 41]. Rheumatoid lung nodules are pathologically identical to subcutaneous nodules and are the only pulmonary manifestation that is specific for RA [40].

Rheumatoid pulmonary nodules are detected radiologically and are usually not associated with symptoms. Rheumatoid lung nodules need to be distinguished from malignant and infectious nodules. In this regard, it should be noted that rheumatoid lung nodules can demonstrate mild fluorodeoxyglucose (FDG) uptake on positron emission tomography (PET) scanning. Transthoracic needle biopsy or bronchoscopic biopsy and sometimes surgical lung biopsy may be needed to confirm the diagnosis in cases where evolution of the lung lesion(s) causes suspicion regarding the underlying nature.

Rheumatoid lung nodules generally have a benign course. However, these lung nodules that are commonly subpleural in location can cavitate and cause pneumothorax and sometimes a bronchopleural fistula or empyema [38, 63, 65–67].

Caplan's syndrome refers to multiple lung nodules seen in patients with both RA and pneumoconiosis as originally described by Caplan in 1953 [68–72]. It has sometimes been called "rheumatoid pneumoconiosis" [68, 70]. Pneumoconiosis may be related to coal, silica, asbestos, or other inorganic dust exposure. Histopathologically, findings of necrobiotic nodule are seen with the additional presence of inorganic dust particles [40, 68, 73]. In this setting, these nodules can appear relatively rapidly over a course of weeks to a few months and often cavitate, resembling tuberculomas [68, 69]. Most patients with Caplan's syndrome are asymptomatic.

Airway Disease

Rheumatoid arthritis can cause several forms of airway disease including upper airway obstruction (cricoarytenoiditis), bronchiectasis, and small airways disease (bronchiolitis) [31, 33, 40, 43]. HRCT can detect signs of airway abnormalities such as bronchiectasis, air trapping, and bronchial wall thickening in the majority of patients with RA [63, 74, 75].

Upper airway obstruction resulting from cricoarytenoiditis can be life-threatening [76, 77]. Cricoarytenoiditis results from synovitis of the cricoarytenoid joint and generally occurs in patients with long-standing RA and severe articular disease [33]. Cricoarytenoid abnormalities can be seen by laryngoscopy and CT in up to 75 % of patients with RA but is not associated with symptoms in most of these subjects. When cricoarytenoiditis is bilateral and severe causing fixed airflow obstruction, flattening (plateau) is seen in the inspiratory and expiratory limbs of the flow-volume loop on pulmonary function testing [78]. Management of cricoarytenoiditis may require surgical intervention with mobilization of the cricoarytenoid joints. In those patients presenting with acute stridor emergency, tracheostomy may be needed [79].

Bronchiectasis (permanently dilated bronchi) has been reported in up to 30 % in patients with RA [63, 74, 75]. In most of these patients, relevant respiratory symptoms are absent and bronchiectasis does not appear to be clinically significant.

Bronchiolar disease seen in patients with RA is varied. Perhaps the most serious form of bronchiolar disease in this population is constrictive bronchiolitis (also called obliterative bronchiolitis or bronchiolitis obliterans). Although uncommon, constrictive bronchiolitis can gradually progress resulting in worsening airflow obstruction and eventually respiratory failure [51, 78, 80–83]. These patients usually present with persistent exertional dyspnea and cough. Lungs will typically sound clear to auscultation with no crackles or wheezes [51, 81]. Pulmonary function testing reveals evidence of airflow obstruction with air-trapping and hyperinflation. Airflow obstruction is irreversible with no response to inhaled bronchodilator. Diffusing capacity measurement is normal or only mildly reduced. High-resolution CT scan of the chest typically demonstrates a mosaic pattern with patchy areas of air-trapping (areas of hypoattenuation) which becomes more pronounced on expiratory CT imaging (Fig. 3.5) [81, 84]. Management of constrictive bronchiolitis in patients with RA remains difficult because it generally does not respond to currently available therapies including, corticosteroids, immunomodulators, macrolides, etc. [80, 81, 85].

Follicular bronchiolitis is another form of bronchiolar disease that can be seen in patients with RA [51, 86, 87]. Follicular bronchiolitis is

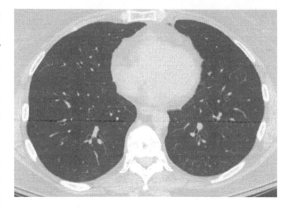

Fig. 3.5 HRCT scan of a 35-year-old woman, non-smoker, with a long history of rheumatoid arthritis and progressive exertional dyspnea over the preceding several months. Mosaic pattern in seen in both lungs due to patchy air trapping. Her FEV1 was 1.84 L (53 % predicted) with an FEV1/FVC ratio of 57.9 %. Six years later, she underwent a double lung transplant for progressive obstructive lung disease. Explant confirmed the diagnosis of constrictive bronchiolitis

associated with small nodular opacities in the lung on HRCT and variable abnormalities on pulmonary function testing [86–88]. In contrast to constrictive bronchiolitis, prognosis is relatively good for patients with follicular bronchiolitis [86–88].

Pulmonary Vascular Disease

Systemic vasculitis can rarely be seen in patients with RA and involve the pulmonary vasculature [40, 89]. This vascular involvement can result in alveolar hemorrhage [90]. Pulmonary hypertension in patients with RA is usually associated with advanced ILD but can sometimes be seen with pulmonary vasculitis in the absence of parenchymal fibrosis [33, 91, 92].

Pleural Disease

Pleural disease is common in patients with RA although it is frequently subclinical. On autopsy, pleural abnormalities can be identified in 38–73 % of patients [33, 40, 93, 94]. The spectrum of pleural involvement in RA includes pleuritis, pleural effusion, empyema, pneumothorax and bronchopleural fistula.

Pleural effusion is more commonly seen in men with longstanding joint disease and subcutaneous nodules [32, 33, 95]. Most rheumatoid pleural effusions are small, unilateral, and asymptomatic [32, 33, 95, 96]. The pleural fluid will typically be exudative by biochemical parameters with a low glucose level (usually <30 mg/dL) and a high rheumatoid factor titer [33, 95, 96]. For persistently symptomatic pleural effusions, treatment with corticosteroids (e.g., prednisone 10–20 mg/day), other immunosuppressive therapies, as well as nonsteroidal anti-inflammatory agents has been reported to be effective [33, 96, 97]. Pleurodesis is rarely needed in patients with rheumatoid pleural effusion [66, 96].

Sometimes, the rheumatoid pleural effusion may display characteristics of pseudochylothorax (also called chyliform, pseudochylous or cholesterol pleural effusion) and appear turbid or milky white with a high cholesterol level (typically >200 mg/dL) [95, 96, 98]. This is seen in the setting of a chronic pleural effusion associated with thickened pleura.

More severe forms of pleural disease are rare and include spontaneous pneumothorax, empyema, fibrothorax, and broncho-pleural fistula [33, 66, 95, 96]. Not uncommonly, management of these complications involves surgical maneuvers.

Conclusions

Rheumatoid arthritis can cause a wide spectrum of intrathoracic manifestations, some of which can lead to progressive respiratory embarrassment and occasionally death. Appropriate management of these disease features depends on establishing their relationship to the underlying RA, since similar presentations can be seen with drug-induced diseases and infectious complications. In addition, management must be tailored to the individual patient context including severity of the pulmonary manifestation and comorbidities. These situations can be complex and require a judicious clinical approach.

References

1. Scott DL, Wolfe F, Huizinga TWJ. Rheumatoid arthritis. Lancet. 2010;376(9746):1094–108.
2. Gabriel SE, Crowson CS, Kremers HM, Doran MF, Turesson C, O'Fallon WM, et al. Survival in rheumatoid arthritis: a population-based analysis of trends over 40 years. Arthritis Rheum. 2003;48(1):54–8.
3. Turesson C, O'Fallon WM, Crowson CS, Gabriel SE, Matteson EL. Occurrence of extraarticular disease manifestations is associated with excess mortality in a community based cohort of patients with rheumatoid arthritis. J Rheumatol. 2002;29(1):62–7.
4. Myasoedova E, Davis 3rd JM, Crowson CS, Gabriel SE. Epidemiology of rheumatoid arthritis: rheumatoid arthritis and mortality. Curr Rheumatol Rep. 2010;12(5):379–85.
5. Turesson C, O'Fallon WM, Crowson CS, Gabriel SE, Matteson EL. Extra-articular disease manifestations in rheumatoid arthritis: incidence trends and risk factors over 46 years. Ann Rheum Dis. 2003;62(8):722–7.
6. McInnes IB, Schett G. The pathogenesis of rheumatoid arthritis. N Engl J Med. 2011;365(23):2205–19.
7. van der Woude D, Houwing-Duistermaat JJ, Toes REM, Huizinga TWJ, Thomson W, Worthington J, et al. Quantitative heritability of anti-citrullinated protein antibody-positive and anti-citrullinated protein antibody-negative rheumatoid arthritis. Arthritis Rheum. 2009;60(4):916–23.
8. Avouac J, Gossec L, Dougados M. Diagnostic and predictive value of anti-cyclic citrullinated protein antibodies in rheumatoid arthritis: a systematic literature review. Ann Rheum Dis. 2006;65(7):845–51.
9. Carlens C, Hergens M-P, Grunewald J, Ekbom A, Eklund A, Hoglund CO, et al. Smoking, use of moist snuff, and risk of chronic inflammatory diseases. Am J Respir Crit Care Med. 2010;181(11):1217–22.
10. Stolt P, Bengtsson C, Nordmark B, Lindblad S, Lundberg I, Klareskog L, et al. Quantification of the influence of cigarette smoking on rheumatoid arthritis: results from a population based case–control study, using incident cases. Ann Rheum Dis. 2003;62(9):835–41.
11. Silman AJ, Newman J, MacGregor AJ. Cigarette smoking increases the risk of rheumatoid arthritis. Results from a nationwide study of disease-discordant twins. Arthritis Rheum. 1996;39(5):732–5.
12. Klareskog L, Stolt P, Lundberg K, Kallberg H, Bengtsson C, Grunewald J, et al. A new model for an etiology of rheumatoid arthritis: smoking may trigger HLA-DR (shared epitope)-restricted immune reactions to autoantigens modified by citrullination. Arthritis Rheum. 2006;54(1):38–46.
13. Turesson C, Matteson EL, Colby TV, Vuk-Pavlovic Z, Vassallo R, Weyand CM, et al. Increased CD4+ T cell

infiltrates in rheumatoid arthritis-associated interstitial pneumonitis compared with idiopathic interstitial pneumonitis. Arthritis Rheum. 2005;52(1):73–9.

14. Atkins SR, Turesson C, Myers JL, Tazelaar HD, Ryu JH, Matteson EL, et al. Morphologic and quantitative assessment of CD20+ B cell infiltrates in rheumatoid arthritis-associated nonspecific interstitial pneumonia and usual interstitial pneumonia. Arthritis Rheum. 2006;54(2):635–41.

15. Bongartz T, Cantaert T, Atkins SR, Harle P, Myers JL, Turesson C, et al. Citrullination in extra-articular manifestations of rheumatoid arthritis. Rheumatology. 2007;46(1):70–5.

16. Brown KK. Rheumatoid lung disease. Proc Am Thorac Soc. 2007;4(5):443–8.

17. Ancochea J, Giron RM, Lopez-Botet M. Production of tumor necrosis factor alpha and interleukin-6 by alveolar macrophages from patients with rheumatoid arthritis and interstitial pulmonary disease. Arch Bronconeumol. 1997;33(7):335–40.

18. Horie S, Nakada K, Minota S, Kano S. High proliferative potential colony-forming cells (HPP-CFCs) in the peripheral blood of rheumatoid arthritis patients with interstitial lung disease. Scand J Rheumatol. 2003; 32(5):273–6.

19. Olson AL, Swigris JJ, Sprunger DB, Fischer A, Fernandez-Perez ER, Solomon J, et al. Rheumatoid arthritis-interstitial lung disease-associated mortality. Am J Respir Crit Care Med. 2011;183(3):372–8.

20. Bongartz T, Nannini C, Medina-Velasquez YF, Achenbach SJ, Crowson CS, Ryu JH, et al. Incidence and mortality of interstitial lung disease in rheumatoid arthritis: a population-based study. Arthritis Rheum. 2010;62(6):1583–91.

21. Maradit-Kremers H, Nicola PJ, Crowson CS, Ballman KV, Gabriel SE. Cardiovascular death in rheumatoid arthritis: a population-based study. Arthritis Rheum. 2005;52(3):722–32.

22. Sihvonen S, Korpela M, Laippala P, Mustonen J, Pasternack A. Death rates and causes of death in patients with rheumatoid arthritis: a population-based study.[Erratum appears in Scand J Rheumatol. 2006 Jul-Aug;35(4):332]. Scand J Rheumatol. 2004;33(4): 221–7.

23. Doran MF, Crowson CS, Pond GR, O'Fallon WM, Gabriel SE. Predictors of infection in rheumatoid arthritis. Arthritis Rheum. 2002;46(9):2294–300.

24. Liang KP, Liang KV, Matteson EL, McClelland RL, Christianson TJH, Turesson C. Incidence of noncardiac vascular disease in rheumatoid arthritis and relationship to extraarticular disease manifestations. Arthritis Rheum. 2006;54(2):642–8.

25. Aletaha D, Neogi T, Silman AJ, Funovits J, Felson DT, Bingham 3rd CO, et al. 2010 Rheumatoid arthritis classification criteria: an American College of Rheumatology/European League Against Rheumatism collaborative initiative. Arthritis Rheum. 2010;62(9):2569–81.

26. Davis III JM, Matteson EL, American College of Rheumatology, European League Against Rheumatism.

27. Felson DT, Smolen JS, Wells G, Zhang B, van Tuyl LHD, Funovits J, et al. American College of Rheumatology/European League Against Rheumatism provisional definition of remission in rheumatoid arthritis for clinical trials. Arthritis Rheum. 2011;63(3):573–86.

28. Emery P, Breedveld FC, Hall S, Durez P, Chang DJ, Robertson D, et al. Comparison of methotrexate monotherapy with a combination of methotrexate and etanercept in active, early, moderate to severe rheumatoid arthritis (COMET): a randomised, double-blind, parallel treatment trial. Lancet. 2008; 372(9636):375–82.

29. Tsuchiya Y, Takayanagi N, Sugiura H, Miyahara Y, Tokunaga D, Kawabata Y, et al. Lung diseases directly associated with rheumatoid arthritis and their relationship to outcome. Eur Respir J. 2011;37(6): 1411–7.

30. Gochuico BR, Avila NA, Chow CK, Novero LJ, Wu H-P, Ren P, et al. Progressive preclinical interstitial lung disease in rheumatoid arthritis. Arch Intern Med. 2008;168(2):159–66.

31. Dawson JK, Fewins HE, Desmond J, Lynch MP, Graham DR. Fibrosing alveolitis in patients with rheumatoid arthritis as assessed by high resolution computed tomography, chest radiography, and pulmonary function tests. [see comment]. Thorax. 2001; 56(8):622–7.

32. Mayberry JP, Primack SL, Muller NL. Thoracic manifestations of systemic autoimmune diseases: radiographic and high-resolution CT findings. Radiographics. 2000;20(6):1623–35.

33. Tanoue LT. Pulmonary manifestations of rheumatoid arthritis. Clin Chest Med. 1998;19(4):667–85, viii.

34. Gabbay E, Tarala R, Will R, Carroll G, Adler B, Cameron D, et al. Interstitial lung disease in recent onset rheumatoid arthritis. Am J Respir Crit Care Med. 1997;156(2 Pt 1):528–35.

35. Weyand CM, Schmidt D, Wagner U, Goronzy JJ. The influence of sex on the phenotype of rheumatoid arthritis. Arthritis Rheum. 1998;41(5):817–22.

36. Rajasekaran BA, Shovlin D, Lord P, Kelly CA. Interstitial lung disease in patients with rheumatoid arthritis: a comparison with cryptogenic fibrosing alveolitis. Rheumatology. 2001;40(9):1022–5.

37. Saag KG, Kolluri S, Koehnke RK, Georgou TA, Rachow JW, Hunninghake GW, et al. Rheumatoid arthritis lung disease. Determinants of radiographic and physiologic abnormalities. Arthritis Rheum. 1996;39(10):1711–9.

38. Yousem SA, Colby TV, Carrington CB. Lung biopsy in rheumatoid arthritis. Am Rev Respir Dis. 1985;131(5):770–7.

39. Lee HK, Kim DS, Yoo B, Seo JB, Rho JY, Colby TV, et al. Histopathologic pattern and clinical features of rheumatoid arthritis-associated interstitial lung disease. Chest. 2005;127(6):2019–27.

40. Colby TV. Pulmonary pathology in patients with systemic autoimmune diseases. Clin Chest Med. 1998;19(4):587–612, vii.

41. Hakala M, Paakko P, Huhti E, Tarkka M, Sutinen S. Open lung biopsy of patients with rheumatoid arthritis. Clin Rheumatol. 1990;9(4):452–60.

42. Kim EJ, Collard HR, King Jr TE. Rheumatoid arthritis-associated interstitial lung disease: the relevance of histopathologic and radiographic pattern. Chest. 2009;136(5):1397–405.

43. Nannini C, Ryu JH, Matteson EL. Lung disease in rheumatoid arthritis. Curr Opin Rheumatol. 2008; 20(3):340–6.

44. Parambil JG, Myers JL, Ryu JH. Diffuse alveolar damage: uncommon manifestation of pulmonary involvement in patients with connective tissue diseases. Chest. 2006;130(2):553–8.

45. Parambil JG, Myers JL, Aubry M-C, Ryu JH. Causes and prognosis of diffuse alveolar damage diagnosed on surgical lung biopsy. Chest. 2007;132(1):50–7.

46. Churg A, Wright JL, Tazelaar HD. Acute exacerbations of fibrotic interstitial lung disease. Histopathology. 2011;58(4):525–30.

47. Mori S, Cho I, Koga Y, Sugimoto M. Comparison of pulmonary abnormalities on high-resolution computed tomography in patients with early versus long-standing rheumatoid arthritis. J Rheumatol. 2008; 35(8):1513–21.

48. Tanaka N, Kim JS, Newell JD, Brown KK, Cool CD, Meehan R, et al. Rheumatoid arthritis-related lung diseases: CT findings. Radiology. 2004;232(1): 81–91.

49. Horton MR. Rheumatoid arthritis associated interstitial lung disease. Crit Rev Comput Tomogr. 2004; 45(5–6):429–40.

50. Cottin V, Cordier J-F. Combined pulmonary fibrosis and emphysema in connective tissue disease. Curr Opin Pulm Med. 2012;18(5):418–27.

51. Ryu JH, Myers JL, Swensen SJ. Bronchiolar disorders. Am J Respir Crit Care Med. 2003;168(11): 1277–92.

52. Ascherman DP. Interstitial lung disease in rheumatoid arthritis. Curr Rheumatol Rep. 2010;12(5):363–9.

53. Young A, Koduri G. Extra-articular manifestations and complications of rheumatoid arthritis. Best Pract Res Clin Rheumatol. 2007;21(5):907–27.

54. Lamblin C, Bergoin C, Saelens T, Wallaert B. Interstitial lung diseases in collagen vascular diseases. Eur Respir J Suppl. 2001;32:69s–80.

55. Saketkoo LA, Espinoza LR. Rheumatoid arthritis interstitial lung disease: mycophenolate mofetil as an antifibrotic and disease-modifying antirheumatic drug. Arch Intern Med. 2008;168(15):1718–9.

56. Vassallo R, Matteson E, Thomas Jr CF. Clinical response of rheumatoid arthritis-associated pulmonary fibrosis to tumor necrosis factor-alpha inhibition. Chest. 2002;122(3):1093–6.

57. Horai Y, Miyamura T, Shimada K, Takahama S, Minami R, Yamamoto M, et al. Eternacept for the treatment of patients with rheumatoid arthritis and concurrent interstitial lung disease. J Clin Pharm Ther. 2012;37(1):117–21.

58. Tournadre A, Ledoux-Eberst J, Poujol D, Dubost J-J, Ristori J-M, Soubrier M. Exacerbation of interstitial lung disease during etanercept therapy: Two cases. Joint Bone Spine. 2008;75(2):215–8.

59. Hagiwara K, Sato T, Takagi-Kobayashi S, Hasegawa S, Shigihara N, Akiyama O. Acute exacerbation of preexisting interstitial lung disease after administration of etanercept for rheumatoid arthritis. J Rheumatol. 2007;34(5):1151–4.

60. Lindsay K, Melsom R, Jacob BK, Mestry N. Acute progression of interstitial lung disease: a complication of etanercept particularly in the presence of rheumatoid lung and methotrexate treatment. Rheumatology. 2006;45(8):1048–9.

61. Matteson EL, Bongartz T, Ryu JH, Crowson CS, Hartman TE, Dellaripa PF. Open-label, pilot study of the safety and clinical effects of rituximab in patients with rheumatoid arthritis-associated interstitial pneumonia. Open J Rheumatol Autoimmune Dis. 2012; 2(3):53–8.

62. Liote H, Liote F, Seroussi B, Mayaud C, Cadranel J. Rituximab-induced lung disease: a systematic literature review. Eur Respir J. 2010;35(3):681–7.

63. Cortet B, Flipo RM, Remy-Jardin M, Coquerelle P, Duquesnoy B, Remy J, et al. Use of high resolution computed tomography of the lungs in patients with rheumatoid arthritis. Ann Rheum Dis. 1995;54(10): 815–9.

64. Walker WC, Wright V. Pulmonary lesions and rheumatoid arthritis. Medicine. 1968;47(6):501–20.

65. Rueth N, Andrade R, Groth S, D'Cunha J, Maddaus M. Pleuropulmonary complications of rheumatoid arthritis: a thoracic surgeon's challenge. Ann Thorac Surg. 2009;88(3):e20–1.

66. Caples SM, Utz JP, Allen MS, Ryu JH. Thoracic surgical procedures in patients with rheumatoid arthritis. J Rheumatol. 2004;31(11):2136–41.

67. Adelman HM, Dupont EL, Flannery MT, Wallach PM. Case report: recurrent pneumothorax in a patient with rheumatoid arthritis. Am J Med Sci. 1994; 308(3):171–2.

68. Schreiber J, Koschel D, Kekow J, Waldburg N, Goette A, Merget R. Rheumatoid pneumoconiosis (Caplan's syndrome). Eur J Intern Med. 2010;21(3):168–72.

69. Arakawa H, Honma K, Shida H, Saito Y, Morikubo H. Computed tomography findings of Caplan syndrome. J Comput Assist Tomogr. 2003;27(5):758–60.

70. Greaves IA. Rheumatoid "pneumoconiosis" (Caplan's syndrome) in an asbestos worker: a 17 years' follow-up. Thorax. 1979;34(3):404–5.

71. Unge G, Mellner C. Caplan's syndrome—a clinical study of 13 cases. Scand J Respir Dis. 1975;56(6): 287–91.

72. Caplan A. Certain unusual radiological appearances in the chest of coal-miners suffering from rheumatoid arthritis. Thorax. 1953;8:28–37.

73. Helmers R, Galvin J, Hunninghake GW. Pulmonary manifestations associated with rheumatoid arthritis. Chest. 1991;100(1):235–8.

74. Perez T, Remy-Jardin M, Cortet B. Airways involvement in rheumatoid arthritis: clinical, functional, and HRCT findings. Am J Respir Crit Care Med. 1998;157 (5 Pt 1):1658–65.

75. Cortet B, Perez T, Roux N, Flipo RM, Duquesnoy B, Delcambre B, et al. Pulmonary function tests and high resolution computed tomography of the lungs in patients with rheumatoid arthritis. Ann Rheum Dis. 1997;56(10):596–600.

76. Geterud A, Bake B, Berthelsen B, Bjelle A, Ejnell H. Laryngeal involvement in rheumatoid arthritis. Acta Otolaryngol. 1991;111(5):990–8.

77. Charlin B, Brazeau-Lamontagne L, Levesque RY, Lussier A. Cricoarytenoiditis in rheumatoid arthritis: comparison of fibrolaryngoscopic and high resolution computerized tomographic findings. J Otolaryngol. 1985;14(6):381–6.

78. Ryu JH, Scanlon PD. Obstructive lung diseases: COPD, asthma, and many imitators. Mayo Clin Proc. 2001;76(11):1144–53.

79. Peters JE, Burke CJ, Morris VH. Three cases of rheumatoid arthritis with laryngeal stridor. Clin Rheumatol. 2011;30(5):723–7.

80. Devouassoux G, Cottin V, Liote H, Marchand E, Frachon I, Schuller A, et al. Characterisation of severe obliterative bronchiolitis in rheumatoid arthritis. Eur Respir J. 2009;33(5):1053–61.

81. Parambil JG, Yi ES, Ryu JH. Obstructive bronchiolar disease identified by CT in the non-transplant population: analysis of 29 consecutive cases. Respirology. 2009;14(3):443–8.

82. Schwarz MI, Lynch DA, Tuder R. Bronchiolitis obliterans: the lone manifestation of rheumatoid arthritis? Eur Respir J. 1994;7(4):817–20.

83. Geddes DM, Webley M, Emerson PA. Airways obstruction in rheumatoid arthritis. Ann Rheum Dis. 1979;38(3):222–5.

84. Devakonda A, Raoof S, Sung A, Travis WD, Naidich D. Bronchiolar disorders: a clinical-radiological diagnostic algorithm. Chest. 2010;137(4):938–51.

85. Ryu JH. Classification and approach to bronchiolar diseases. Curr Opin Pulm Med. 2006;12(2):145–51.

86. Howling SJ, Hansell DM, Wells AU, Nicholson AG, Flint JD, Muller NL. Follicular bronchiolitis: thin-section CT and histologic findings. Radiology. 1999;212(3):637–42.

87. Hayakawa H, Sato A, Imokawa S, Toyoshima M, Chida K, Iwata M. Bronchiolar disease in rheumatoid arthritis. Am J Respir Crit Care Med. 1996;154(5): 1531–6.

88. Aerni MR, Vassallo R, Myers JL, Lindell RM, Ryu JH. Follicular bronchiolitis in surgical lung biopsies: clinical implications in 12 patients. Respir Med. 2008;102(2):307–12.

89. Genta MS, Genta RM, Gabay C. Systemic rheumatoid vasculitis: a review. Semin Arthritis Rheum. 2006;36(2):88–98.

90. Schwarz MI, Zamora MR, Hodges TN, Chan ED, Bowler RP, Tuder RM. Isolated pulmonary capillaritis and diffuse alveolar hemorrhage in rheumatoid arthritis and mixed connective tissue disease. Chest. 1998;113(6):1609–15.

91. Morikawa J, Kitamura K, Habuchi Y, Tsujimura Y, Minamikawa T, Takamatsu T. Pulmonary hypertension in a patient with rheumatoid arthritis. Chest. 1988;93(4):876–8.

92. Kay JM, Banik S. Unexplained pulmonary hypertension with pulmonary arthritis in rheumatoid disease. Br J Dis Chest. 1977;71(1):53–9.

93. Franquet T. High-resolution CT, of lung disease related to collagen vascular disease. Radiol Clin North Am. 2001;39(6):1171–87.

94. Gauhar UA, Gaffo AL, Alarcon GS. Pulmonary manifestations of rheumatoid arthritis. Semin Respir Crit Care Med. 2007;28(4):430–40.

95. Joseph J, Sahn SA. Connective tissue diseases and the pleura. Chest. 1993;104(1):262–70.

96. Balbir-Gurman A, Yigla M, Nahir AM, Braun-Moscovici Y. Rheumatoid pleural effusion. Semin Arthritis Rheum. 2006;35(6):368–78.

97. Avnon LS, Abu-Shakra M, Flusser D, Heimer D, Sion-Vardy N. Pleural effusion associated with rheumatoid arthritis: what cell predominance to anticipate? Rheumatol Int. 2007;27(10): 919–25.

98. Ryu JH, Tomassetti S, Maldonado F. Update on uncommon pleural effusions. Respirology. 2011; 16(2):238–43.

Interstitial Lung Disease in Systemic Sclerosis

4

Nargues Weir and Virginia Steen

Introduction

Scleroderma is a multisystem autoimmune disease characterized by progressive fibrosis of the skin and internal organs. The incidence in the United States and among European countries ranges between 4 and 19 new cases per million persons each year, but the prevalence varies widely, with the last estimate in the US being 276 cases per million [1, 2]. The disease presents in the fifth or sixth decade of life and more commonly among women, with African-Americans presenting younger than Caucasians [1, 3–5]. Fibrotic lung disease is prevalent with estimates of 74 % diagnosis at autopsy [6] and interstitial lung disease (ILD) is now established as the leading cause of death in scleroderma [7–9].

Risk Factors

Skin thickening is a risk factor for overall mortality in scleroderma, but there is no association between skin involvement and ILD [9, 10].

N. Weir, M.D.
Department of Medicine, NIH-Inova Advanced Lung Disease Program, Falls Church, VA, USA
e-mail: Nargues.weir@inova.org

V. Steen, M.D. (✉)
Department of Medicine, Georgetown University Medical Center, Washington, DC, USA
e-mail: steenv@georgetown.edu

Patients with scleroderma-specific autoantibodies, particularly anti-topoisomerase, anti U1-RNP (often associated with mixed connective tissue disease patients), and ANAs with a nucleolar pattern, anti U3-RNP and anti Th/To, are much more likely to have significant pulmonary fibrosis compared to patients with anti-centromere or anti-RNA polymerase III antibodies [11–13].

Abnormal pulmonary function tests (PFTs) may be the most helpful risk factors for identifying ILD in scleroderma and thus, PFTs should be performed at the first evaluation. A low forced vital capacity (FVC) and/or diffusion capacity for carbon monoxide (DLco) at presentation or within the first 2 years of scleroderma [14, 15] predict progressive ILD. Progressive deterioration of FVC and DLco are also indicative of poor outcomes and development of end-stage lung disease [16, 17]. Patients with fibrotic lung disease tend to have more significant dyspnea at presentation (New York Heart Association Class III or IV) and have crackles on lung exam [18]. Other risk factors for progressive lung fibrosis that have borne out in cohort studies include male gender [9], African-American race [19], diffuse disease subtype [4], digital ulcers [5], the presence of proteinuria [15], anti-topoisomerase antibody [19], and shorter disease duration. Smoking has been previously linked with rapid progression and more severe restriction in cohorts [20], but many recent studies have countered this association, demonstrating equally severe restriction among nonsmokers [19, 21–23].

P.F. Dellaripa et al. (eds.), *Pulmonary Manifestations of Rheumatic Disease: A Comprehensive Guide*,
DOI 10.1007/978-1-4939-0770-0_4, © Springer Science+Business Media New York 2014

Diagnosis

Exertional dyspnea and cough are common symptoms of ILD, but because of the high prevalence and morbidity and mortality associated with lung involvement, screening is recommended for all patients with scleroderma by initial and periodic PFTs regardless of symptoms [24]. The most sensitive markers of PFTs for restrictive lung disease are the FVC and the diffusion capacity for carbon monoxide (DLco) [25]. The latter is more sensitive for detection of early disease [18, 26, 27], although an isolated reduction of DLco is more commonly associated with progressive pulmonary vascular disease [28]. However, given the prevalence of concomitant pulmonary vascular disease, which is also associated with reduced DLco, the specificity for ILD is reduced in scleroderma [28]. Given this comorbid issue, a FVC%/DLco% ratio of greater than 1.6 is sometimes helpful to determine the presence of pulmonary hypertension as opposed to early ILD [8, 29]. Screening is performed biannually and abnormal values are debatable, with values used in practice and in clinical trials ranging anywhere from FVC ≤70 % to FVC ≤80 % predicted, or utilizing a decrement in FVC by ≥10 % [30]. Values for diffusion capacity are more traditionally considered abnormal when DLco ≤80 % predicted or a decrement by ≥15 % is noted [31–33]. However, given the variability seen in PFTs, a more reliable method of diagnosis is required, namely computed tomography, with high resolution imaging.

High-resolution computed tomography (HRCT) scanning of the chest is much more sensitive than plain chest radiography or standard computed tomography [30, 34], and it is considered to be the gold standard for diagnosing ILD, in scleroderma and other ILDs. It allows for low sampling rate with very low radiation dose exposure making this the ideal noninvasive diagnostic tool [35]. It correlates well with PFTs and other clinical markers of function in scleroderma [21, 36]. Early changes of ILD on HRCT are ground-glass opacities, followed by interseptal thickening, and reticular or reticulonodular changes [18, 21, 37]. More advanced or fibrotic changes seen on HRCT include traction bronchiectasis which is a sign of architectural distortion, cystic changes, and frank honeycombing [18, 21] These changes typically begin at the peripheral, posterior, and basal lung zones, and progress centrally, anteriorly, and caudally [18].

The findings of ground-glass opacity (GGO) had initially been associated with reversible disease based on several clinicopathologic studies [38, 39]. However, later studies have questioned this assertion. GGOs have been more recently associated with fibrosis, progression of disease, and lack of response to treatment in other series [40]. While there is evidence of association between GGO and alveolar inflammation [21, 41], this cellularity neither predicts progression of disease nor response to therapy [41, 42].

Pathogenesis

Diagnosis of ILD is made predominantly on PFTs and confirmed by HRCT. Surgical lung biopsies are not routinely pursued unless the presentation or radiographic appearance is atypical. Pathologically, surgical biopsies show inflammation and fibrosis, in the lower lobes more so than the upper lobes, with rare involvement of the pleura [43]. Focal peribronchial lymphoid hyperplasia and occasional follicular bronchiolitis can also be seen [43]. While pathologically it can be indistinguishable from idiopathic pulmonary fibrosis (IPF), matched scleroderma patients have milder restriction on PFTS [43], less breathlessness, hypoxia, and functional impairment [44], and significantly better survival compared with IPF [45]. Survival remains between 77 and 86 % at 5 years [16, 45, 46].

While bronchoalveolar lavage (BAL) still retains a function in research [47], there is no currently established clinical role for BAL in the diagnosis of scleroderma fibrotic lung disease [48]. Confirmation of alveolitis by both BAL and surgical lung biopsy has been investigated for diagnostic purposes and notably there is good correlation with HRCT findings [38, 39]. There is much conflicting data as to whether BAL cellularity can predict response to therapy or even be altered with therapy [41, 42]. Therefore, BAL currently remains a valuable research tool to expand our understanding of the inflammatory, fibrotic, oxidant, and other natures of the lower respiratory tract.

The vast majority of scleroderma ILD is nonspecific interstitial pneumonitis (NSIP) [16]. Fibrotic NSIP appears to be more prevalent than cellular NSIP in the largest published surgical series [16]. PFTs and survival did not differ between the NSIP subtypes in that report, nor did survival differ between NSIP and usual interstitial pneumonitis (UIP) [16]. Therefore, surgical lung biopsy is not routinely recommended since the pathological subtype of scleroderma ILD does not impact survival. Second in prevalence is UIP, followed by end-stage lung disease. Less commonly seen are respiratory bronchiolitis-ILD and centrilobular fibrosis [49]. Survival in scleroderma ILD overall is better than in IPF, even when it is indistinguishable by PFTs, HRCT, or pathology [44, 50].

Lastly, thoracic malignancy ought to be mentioned when discussing scleroderma lung disease. While 13 % of scleroderma mortality is attributed to cancer deaths, lung cancer is the leading cause of cancer in scleroderma and many of the primary causes are indeed thoracic in etiology [51, 52]. Among these, non-small cell carcinoma of the lung is the most common, but small cell carcinoma of the lung, lymphoma, breast cancer, and esophageal cancer are also seen [51]. Lung cancers are strongly associated with cigarette smoking in scleroderma, related to a sevenfold risk of malignancy in these patients [53]. Pulmonary fibrosis in itself however does not increase the risk for lung cancer [53].

Treatment

The natural history of ILD is quite variable and stability is the rule for many patients. The decision to treat should be based on the likelihood that patients have the potential to respond to the immunosuppressive agents being used today. Thus, the presence of more than 20 % of the lung involved in the HRCT, early disease, and progression of FVC during serial PFTs is more helpful than symptoms or the mere presence of interstitial changes on HRCT [54]. The treatment

of lung disease is the same in limited and diffuse disease, and is predicated upon the large trials that have been completed within the past decade. The first large study of cyclophosphamide demonstrated a modest yet significant improvement in FVC compared to placebo without improvement in DLco [55]. In addition to the small but statistical difference in the FVC, the study showed improvement in other measures of clinical importance in the cyclophosphamide group. This difference from the placebo group correlated most closely with more fibrosis on HRCT as opposed to findings of ground glass or alveolitis on BAL. Another randomized controlled trial using intravenous cyclophosphamide in combination with other drug interventions similarly found a small improvement in FVC (not significant) but again without improvement in diffusion impairment [56]. Cough improved significantly in the treatment group of the Scleroderma Lung Study, but this improvement did not correlate with improvement in FVC [57]. This improvement disappeared after cyclophosphamide was discontinued. Also in the Scleroderma Lung Study, fibrotic scores on HRCT stabilized in the cyclophosphamide group compared with significant progression in the placebo group, and these radiographic changes correlated with PFTs and dyspnea scores [58, 59]. The addition of corticosteroids at varying doses has been studied as well, but rarely in a controlled fashion and generally is not used in scleroderma lung disease [56, 60, 61]. Other drugs that are used but have been studied in only limited settings include azathioprine (mostly for maintenance therapy) [56, 62], and mycophenolate mofetil [63, 64]. A large ongoing trial comparing mycophenolate mofetil to cyclophosphamide should be helpful in future treatment.

Future Directions in Scleroderma ILD

Future biomarkers for screening and monitoring scleroderma lung disease may include IL-15 [65] and plasma homocysteine [66]. More recently, both serum KL-6 and serum surfactant protein D (SP-D) have been shown to correlate with fibrotic lung scores in scleroderma patients making them promising biomarkers [67, 68]. Both levels are elevated in scleroderma patients compared with healthy controls and correlate progressively with worsening lung fibrosis. BAL detection of impaired hepatocyte growth factor and CCL18 may help detect those at greater risk for ILD [69]. Exhaled alveolar nitric oxide may be able to detect very early ILD [70, 71]. Imaging modalities like ultrasound can detect thickened interlobular septa and has the advantage of portability and being free from exposure to ionizing radiation [72]. Ultrasound may allow for more frequent imaging and universal screening. Future interventions that are being investigated include imatinib [73, 74], *N*-acetylcysteine [75, 76], anti-IL-6 receptor antibody [77], and rituximab [78–80].

The following cases demonstrate some of the difficulties and challenges in managing patients with scleroderma and lung disease.

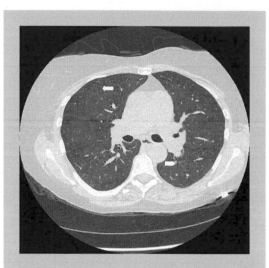

Fig. 4.1 HRCT in early scleroderma demonstrates subtle reticulonodular changes (*arrowhead*) with traction bronchiectasis (*arrow*)

Case Vignette 1: Limited Scleroderma with Aggressive Interstitial Lung Disease

A 48-year-old Caucasian woman has had 3 years of Raynaud's and 18 months of hand swelling, with numbness and tingling. She also had gastroesophageal reflux disease (GERD) but denied any shortness of breath or cough. She was seen by a rheumatologist and found to have skin thickening limited to her hands and fingers, a positive anti-topoisomerase (Scl 70) antibody and had PFTs showing a FVC% predicted of 70 % and a DLCO% predicted of 68 %. Chest X-ray reportedly showed mild atelectasis. HRCT showed subtle reticulonodular changes (Fig. 4.1). She was started on nifedipine, omeprazole, and naproxyn and was instructed to return in 6 months. At her return visit, she had new digital ulcers, increased fatigue, increased hyperpigmentation but no change in her limited skin thickening, but she also had a tendon

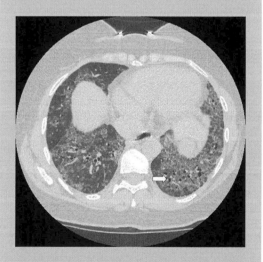

Fig. 4.2 HRCT in scleroderma demonstrating the lung bases are diffusely involved not only with ground-glass opacities but also with fibrotic changes as evidenced by cystic honey-combed changes adjacent to the diaphragm. Traction bronchiectasis (*arrow*) is again appreciated

friction rub on her right Achilles tendon. Repeat PFTs at this time showed a FVC% predicted of 63 % and a DLCO% predicted of 65 %, and the high resolution CT scan showed typical basilar interstitial fibrosis (Fig. 4.2).

(continued)

Case Vignette 1 (continued)

Although typically limited cutaneous scleroderma patients are less likely to present with or develop ILD compared with diffuse patients [18], there are several groups of limited scleroderma who develop ILD which is indistinguishable from that seen in diffuse scleroderma. Patients such as this one who have a anti-topoisomerase or Scl-70 autoantibody, early disease and even a tendon friction rub but who do not have diffuse cutaneous skin thickening are particularly at risk. More than 25 % of Scl-70 patients do not get diffuse skin disease but they can get severe lung disease similar to other Scl-70 patients. Likewise, limited cutaneous patients with a nucleolar pattern ANA are at high risk and these patients should be carefully followed and screened for ILD. Only limited cutaneous patients with anti-centromere antibody are very unlikely to develop significant ILD, although they may have some changes on HRCT and have intermittent aspiration pneumonias causing other problems.

The pathologic lung changes in limited disease are identical to what is seen in diffuse disease, with the majority of the pathologic diagnoses being NSIP, and the second most frequent being UIP [81]. While lung involvement in limited disease has traditionally been described as milder and slower in progression, 40 % of the patients in the Scleroderma Lung Study had limited disease. Their PFTs were equally impaired as the patients with diffuse disease, and they demonstrated similar response to therapy with even worse fibrosis noted within the limited subgroup [82]. Therefore, there are limited cutaneous scleroderma patients, particularly those with anti Scl 70 or a nucleolar antibody, who have severe disease and progression similar to those with classic diffuse cutaneous disease.

Case Vignette 2: End-Stage Pulmonary Fibrosis

A 58-year-old African-American man developed Raynaud's syndrome, swollen hands and legs, muscle weakness, and shortness of breath 6 years prior to presentation. Initial evaluation revealed diffuse scleroderma, positive ANA with a nucleolar pattern, and ILD with restrictive PFTs. His FVC% predicted was 65 % and his DLCO% predicted was 55 %. He was treated with intravenous cyclophosphamide for 6 months and then transitioned to oral mycophenolate. Although initially his PFTs and HRCT scan stabilized, over the next 4 years he had slow but persistent progression of his ILD, and his most recent FVC% predicted was 45 % and DLCO% predicted was 25 %. He has recently developed increasing shortness of breath, has become oxygen dependent, with complaints of severe cough. His HRCT (Figs. 4.3 and 4.4) does not reveal significant progression in interstitial disease over

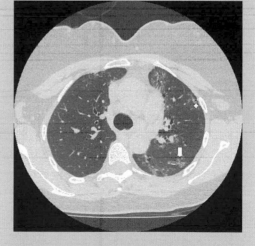

Fig. 4.3 HRCT images from upper thorax of diffuse scleroderma demonstrate less fibrotic changes but still some ground-glass opacities (*arrow*) and subpleural cystic changes (*star*). Increased interstitial markings are seen proximally and distally but sparing the pleural edge

(continued)

Case Vignette 2 (continued)

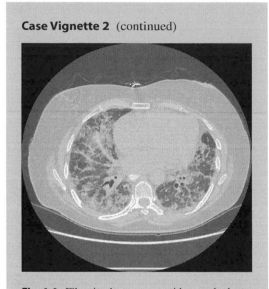

Fig. 4.4 Fibrotic changes are evident at the bases of the lungs with mild cardiomegaly. No honeycombing is seen but traction bronchiectasis is noted

the past year, but there was some increase in heart size. An echocardiogram showed a left ventricular ejection fraction of 60 %, and a right ventricular systolic pressure of 50 mmHg. He is referred for further evaluation and treatment of his scleroderma lung disease.

This patient clearly has severe end-stage lung disease which progressed in spite of being treated aggressively. It is unlikely that further immunosuppressive therapy will have much of a chance to reverse this process and it may be that the risk of infection with such drugs outweighs any potential benefit. He may have developed some secondary pulmonary hypertension from his ILD and/or hypoxia, or he could have some cardiac myofibrosis from his scleroderma causing pulmonary venous hypertension. It is not known whether treatment for the pulmonary hypertension at this point would be helpful but a right heart catheterization should be done to determine the extent and type of pulmonary hyperten-

sion present. Cardiopulmonary exercise training with oxygen supplementation may be helpful in improving his functional capacity [83]. Importantly, aggressive treatment of reflux to prevent aspiration and immunization to prevent infection is extremely important. Cough is his biggest problem and is very challenging to treat. While anti reflux, and antitussive treatment should be tried, there are no easy answers for this problem. Common treatments for palliation of cough in ILD include benzonatate, bronchodilators, and opiates. Lung transplantation has been successfully performed in scleroderma patients [84, 85] although esophageal reflux and disability from other multisystem disease may exclude such patients as this one. The outcomes in select patients at these centers are similar to other ILDs [86].

Case Vignette 3: Atypical Lung Problems
A 69-year-old Caucasian woman has had Raynaud's syndrome for more than 20 years. She has had GERD for that duration as well. Over the past several years she has had several episodes of bronchitis and/or pneumonias associated with cough and increasing dyspnea, and this has become more persistent in the past 6 months. She was seen by a pulmonologist who noticed that she had swollen hands and some telangiectasia, and PFTs showed mild restrictive disease with a FVC of 75 % but a DLCO of 45 %. A HRCT showed asymmetric interstitial fibrosis with mild fibrotic changes in the right upper lobe and lingual and less involvement of the left lower lobe with centrilobular fibrosis as well as a markedly dilated esophagus (Fig. 4.5). An echocardiogram was normal without any evidence of pulmonary hypertension. An anti-centromere antibody was positive and she was referred for the new diagnosis of

(continued)

Case Vignette 3 (continued)

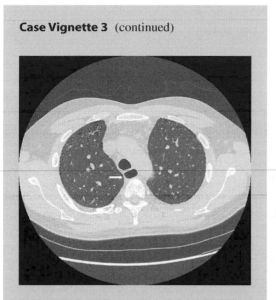

Fig. 4.5 HRCT images in scleroderma GERD show distended esophagus (*arrow*) equal to the size of the trachea. Subpleural cysts are seen anteriorly bilaterally indicative of interstitial lung disease

scleroderma with ILD and the question of whether she should be treated with cyclophosphamide was raised.

This case demonstrates how important the clinical phenotype is in diagnosing lung disease in scleroderma. This lady actually had long standing anti-centromere antibody without significant scleroderma pulmonary fibrosis, but she had developed some secondary fibrotic changes most likely related to recurrent aspiration and/or prior pneumonias. The severe decrease in her DLco more likely represents her potential for future pulmonary vasculopathy than reflecting an active fibrotic lung process. One of the salient features of scleroderma is esophageal dysmotility and accompanying GERD [87]. It is debatable whether GERD is equally prevalent among limited and diffuse scleroderma subtypes [25, 88], but it is equally symptomatic and asymptom-

atic among those with and without fibrotic lung disease [25, 89]. There is no difference in autoantibodies between scleroderma patients with and without GERD in large cohorts [27, 90–92]. While HRCT fibrotic scores correlate well with frequency of reflux events, there is no correlation between extent of fibrosis and presence or absence of hiatal hernia. GERD, as measured by manometry, is associated in some series with both progressive decline in PFTs and development of parenchymal abnormalities on HRCT scans typical of fibrotic lung disease [27]. Once end-stage lung disease develops, GERD is present in all scleroderma patients with ILD, regardless of symptoms [93]. While GERD is highly prevalent in scleroderma, not all patients with GERD develop ILD [25, 89], suggesting that other features, perhaps autoantibody phenotypes, have closer associations with the development of fibrotic disease than the presence of GERD.

Screening for GERD can begin with the HRCT, since esophageal dilatation has a positive predictive value of 83 % for the diagnosis of scleroderma [94] and is helpful, particularly when attempting to differentiate the cause of ILD [95]. HRCT evidence of esophageal dilatation has been associated with reduced DLco but not fibrotic scores based on one study, and this may be due to the strong coexistence of pulmonary vasculopathy and esophageal disease in limited scleroderma [96]. Although the gold standard of diagnosing GERD is manometry, this is rarely necessary in scleroderma because the prevalence of GERD is so high.

The best pathologic description of lung disease associated with scleroderma GERD was reported by de Souza et al. [49]. They prospectively evaluated 28 patients with scleroderma ILD with surgical lung

(continued)

Case Vignette 3 (continued)

biopsies as well as radiographic, esophageal, and PFT assessments. They described centrilobular fibrosis in addition to NSIP and rarely UIP. Those patients with isolated centrilobular fibrosis were found to have foreign bodies and intraluminal basophilic content. Centrilobular fibrosis was associated with esophageal abnormalities, respiratory symptoms, and moderate lung restriction.

Treatment for GERD and esophageal dysmotility is primarily early initiation and long-term use of proton-pump inhibitors which decrease acid reflux and the complications of esophageal disease, such as strictures, Barrett's esophagus, and adenocarcinoma. Behavioral interventions are imperative since dysfunctional motility leads to nonacid reflux as well. Elevation of the chest and head of the bed, avoiding laying down for 4 h after eating, and eating smaller more frequent meals to avoid distending the stomach and exacerbating reflux are some of these key measures [97]. Motility agents may also be necessary. Metoclopromide improves gastric dysmotility but does not impact esophageal aperistalsis, and the central nervous system side effects limit its use. Other medications not approved for use by the FDA in the US, such as domperidone, are sometimes used out of compassionate need [98]. Avoiding offending foods and medications that impact gastrointestinal motility are also important. While surgical procedures for reflux in general have been very helpful, they are associated with significant morbidity and a high rate of complications particularly in scleroderma patients [99]. Certainly, when assessing for lung transplantation, surgical evaluation for gastroesophageal disease in scleroderma is warranted given its implications on post-transplant complications and survival [100].

Conclusion

ILD is prevalent in systemic sclerosis and is associated with significant morbidity and mortality. Therefore, it is important to screen patients annually and to have a low threshold for diagnostic imaging for confirmation of abnormal PFTs and symptoms. Treatment is available today with ongoing large clinical trials to better define optimal management.

References

1. Mayes MD, et al. Prevalence, incidence, survival, and disease characteristics of systemic sclerosis in a large US population. Arthritis Rheum. 2003;48(8): 2246–55.
2. Vonk MC, et al. Systemic sclerosis and its pulmonary complications in The Netherlands: an epidemiological study. Ann Rheum Dis. 2009;68(6):961–5.
3. Arnett FC, et al. Familial occurrence frequencies and relative risks for systemic sclerosis (scleroderma) in three United States cohorts. Arthritis Rheum. 2001;44(6):1359–62.
4. Simeon-Aznar CP, et al. Registry of the Spanish network for systemic sclerosis: clinical pattern according to cutaneous subsets and immunological status. Semin Arthritis Rheum. 2012;41(6): 789–800.
5. Khimdas S, et al. Associations with digital ulcers in a large cohort of systemic sclerosis: results from the Canadian Scleroderma Research Group registry. Arthritis Care Res (Hoboken). 2011;63(1): 142–9.
6. D'Angelo WA, et al. Pathologic observations in systemic sclerosis (scleroderma). A study of fifty-eight autopsy cases and fifty-eight matched controls. Am J Med. 1969;46(3):428–40.
7. Arias-Nunez MC, et al. Systemic sclerosis in northwestern Spain: a 19-year epidemiologic study. Medicine (Baltimore). 2008;87(5):272–80.
8. Steen V. Predictors of end stage lung disease in systemic sclerosis. Ann Rheum Dis. 2003;62(2):97–9.
9. Ioannidis JP, et al. Mortality in systemic sclerosis: an international meta-analysis of individual patient data. Am J Med. 2005;118(1):2–10.
10. Domsic RT, et al. Skin thickness progression rate: a predictor of mortality and early internal organ involvement in diffuse scleroderma. Ann Rheum Dis. 2011;70(1):104–9.
11. Graf SW, et al. South Australian Scleroderma Register: autoantibodies as predictive biomarkers of phenotype and outcome. Int J Rheum Dis. 2012; 15(1):102–9.

12. Greidinger EL, et al. African-American race and antibodies to topoisomerase I are associated with increased severity of scleroderma lung disease. Chest. 1998;114(3):801–7.

13. Steen VD. Autoantibodies in systemic sclerosis. Semin Arthritis Rheum. 2005;35(1):35–42.

14. Plastiras SC, et al. Scleroderma lung: initial forced vital capacity as predictor of pulmonary function decline. Arthritis Rheum. 2006;55(4):598–602.

15. Morgan C, et al. Predictors of end stage lung disease in a cohort of patients with scleroderma. Ann Rheum Dis. 2003;62(2):146–50.

16. Bouros D, et al. Histopathologic subsets of fibrosing alveolitis in patients with systemic sclerosis and their relationship to outcome. Am J Respir Crit Care Med. 2002;165(12):1581–6.

17. Steen VD, et al. Severe restrictive lung disease in systemic sclerosis. Arthritis Rheum. 1994;37(9):1283–9.

18. Launay D, et al. High resolution computed tomography in fibrosing alveolitis associated with systemic sclerosis. J Rheumatol. 2006;33(9):1789–801.

19. Assassi S, et al. Predictors of interstitial lung disease in early systemic sclerosis: a prospective longitudinal study of the GENISOS cohort. Arthritis Res Ther. 2010;12(5):R166.

20. Steen VD, et al. Pulmonary involvement in systemic sclerosis (scleroderma). Arthritis Rheum. 1985;28(7):759–67.

21. Goldin JG, et al. High-resolution CT scan findings in patients with symptomatic scleroderma-related interstitial lung disease. Chest. 2008;134(2):358–67.

22. Hudson M, et al. Cigarette smoking in patients with systemic sclerosis. Arthritis Rheum. 2011;63(1):230–8.

23. Quadrelli SA, et al. Patterns of pulmonary function in smoking and nonsmoking patients with progressive systemic sclerosis. Rheumatol Int. 2009;29(9):995–9.

24. Lopes AJ, et al. Systemic sclerosis-associated interstitial pneumonia: evaluation of pulmonary function over a five-year period. J Bras Pneumol. 2011;37(2):144–51.

25. Savarino E, et al. [Possible connection between gastroesophageal reflux and interstitial pulmonary fibrosis in patients with systemic sclerosis]. Recenti Prog Med. 2009;100(11):512–6.

26. Bellia M, et al. HRCT and scleroderma: semiquantitative evaluation of lung damage and functional abnormalities. Radiol Med. 2009;114(2):190–203.

27. Marie I, et al. Esophageal involvement and pulmonary manifestations in systemic sclerosis. Arthritis Rheum. 2001;45(4):346–54.

28. Steen VD, et al. Isolated diffusing capacity reduction in systemic sclerosis. Arthritis Rheum. 1992;35(7):765–70.

29. Launay D, et al. Clinical characteristics and survival in systemic sclerosis-related pulmonary hypertension associated with interstitial lung disease. Chest. 2011;140(4):1016–24.

30. Steele R, et al. Clinical decision rule to predict the presence of interstitial lung disease in systemic sclerosis. Arthritis Care Res (Hoboken). 2012;64(4):519–24.

31. Lung function testing: selection of reference values and interpretative strategies. American Thoracic Society. Am Rev Respir Dis. 1991;144(5):1202–18.

32. Goh NS, et al. Bronchoalveolar lavage cellular profiles in patients with systemic sclerosis-associated interstitial lung disease are not predictive of disease progression. Arthritis Rheum. 2007;56(6):2005–12.

33. Latsi PI, et al. Fibrotic idiopathic interstitial pneumonia: the prognostic value of longitudinal functional trends. Am J Respir Crit Care Med. 2003;168(5):531–7.

34. Schurawitzki H, et al. Interstitial lung disease in progressive systemic sclerosis: high-resolution CT versus radiography. Radiology. 1990;176(3):755–9.

35. Winklehner A, et al. Screening for interstitial lung disease in systemic sclerosis: the diagnostic accuracy of HRCT image series with high increment and reduced number of slices. Ann Rheum Dis. 2012;71(4):549–52.

36. Ooi GC, et al. Interstitial lung disease in systemic sclerosis. Acta Radiol. 2003;44(3):258–64.

37. Daimon T, et al. Nonspecific interstitial pneumonia associated with collagen vascular disease: analysis of CT features to distinguish the various types. Intern Med. 2009;48(10):753–61.

38. Remy-Jardin M, et al. Pulmonary involvement in progressive systemic sclerosis: sequential evaluation with CT, pulmonary function tests, and bronchoalveolar lavage. Radiology. 1993;188(2):499–506.

39. Wells AU, et al. High resolution computed tomography as a predictor of lung histology in systemic sclerosis. Thorax. 1992;47(9):738–42.

40. Shah RM, Jimenez S, Wechsler R. Significance of ground-glass opacity on HRCT in long-term follow-up of patients with systemic sclerosis. J Thorac Imaging. 2007;22(2):120–4.

41. Strange C, et al. Bronchoalveolar lavage and response to cyclophosphamide in scleroderma interstitial lung disease. Am J Respir Crit Care Med. 2008;177(1):91–8.

42. Mittoo S, et al. Persistence of abnormal bronchoalveolar lavage findings after cyclophosphamide treatment in scleroderma patients with interstitial lung disease. Arthritis Rheum. 2007;56(12):4195–202.

43. Harrison NK, et al. Structural features of interstitial lung disease in systemic sclerosis. Am Rev Respir Dis. 1991;144(3 Pt 1):706–13.

44. Wells AU, et al. Functional impairment in lone cryptogenic fibrosing alveolitis and fibrosing alveolitis associated with systemic sclerosis: a comparison. Am J Respir Crit Care Med. 1997;155(5):1657–64.

45. Wells AU, et al. Fibrosing alveolitis associated with systemic sclerosis has a better prognosis than lone cryptogenic fibrosing alveolitis. Am J Respir Crit Care Med. 1994;149(6):1583–90.

46. Su R, et al. An analysis of connective tissue disease-associated interstitial lung disease at a US Tertiary Care Center: better survival in patients with systemic sclerosis. J Rheumatol. 2011;38(4):693–701.

47. Schmidt K, et al. Bronchoalveoloar lavage fluid cytokines and chemokines as markers and predictors for the outcome of interstitial lung disease in systemic sclerosis patients. Arthritis Res Ther. 2009; 11(4):R111.

48. Kinder BW, King Jr TE. Prognostic significance of bronchoalveolar lavage cellular analysis in scleroderma lung disease. Am J Respir Crit Care Med. 2008;177(11):1292–3, author reply 1293.

49. de Souza RB, et al. Centrilobular fibrosis: an under-recognized pattern in systemic sclerosis. Respiration. 2009;77(4):389–97.

50. Wells AU, et al. Fibrosing alveolitis in systemic sclerosis. Bronchoalveolar lavage findings in relation to computed tomographic appearance. Am J Respir Crit Care Med. 1994;150(2):462–8.

51. Tyndall AJ, et al. Causes and risk factors for death in systemic sclerosis: a study from the EULAR Scleroderma Trials and Research (EUSTAR) database. Ann Rheum Dis. 2010;69(10):1809–15.

52. Kuo CF, et al. Cancer risk among patients with systemic sclerosis: a nationwide population study in Taiwan. Scand J Rheumatol. 2012;41(1):44–9.

53. Pontifex EK, Hill CL, Roberts-Thomson P. Risk factors for lung cancer in patients with scleroderma: a nested case–control study. Ann Rheum Dis. 2007; 66(4):551–3.

54. Goh NS, et al. Interstitial lung disease in systemic sclerosis: a simple staging system. Am J Respir Crit Care Med. 2008;177(11):1248–54.

55. Tashkin DP, et al. Cyclophosphamide versus placebo in scleroderma lung disease. N Engl J Med. 2006; 354(25):2655–66.

56. Hoyles RK, et al. A multicenter, prospective, randomized, double-blind, placebo-controlled trial of corticosteroids and intravenous cyclophosphamide followed by oral azathioprine for the treatment of pulmonary fibrosis in scleroderma. Arthritis Rheum. 2006;54(12):3962–70.

57. Theodore AC, et al. Correlation of cough with disease activity and treatment with cyclophosphamide in scleroderma interstitial lung disease: findings from the Scleroderma Lung Study. Chest. 2012; 142(3):614–21.

58. Goldin J, et al. Treatment of scleroderma-interstitial lung disease with cyclophosphamide is associated with less progressive fibrosis on serial thoracic high-resolution CT scan than placebo: findings from the scleroderma lung study. Chest. 2009;136(5): 1333–40.

59. Kim HJ, et al. Quantitative texture-based assessment of one-year changes in fibrotic reticular patterns on HRCT in scleroderma lung disease treated with oral cyclophosphamide. Eur Radiol. 2011;21(12): 2455–65.

60. Griffiths B, et al. Systemic sclerosis and interstitial lung disease: a pilot study using pulse intravenous methylprednisolone and cyclophosphamide to assess the effect on high resolution computed tomography scan and lung function. J Rheumatol. 2002;29(11): 2371–8.

61. Wanchu A, et al. High-dose prednisolone and bolus cyclophosphamide in interstitial lung disease associated with systemic sclerosis: a prospective open study. Int J Rheum Dis. 2009;12(3):239–42.

62. Paone C, et al. Twelve-month azathioprine as maintenance therapy in early diffuse systemic sclerosis patients treated for 1-year with low dose cyclophosphamide pulse therapy. Clin Exp Rheumatol. 2007; 25(4):613–6.

63. Gerbino AJ, Goss CH, Molitor JA. Effect of mycophenolate mofetil on pulmonary function in scleroderma-associated interstitial lung disease. Chest. 2008;133(2):455–60.

64. Koutroumpas A, et al. Mycophenolate mofetil in systemic sclerosis-associated interstitial lung disease. Clin Rheumatol. 2010;29(10):1167–8.

65. Wuttge DM, et al. Serum IL-15 in patients with early systemic sclerosis: a potential novel marker of lung disease. Arthritis Res Ther. 2007;9(5):R85.

66. Caramaschi P, et al. Homocysteine plasma concentration is related to severity of lung impairment in scleroderma. J Rheumatol. 2003;30(2):298–304.

67. Bonella F, et al. Surfactant protein D and KL-6 serum levels in systemic sclerosis: correlation with lung and systemic involvement. Sarcoidosis Vasc Diffuse Lung Dis. 2011;28(1):27–33.

68. Takahashi T, et al. Dynamics of serum angiopoietin-2 levels correlate with efficacy of intravenous pulse cyclophosphamide therapy for interstitial lung disease associated with systemic sclerosis. Mod Rheumatol. 2013;23(5):884–90.

69. Bogatkevich GS, et al. Impairment of the antifibrotic effect of hepatocyte growth factor in lung fibroblasts from African Americans: possible role in systemic sclerosis. Arthritis Rheum. 2007;56(7):2432–42.

70. Wuttge DM, et al. Increased alveolar nitric oxide in early systemic sclerosis. Clin Exp Rheumatol. 2010;28(5 Suppl 62):S5–9.

71. Hua-Huy T, et al. Increased alveolar concentration of nitric oxide is related to serum-induced lung fibroblast proliferation in patients with systemic sclerosis. J Rheumatol. 2010;37(8):1680–7.

72. Delle Sedie A, et al. Ultrasound lung comets in systemic sclerosis: a useful tool to detect lung interstitial fibrosis. Clin Exp Rheumatol. 2010;28 (5 Suppl 62):S54.

73. Spiera RF, et al. Imatinib mesylate (Gleevec) in the treatment of diffuse cutaneous systemic sclerosis: results of a 1-year, phase IIa, single-arm, open-label clinical trial. Ann Rheum Dis. 2011;70(6): 1003–9.

74. Divekar AA, et al. Treatment with imatinib results in reduced IL-4-producing T cells, but increased CD4(+) T cells in the broncho-alveolar lavage of patients with systemic sclerosis. Clin Immunol. 2011;141(3):293–303.

75. Rosato E, et al. Long-term N-acetylcysteine therapy in systemic sclerosis interstitial lung disease: a retrospective study. Int J Immunopathol Pharmacol. 2011;24(3):727–33.

76. Failli P, et al. Effect of N-acetyl-L-cysteine on peroxynitrite and superoxide anion production of lung alveolar macrophages in systemic sclerosis. Nitric Oxide. 2002;7(4):277–82.

77. Shima Y, et al. The skin of patients with systemic sclerosis softened during the treatment with anti-IL-6 receptor antibody tocilizumab. Rheumatology. 2010;49(12):2408–12.

78. Daoussis D, et al. Experience with rituximab in scleroderma: results from a 1-year, proof-of-principle study. Rheumatology. 2010;49(2):271–80.

79. Yoo WH. Successful treatment of steroid and cyclophosphamide-resistant diffuse scleroderma-associated interstitial lung disease with rituximab. Rheumatol Int. 2012;32(3):795–8.

80. Haroon M, et al. Cyclophosphamide-refractory scleroderma-associated interstitial lung disease: remarkable clinical and radiological response to a single course of rituximab combined with high-dose corticosteroids. Ther Adv Respir Dis. 2011;5(5): 299–304.

81. Fischer A, et al. Unique characteristics of systemic sclerosis sine scleroderma-associated interstitial lung disease. Chest. 2006;130(4):976–81.

82. Clements PJ, et al. Scleroderma lung study (SLS): differences in the presentation and course of patients with limited versus diffuse systemic sclerosis. Ann Rheum Dis. 2007;66(12):1641–7.

83. Huppmann P, et al. Effects of in-patient pulmonary rehabilitation in patients with interstitial lung disease. Eur Respir J. 2013;42(2):444–53.

84. Schachna L, et al. Lung transplantation in scleroderma compared with idiopathic pulmonary fibrosis and idiopathic pulmonary arterial hypertension. Arthritis Rheum. 2006;54(12):3954–61.

85. Saggar R, et al. Systemic sclerosis and bilateral lung transplantation: a single centre experience. Eur Respir J. 2010;36(4):893–900.

86. Massad MG, et al. Outcomes of lung transplantation in patients with scleroderma. World J Surg. 2005; 29(11):1510–5.

87. Wipff J, et al. Prevalence of Barrett's esophagus in systemic sclerosis. Arthritis Rheum. 2005;52(9):2882–8.

88. Nishimagi E, et al. Characteristics of patients with early systemic sclerosis and severe gastrointestinal tract involvement. J Rheumatol. 2007;34(10):2050–5.

89. Gilson M, et al. Prognostic factors for lung function in systemic sclerosis: prospective study of 105 cases. Eur Respir J. 2010;35(1):112–7.

90. Liu X, et al. Prevalence and clinical importance of gastroesophageal reflux in Chinese patients with systemic sclerosis. Clin Exp Rheumatol. 2012;30 (2 Suppl 71):S60–6.

91. Savarino E, et al. Gastroesophageal reflux and pulmonary fibrosis in scleroderma: a study using pH-impedance monitoring. Am J Respir Crit Care Med. 2009;179(5):408–13.

92. Marie I, et al. Delayed gastric emptying determined using the 13C-octanoic acid breath test in patients with systemic sclerosis. Arthritis Rheum. 2012; 64(7):2346–55.

93. D'Ovidio F, et al. Prevalence of gastroesophageal reflux in end-stage lung disease candidates for lung transplant. Ann Thorac Surg. 2005;80(4):1254–60.

94. Vonk MC, et al. Oesophageal dilatation on high-resolution computed tomography scan of the lungs as a sign of scleroderma. Ann Rheum Dis. 2008; 67(9):1317–21.

95. Bhalla M, et al. Chest CT in patients with scleroderma: prevalence of asymptomatic esophageal dilatation and mediastinal lymphadenopathy. AJR Am J Roentgenol. 1993;161(2):269–72.

96. Pandey AK, et al. Oesophageal dilatation on high-resolution CT chest in systemic sclerosis: what does it signify? J Med Imaging Radiat Oncol. 2011; 55(6):551–5.

97. Ebert EC. Esophageal disease in progressive systemic sclerosis. Curr Treat Options Gastroenterol. 2008;11(1):64–9.

98. Ndraha S. Combination of PPI with a prokinetic drug in gastroesophageal reflux disease. Acta Med Indones. 2011;43(4):233–6.

99. Kent MS, et al. Comparison of surgical approaches to recalcitrant gastroesophageal reflux disease in the patient with scleroderma. Ann Thorac Surg. 2007;84(5):1710–5. discussion 1715–6.

100. Hoppo T, et al. Antireflux surgery preserves lung function in patients with gastroesophageal reflux disease and end-stage lung disease before and after lung transplantation. Arch Surg. 2011;146(9):1041–7.

Inflammatory Myopathy/ Anti synthetase Syndrome

5

Cheilonda Johnson, Chester V. Oddis, and Sonye K. Danoff

Abbreviations

ARS	Aminoacyl transfer RNA synthetase
CADM	Clinically amyopathic dermatomyositis
CAM	Cancer-associated myositis
CK	Creatine kinase
CTD	Connective tissue disease
DAD	Diffuse alveolar damage
DLCO	Diffusing capacity of the lung for carbon monoxide
DM	Dermatomyositis
FEV_1	Forced expiratory volume in 1 s
FVC	Forced vital capacity
HRCT	High resolution chest tomography
IBM	Inclusion body myositis
IIM	Idiopathic inflammatory myopathy
ILD	Interstitial lung disease
kDa	Kilodalton
MAA	Myositis-associated autoantibodies
MDAS	Melanoma differentiation associated gene 5
MEP	Maximal expiratory pressure
MIP	Maximal inspiratory pressure
MSA	Myositis-specific autoantibodies
6MWT	Six-minute-walk test
NSIP	Nonspecific interstitial pneumonia
OP	Organizing pneumonia
PFT	Pulmonary function test
PM	Polymyositis
PR	Pulmonary rehabilitation
TLC	Total lung capacity
tRNA	Transfer ribonucleic acid
UIP	Usual interstitial pneumonia

C. Johnson, M.D., M.H.S.
S.K. Danoff, M.D., Ph.D. (✉)
Division of Pulmonary/Critical Care Medicine,
Department of Medicine, Johns Hopkins University
School of Medicine, Baltimore, MD, USA
e-mail: Cjohn164@jhmi.edu; sdanoff@jhmi.edu

C.V. Oddis, M.D.
Division of Rheumatology, Department of Medicine,
University of Pittsburgh Medical Center,
Pittsburgh, PA, USA
e-mail: Cvo5@pitt.edu

P.F. Dellaripa et al. (eds.), *Pulmonary Manifestations of Rheumatic Disease: A Comprehensive Guide*,
DOI 10.1007/978-1-4939-0770-0_5, © Springer Science+Business Media New York 2014

Case Vignette 1

A 35-year-old woman presented to her primary care provider with a bilateral, erythematous hand rash (Fig. 5.1). She also noted painful fissures along the edges of her nail beds that increased during cold weather. A skin biopsy of the affected area revealed interface dermatitis.

Over the next 12 months, she developed proximal muscle weakness and a small joint inflammatory arthritis. A muscle biopsy showed perivascular inflammation consistent with dermatomyositis and she possessed the anti-Jo-1 autoantibody. The patient improved over several months after glucocorticoid therapy which was then tapered and discontinued. Her muscle weakness recurred and she developed dyspnea with exertion. A high resolution CT (HRCT) scan of the chest revealed diffuse ground-glass opacities and pulmonary function tests (PFTs) revealed mild restriction with a moderate to severely reduced diffusing capacity of the lung for carbon monoxide (DLCO). Bronchoscopy ruled out infection and an open lung biopsy showed organizing pneumonia (OP). Prednisone was restarted in combination with azathioprine. Over the following year, dermatologic, muscular, and pulmonary symptoms improved (Fig. 5.2) and prednisone was tapered off. The patient remained stable on low-dose azathioprine.

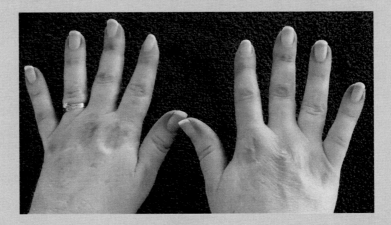

Fig. 5.1 Bilateral erythematous rash of Gottron papules

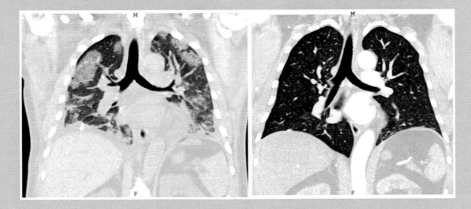

Fig. 5.2 Resolution of pulmonary infiltrates with treatment

Overview

Dermatomyositis (DM) and polymyositis (PM) are idiopathic inflammatory myopathies (IIMs), a rare heterogeneous group of acquired autoimmune muscle disorders that frequently affect the lungs. DM is a complement-mediated microangiopathy of muscle where B cells and the late component of complement are found in the perimysial and perivascular tissue. Characteristic skin changes, including Gottron's papules, occur with muscle weakness (Fig. 5.1) [1, 2]. PM is a T-cell mediated disorder also leading to muscle weakness [1]. Skin findings notwithstanding, both diseases have similar muscular and extramuscular manifestations. As a result, for the remainder of the chapter the terms myositis and IIM will collectively refer to DM and PM unless otherwise specified.

Patients with myositis typically present with symmetric proximal muscle weakness progressing over weeks to months [3]. Although many classification criteria exist for IIM, those of Bohan and Peter remain the most clinically useful [4–7]. The essential elements include proximal muscle weakness on physical examination, elevated serum muscle enzymes (CPK), an abnormal electromyogram (EMG), a muscle biopsy consistent with myositis, and (in the case of DM) characteristic rashes (Table 5.1). Despite the muscle-focused criteria proposed by Bohan and Peter, myositis affects multiple organs with the lung being the most common site of extramuscular involvement [8] and a significant source of morbidity and mortality [9]. Multiple pulmonary manifestations may occur (Table 5.2); however, this chapter will focus on interstitial lung disease (ILD), the most common and devastating pulmonary manifestation in patients with myositis [10].

Epidemiology

The reported prevalence of myositis-associated ILD (myositis-ILD) ranges from 5 to 78 % depending on the population and diagnostic criteria utilized [2, 3, 8–10]. Although the frequency of ILD is similar in PM and DM, patients with DM-ILD generally do worse with more frequent severe treatment-refractory disease [8, 11].

The diagnosis of myositis-ILD has significant prognostic implications as this complication portends a poorer survival than in patients with myositis alone [2, 8]. Overall, however, myositis-ILD patients respond favorably to treatment with

Table 5.1 Polymyositis/dermatomyositis diagnostic criteria

Bohan and Peter [4, 5]				Dalakas and Hohlfeld [6]			
1. Symmetric myopathic muscle weakness				1. Symmetric myopathic muscle weakness			
2. Muscle biopsy with microfiber necrosis, phagocytosis, regeneration, fiber diameter variation, and inflammatory exudate				2. Muscle biopsy findings			
				(a) CD8/MHC-I complexes			
				(b) MHC-I expression only			
				(c) Perifasicular, perimysial, or perivascular infiltrates			
3. Elevated serum skeletal muscle enzymes				3. Elevated serum skeletal muscle enzymes			
4. Myopathic electromyographic findings				4. Myopathic electromyographic findings			
				5. Rash or calcinosis			
				(a) Present			
				(b) Absent			
Polymyositis		Dermatomyositis		Polymyositis		Dermatomyositis	
Definite	Probable	Definite	Probable	Definite	Probable	Definite	Probable
All 4 criteria	2–3 criteria	3–4 criteria+DM rash	2 criteria+DM rash	1, 2a, 3–4, 5b	1, 2b, 3–4, 5b	1, 2c, 3–4, 5a	1, 2c, 3–4, 5b

Adapted from with permission from Kalluri M, Oddis CV. Pulmonary manifestations of the idiopathic inflammatory myopathies. Clinics in Chest Medicine. 2010;31(3):501–12

Table 5.2 Pulmonary manifestations of myositis

Pulmonary parenchyma	Pulmonary vasculature	Extra-parenchymal
ILD	Pulmonary hypertension	Diaphragm muscle weakness
Pneumonia	Pulmonary capillaritis/diffuse alveolar damage	Intercostal muscle weakness
Drug-induced ILD		Pneumothorax
		Pneumomediastinum
		Dysphagia (aspiration)
		Myocarditis (pulmonary edema)
		Cardiomyopathy (pulmonary edema)

1-, 5-, and 10-year survival rates around 94 %, 90 %, and 87 % respectively [2, 12]. Factors predicting a poor prognosis include the acute onset of dyspnea, a pulmonary histology consistent with usual interstitial pneumonia (UIP), DM with a clinical microangiopathy or digital infarcts, clinically amyopathic DM (CADM), and an initial DLCO and FVC less than 45 and 60 %, respectively [2].

Clinical Manifestations

Patients typically present with dyspnea with or without cough but the presentation and course is highly variable from a mild, subacute, or chronic course to the rapid onset of acute respiratory failure necessitating mechanical ventilation. Further, ILD can precede, occur concomitantly with, or follow the diagnosis of IIM. As is illustrated in Case Vignette 1, ILD may follow the onset of skin or muscle disease and surveillance for respiratory disease is important even in the face of improvement of more typical manifestations of disease.

PFTs typically show a restrictive pattern with a reduced total lung capacity (TLC), FVC, FEV_1, and normal or increased FEV_1/FVC ratio [2] with a low DLCO [2].

Radiographic and Histopathologic Findings

HRCT typically demonstrates reticular ground-glass opacities without honeycomb changes (Fig. 5.3) which correspond to a nonspecific interstitial pneumonia (NSIP) histopathology

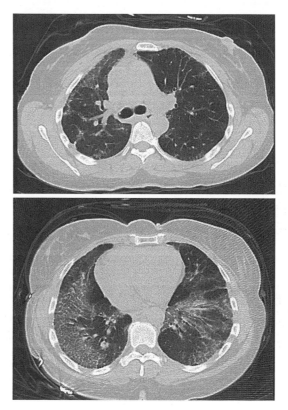

Fig. 5.3 High-resolution chest CT imaging in a patient presenting with myositis-associated ILD. CT findings include diffuse ground-glass opacities

[2, 8]. A honeycombing pattern typical of UIP can also be seen [8].

Lung biopsy is generally not necessary in the patient with established myositis since HRCT findings correlate with open lung biopsy findings [2]. When lung biopsy is required, a surgical lung biopsy is preferred over a transbronchial approach [2]. The most common histologic subtype is NSIP followed by UIP, diffuse alveolar damage (DAD), and OP [2, 8].

Autoantibodies

The presence of autoantibodies recognizing intracellular antigens correspond to distinct clinical phenotypes in the myositis spectrum and have important implications in the pathogenesis and treatment of the disease [3, 13, 14]. Myositis autoantibodies fall into two categories: myositis-specific autoantibodies (MSAs) and myositis-associated autoantibodies (MAAs) (Table 5.3) [13]. MSAs are almost exclusively seen in IIM and 60–80 % of patients with myositis have at least one [3, 14], while MAAs are more frequently seen in myositis overlapping with another connective tissue disease (CTD) [13]. The MSAs seen with myositis-ILD are discussed next.

Antisynthetase Autoantibodies

The most common MSAs, the antisynthetase autoantibodies, are directed against the aminoacyl transfer RNA synthetases (ARSs) which catalyze the attachment of amino acids to their cognate tRNA [3, 13]. To date, antibodies to 8 ARS have been identified (Table 5.3). Anti-Jo-1 (anti-histidyl tRNA synthetase) is the most common with a frequency of 20–30 % in PM and DM patients [2, 3, 13, 15]. The non-Jo-1 anti synthetase autoantibodies (Table 5.2) are collectively found in 20 % of IIM patients [3, 13, 15]. Patients with anti synthetase antibodies have some or all of the features of the anti synthetase syndrome which includes fever, myositis, Raynaud phenomenon, polyarthritis, "mechanic hands," and ILD (Table 5.3). Generally, such patients respond favorably to glucocorticoid therapy, although relapses are common [3, 13]. In longitudinal analyses, anti-Jo-1 autoantibody levels have been shown to correlate with muscle, joint, pulmonary, and global disease activity [16, 17] and may be useful for monitoring disease activity and response to therapy [16, 17]. Although the presence of one of the eight anti-ARS autoantibodies is generally associated with some or all of the features of the anti synthetase syndrome, the

Table 5.3 Myositis-specific autoantibodies

	Target autoantigen	Clinical association
Myositis-specific autoantibody		
Anti synthetase autoantibodies	Aminoacyl transfer RNA synthetase	Antisynthetase syndrome: myositis, interstitial lung disease, Raynaud phenomenon, arthritis, Mechanic's hands, fever
• Anti-Jo-1	Histidyl	
• PL-12	Alanyl	
• PL-7	Theronyl	
• EJ	Glycyl	
• OJ	Isoleucyl	
• KS	Asparaginyl	
• Ha	Tyrosyl	
• Zo	Phenylalanyl	
Anti-SRP	Signal recognition protein	Necrotizing myopathy
Anti-Mi-2	Nucleosome remodeling deacetylase complex (NuRD)	DM
Anti-p-155/140	Transcriptional intermediary factor 1 gamma (TIF1-γ)	DM and malignancy
Anti-SUMO-1	Small ubiquitin-like modifier 1 (SUMO-1)	DM
Anti-CADM-140	Melanoma differentiation-associated gene 5 (MDA-5)	CADM and ILD
Anti-p140	Nuclear matrix protein 2 (NXP2)	DM and ILD
Anti-200/100	3-hydroxy-3methylglutarly-coenzyme A reductase	Necrotizing myopathy

Adapted with permission from Betteridge ZE, Gunawardena H, McHugh NJ. Novel autoantibodies and clinical phenotypes in adult and juvenile myositis. Arthritis research & therapy. 2011;13(2):209

myositis subtype (PM vs. DM), CK levels, lung involvement, and myositis severity may vary (Table 5.3) [3, 13].

Dermatomyositis-Specific Autoantibodies

Anti-p-155/140 Autoantibodies

Autoantibodies directed against a 155/140 kDa doublet corresponding to transcription intermediary factor 1-gamma (TIF1-γ) (Table 5.3), are found in up to 20 % of patients with DM and are associated with an increased risk of cancer-associated myositis (CAM) [18, 19].

Anti-SUMO-1

Anti-SUMO-1 (small ubiquitin-like modifier 1) is found in 8 % of patients with DM and is associated with malignancy and ILD [3, 13]. Interestingly, in one series most patients with anti-SUMO-1, demonstrated skin manifestations before myositis and ILD [3, 20].

Anti-MDA5

Clinically amyopathic dermatomyositis (CADM) is a rare but important myositis subset where patients have skin findings consistent with DM without clinically apparent muscle involvement [2]. CADM has been shown to be associated with acute and rapidly progressive ILD and the antigenic target has been identified as an RNA helicase encoded by melanoma differentiation-associated gene 5 (MDAS) [21]. CADM is discussed in more detail after Case Vignette 3.

Therapy

There are no randomized controlled trials evaluating the treatment of myositis-ILD. Glucocorticoids are the mainstay of empiric therapy and most patients respond to some degree for a period of time [1, 8]. Other immunosuppressive therapies may be used initially in patients with ILD but are also often required as second-line agents in patients who fail to respond to glucocorticoids [8].

Table 5.4 Treatment of myositis-associated interstitial lung disease

Drug/dosage	Clinical scenario
Glucocorticoids Prednisone 1 mg/kg/day Methylprednisolone 1 g IV×3 days	First line therapy for myositis-ILD
Cyclophosphamide (CYC) 1–2 mg/kg/day	Acute or refractory myositis-ILD
Calcineurin inhibitors Cyclosporine 2–5 mg/kg/day Tacrolimus (based on trough levels)	Refractory myositis-ILD
Rituximab 1 g every other week×2 doses	Refractory antisynthetase syndrome
Methotrexate 15–25 mg/week	Refractory PM/DM; controversial in ILD
Azathioprine 2–3 mg/kg/day	Second-line therapy, maintenance after CYC
Mycophenolate mofetil 1 g/twice daily	Steroid sparing agent in progressive disease
Intravenous immunoglobulin (IVIG)	Salvage therapy

Adapted with permission from Kalluri M, Oddis CV. Pulmonary manifestations of the idiopathic inflammatory myopathies. Clinics in chest medicine. 2010;31(3): 501–12

A summary of therapies utilized in the treatment of myositis-ILD is provided in Table 5.4.

Some of the agents used to treat myositis can also cause ILD. Methotrexate can cause an acute pneumonitis with fever often within the first year of use. It is very effective for myositis and can be used in anti-Jo-1 positive patients with milder, stable forms of ILD, but it should be avoided if the lung disease is active [2, 8].

Adjunctive Therapy

Pulmonary rehabilitation (PR) is recommended as adjunctive therapy for patients with chronic lung diseases [22, 23]. PR involves exercise training, behavior modification, and respiratory therapy and has been shown to improve the six-minute-walk test (6MWT) distance and quality of life in patients with ILD [22, 24].

Annual influenza and pneumococcal vaccination based on standard guidelines are recommended to reduce the risk of pulmonary infection in patients with chronic lung disease and those on immunosuppressive treatment [25–27].

Oxygen therapy provides symptomatic benefit to patients with chronic lung diseases and should be provided to any patient with resting or exertional hypoxemia [28].

Case Vignette 2
A 55-year-old African American woman who was a varsity college athlete was well and physically active until 9 months prior to her clinical evaluation when she noted dyspnea while shopping. She was admitted to a hospital and given IV antibiotics for presumptive pneumonia and an HRCT showed diffuse ground-glass opacities. Her dyspnea persisted, and 1 month later she underwent an open lung biopsy that revealed UIP. Over the next several months, her dyspnea worsened and proximal lower extremity muscle weakness developed to the degree that she had to use her arms to pull on the banister as she walked up steps. She then developed dry eyes and a dry mouth. On presentation to a tertiary care ILD clinic approximately 9 months after symptom onset, she was tachypneic and tachycardic with a normal oxygen saturation at rest. Her physical examination revealed dry bibasilar crackles, a loud P2 and bilateral lower extremity edema. Her manual muscle testing was notable for 4/5 strength of the deltoids and hip flexors but normal distal muscle strength. Her skin exam was notable for periungual erythema, but no Gottron papules or heliotrope rash. Her PFTs showed severe restriction and a markedly reduced DLCO. She had a negative ANA and anti-Jo-1, but the serum rheumatoid factor was elevated at 122 (nL < 80) and she possessed a high titer positive anti-PL-12 autoantibody. The patient was treated with pulse intravenous methylprednisolone followed by a tapering

dose of oral prednisone as well as azathioprine. One year following presentation, the patient is minimally limited by dyspnea or muscle weakness, but continues to have reduced lung volume and DLCO.

Screening

As described in Case Vignette 2, ILD in this case associated with antisynthetase antibodies, can precede myositis. Thus, a high index of suspicion and initial assessment for occult rheumatologic disease is warranted in patients presenting with ILD [29], and a search for subtle manifestations of an underlying CTD such as dermatologic features, Raynaud phenomenon, and arthritis should be considered. In a series of 114 consecutive patients referred to an ILD clinic, 15 % were diagnosed with a new CTD, a significant proportion of which had myositis [29]. In this series the only demographic predictor associated with an underlying CTD was younger age [29]. Consequently, we recommend screening for undiagnosed CTD in patients presenting with ILD to include a thorough review of systems for CTD as well as an ANA, CK, aldolase, and myositis antibodies [29].

Case Vignette 3
A 42-year-old African American woman presented to the emergency department with a 2-month history of muscle weakness and rash on her hands and back. She noted a new onset Raynaud phenomenon and a 20-lb weight loss. She was tachypneic and hypoxemic at rest. Pulmonary auscultation, revealed bilateral crackles and she had profound muscle weakness and ulcerative lesions on the metacarpophalangeal (MCP) joints, creases of the palms, elbows, and ear pinnae. Her HRCT showed diffuse ground-glass opacities. Initial laboratory studies revealed a CK of 452, an elevated AST and ALT with negative hepatitis serologies, an

(continued)

Case Vignette 3 (continued)

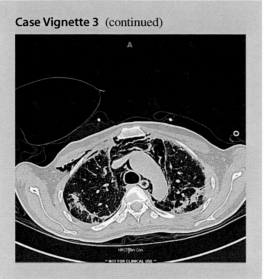

Fig. 5.4 Extensive pneumomediastinum with an extension to the chest wall

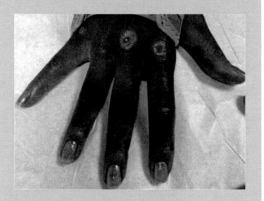

Fig. 5.5 Erosive skin lesions on dorsum of hand characteristic of MDA5 phenotype

ANA of 1:40 and a negative anti-Jo-1 and anti-topoisomerase. Serum immunoprecipitation revealed the presence of the anti-MDA5 autoantibody. She was treated with pulse methylprednisolone but she developed pneumomediastinum with an extension into the soft tissue of the chest and neck (Fig. 5.4).

She was placed on oral glucocorticoids and azathioprine and discharged. Worsening dyspnea and skin lesions recurred due to non-compliance and she was again treated with pulse methylprednisolone and placed on oral immunosuppression. She slowly improved with resolution of the erosive skin lesions (Fig. 5.5) and improved exercise tolerance.

MDA5

Originally described in a cohort of Japanese patients with rapidly progressive ILD in the setting of newly diagnosed CADM [21], MDA5 antibody associated disease has now been described in a wider range of patients with DM as Case Vignette 3 illustrates [30]. The clinical presentation is frequently heralded by the appearance of cutaneous erosive lesions at the MCP joints (Fig. 5.5) along with painful punctate lesions on the palms at the creases of the fingers. The pulmonary manifestations may mimic those of the anti synthetase syndrome, but the autoantigen being targeted is melanoma differentiation-associated gene 5 which is not in the tRNA synthetase family. This autoantibody accounts for approximately 8–13 % of DM patients in two separate US tertiary referral centers [30].

Cancer-Associated Myopathy

The association between IIMs and malignancy has been described for decades with recent large epidemiologic studies confirming the increased risk [31].

Epidemiology

The estimated prevalence of malignancy in patients with myositis is 10–30 % [31]. The vast majority of cancers are detected after the diagnosis of myositis, with the peak incidence within the first year [31, 32]. Overall for most cancer types, the risk extends to the first 5 years after diagnosis before returning to baseline rates [31, 32].

The mean age of onset of CAM is the fifth and sixth decades of life but the age range varies widely [31, 32]. CAM occurs in both men and women with slightly increased risk in men [31].

Adenocarcinoma is the most common, representing 70 % of associated malignancies [31, 33]. This is driven largely by the significantly increased risk in patients with DM where adenocarcinomas predominate. By contrast, hematologic malignancies are the greatest risk among polymyositis

Table 5.5 Malignancies associated with idiopathic inflammatory myopathies

Dermatomyositis	Polymyositis
• Lung cancer	• Non-Hodgkin lymphoma
• Ovarian cancer	• Lung cancer
• Cervical cancer	• Bladder cancer
• Colorectal cancer	
• Gastric cancer	
• Breast cancer	
• Pancreatic cancer	
• Lymphoma	

patients (Table 5.5) [31, 32]. The epidemiology varies by race/ethnicity. Adenocarcinoma of ovary, lung, and gastrointestinal tract predominate in Western nations, while nasopharyngeal carcinoma is more common in Southeast Asia, Southern China, and Northern Africa [31, 34].

As would be expected, 1- and 5-year survival rates are worse in cancer patients with CAM than in patients without CAM [31]. In patients with DM, a simultaneous diagnosis of CAM and DM results in a more severe disease [31].

Risk Factors

The most significant risk factor is DM [31]. Older age, male sex, severe muscle weakness, treatment resistance, skin ulceration or necrosis, periungual erythema, and the V or shawl sign are all associated with occult malignancy [31, 33]. By contrast, the presence of antisynthetase antibodies and ILD appear to have a protective effect but cases have been reported [31]; therefore, the presence of antisynthetase syndrome should not eliminate screening for malignancy in the appropriate clinical setting [31]. Similarly patients with positive MAAs or MSAs develop CAM less frequently but CAM still occurs [31]. One auto-antibody anti-p155/140, however, is associated with a higher frequency of CAM in patients with dermatomyositis [31, 33].

Pathophysiology

Many theories have been proposed but the exact mechanism is unknown. The first is that CAM represents a paraneoplastic syndrome where the tumor itself produces some bioactive mediator that results in an immune response against the skin and muscle [31]. Others hypothesize a causal role between immune compromise and tumor development [31]. Furthermore, the use of cytotoxic agents to treat IIMs could induce malignant transformation [31]. Perhaps, a shared environmental exposure could be both carcinogenic and immunogenic [31]. Finally some propose that an immune response to the tumor itself results in cross-reactivity with skin and muscle antigens [31, 35].

Screening for Malignancy

Due to unclear consensus guidelines, screening practices vary by clinician. Some restrict to age appropriate malignancy screening with additional studies only if dictated by symptoms [31]. While others perform more detailed evaluations, including computed tomography (CT) scanning, positron emission tomography (PET) scans, upper and lower endoscopy, tumor markers, and bone marrow biopsies, regardless of symptoms [31].

Treatment

Treatment of the underlying malignancy can result in myositis remission but patients frequently require treatment with long-term immunosuppression even after cancer remission [31, 36]. Additionally, tumor recurrence can result in recurrent myositis symptoms even after years of quiescence [31, 36].

References

1. Dalakas MC. Pathogenesis and therapies of immune-mediated myopathies. Autoimmunity Rev. 2012; 11(3):203–6.
2. Kalluri M, Oddis CV. Pulmonary manifestations of the idiopathic inflammatory myopathies. Clin Chest Med. 2010;31(3):501–12.
3. Mammen AL. Autoimmune myopathies: autoantibodies, phenotypes and pathogenesis. Nat Rev Neurol. 2011;7(6):343–54.
4. Bohan A, Peter JB. Polymyositis and dermatomyositis (second of two parts). N Engl J Med. 1975; 292(8): 403–7.

5. Bohan A, Peter JB. Polymyositis and dermatomyositis (first of two parts). N Engl J Med. 1975; 292(7):344–7.
6. Dalakas MC, Hohlfeld R. Polymyositis and dermatomyositis. Lancet. 2003;362(9388):971–82.
7. Love LA, Leff RL, Fraser DD, Targoff IN, Dalakas M, Plotz PH, et al. A new approach to the classification of idiopathic inflammatory myopathy: myositis-specific autoantibodies define useful homogeneous patient groups. Medicine. 1991;70(6):360–74.
8. Mimori T, Nakashima R, Hosono Y. Interstitial lung disease in myositis: clinical subsets, biomarkers, and treatment. Curr Rheumatol Rep. 2012;14(3):264–74.
9. Solomon J, Swigris JJ, Brown KK. Myositis-related interstitial lung disease and antisynthetase syndrome. J Bras Pneumol. 2011;37(1):100–9.
10. Labirua A, Lundberg IE. Interstitial lung disease and idiopathic inflammatory myopathies: progress and pitfalls. Curr Opin Rheumatol. 2010;22(6):633–8.
11. Yamasaki Y, Yamada H, Ohkubo M, Yamasaki M, Azuma K, Ogawa H, et al. Longterm survival and associated risk factors in patients with adult-onset idiopathic inflammatory myopathies and amyopathic dermatomyositis: experience in a single institute in Japan. J Rheumatol. 2011;38(8):1636–43.
12. Marie I, Hachulla E, Cherin P, Dominique S, Hatron PY, Hellot MF, et al. Interstitial lung disease in polymyositis and dermatomyositis. Arthritis Rheum. 2002;47(6):614–22.
13. Betteridge ZE, Gunawardena H, McHugh NJ. Novel autoantibodies and clinical phenotypes in adult and juvenile myositis. Arthritis Res Ther. 2011; 13(2):209.
14. Gunawardena H, Betteridge ZE, McHugh NJ. Myositis-specific autoantibodies: their clinical and pathogenic significance in disease expression. Rheumatology (Oxford). 2009;48(6):607–12.
15. Hirakata M. Autoantibodies to aminoacyl-tRNA synthetases. Intern Med. 2005;44(6):527–8.
16. Miller FW, Twitty SA, Biswas T, Plotz PH. Origin and regulation of a disease-specific autoantibody response. Antigenic epitopes, spectrotype stability, and isotype restriction of anti-Jo-1 autoantibodies. J Clin Invest. 1990;85(2):468–75.
17. Stone KB, Oddis CV, Fertig N, Katsumata Y, Lucas M, Vogt M, et al. Anti-Jo-1 antibody levels correlate with disease activity in idiopathic inflammatory myopathy. Arthritis Rheum. 2007;56(9):3125–31.
18. Kaji K, Fujimoto M, Hasegawa M, Kondo M, Saito Y, Komura K, et al. Identification of a novel autoantibody reactive with 155 and 140 kDa nuclear proteins in patients with dermatomyositis: an association with malignancy. Rheumatology (Oxford). 2007;46(1): 25–8.
19. Targoff IN, Mamyrova G, Trieu EP, Perurena O, Koneru B, O'Hanlon TP, et al. A novel autoantibody to a 155-kd protein is associated with dermatomyositis. Arthritis Rheum. 2006;54(11):3682–9.
20. Betteridge ZE, Gunawardena H, Chinoy H, North J, Ollier WE, Cooper RG, et al. Clinical and human leucocyte antigen class II haplotype associations of autoantibodies to small ubiquitin-like modifier enzyme, a dermatomyositis-specific autoantigen target, in UK Caucasian adult-onset myositis. Ann Rheum Dis. 2009;68(10):1621–5.
21. Sato S, Hoshino K, Satoh T, Fujita T, Kawakami Y, Kuwana M. RNA helicase encoded by melanoma differentiation-associated gene 5 is a major autoantigen in patients with clinically amyopathic dermatomyositis: association with rapidly progressive interstitial lung disease. Arthritis Rheum. 2009;60(7): 2193–200.
22. Huppmann P, Sczepanski B, Boensch M, Winterkamp S, Schonheit-Kenn U, Neurohr C, et al. Effects of in-patient pulmonary rehabilitation in patients with interstitial lung disease. Eur Respir J. 2013;42(2): 444–53.
23. Garvey C. Interstitial lung disease and pulmonary rehabilitation. J Cardiopulm Rehabil Prev. 2010; 30(3):141–6.
24. Holland AE, Hill CJ, Glaspole I, Goh N, McDonald CF. Predictors of benefit following pulmonary rehabilitation for interstitial lung disease. Respir Med. 2012;106(3):429–35.
25. Kelly C, Saravanan V. Treatment strategies for a rheumatoid arthritis patient with interstitial lung disease. Expert Opin Pharmacother. 2008;9(18):3221–30.
26. CDC. Prevention and control of influenza with vaccines: recommendations of the Advisory Committee on Immunization Practices (ACIP)—United States, 2012–13 influenza season. MMWR Morb Mortal Wkly Rep. 2012;61(32):613–8.
27. Centers for Disease Control and Prevention (CDC); Advisory Committee on Immunization Practices. Updated recommendations for prevention of invasive pneumococcal disease among adults using the 23-valent pneumococcal polysaccharide vaccine (PPSV23). MMWR Morb Mortal Wkly Rep. 2010; 59(34):1102–6.
28. Swinburn CR, Mould H, Stone TN, Corris PA, Gibson GJ. Symptomatic benefit of supplemental oxygen in hypoxemic patients with chronic lung disease. Am Rev Respir Dis. 1991;143(5 Pt 1):913–5.
29. Mittoo S, Gelber AC, Christopher-Stine L, Horton MR, Lechtzin N, Danoff SK. Ascertainment of collagen vascular disease in patients presenting with interstitial lung disease. Respir Med. 2009;103(8): 1152–8.
30. Fiorentino D, Chung L, Zwerner J, Rosen A, Casciola-Rosen L. The mucocutaneous and systemic phenotype of dermatomyositis patients with antibodies to MDA5 (CADM-140): a retrospective study. J Am Acad Dermatol. 2011;65(1):25–34.
31. Aggarwal R, Oddis CV. Paraneoplastic myalgias and myositis. Rheum Dis Clin North Am. 2011;37(4): 607–21.
32. Hill CL, Zhang Y, Sigurgeirsson B, Pukkala E, Mellemkjaer L, Airio A, et al. Frequency of specific cancer types in dermatomyositis and polymyositis: a population-based study. Lancet. 2001;357(9250): 96–100.

33. Azar L, Khasnis A. Paraneoplastic rheumatologic syndromes. Curr Opin Rheumatol. 2013;25:44–9.
34. Zahr ZA, Baer AN. Malignancy in myositis. Curr Rheumatol Rep. 2011;13(3):208–15.
35. Suber TL, Casciola-Rosen L, Rosen A. Mechanisms of disease: autoantigens as clues to the pathogenesis of myositis. Nat Clin Pract Rheumatol. 2008;4(4): 201–9.
36. Andras C, Ponyi A, Constantin T, Csiki Z, Szekanecz E, Szodoray P, et al. Dermatomyositis and polymyositis associated with malignancy: a 21-year retrospective study. J Rheumatol. 2008;35(3):438–44.

Pulmonary Manifestations of Systemic Lupus Erythematosus (SLE)

6

Shikha Mittoo and Jeffrey J. Swigris

Introduction

Systemic lupus erythematosus (SLE) is a systemic inflammatory disease, characterized serologically by an autoantibody response to nucleic antigens and clinically by injury and/or malfunction in any organ system. During their disease course, up to 50 % of SLE patients will develop pulmonary manifestations [1]. These include pleuritis (with or without effusion), inflammatory and fibrotic forms of interstitial lung disease, alveolar hemorrhage, shrinking lung syndrome, pulmonary hypertension, airways disease, and thromboembolic disease. Table 6.1 summarizes relevant clinical factors and frequency of the major pulmonary manifestations of SLE discussed in this chapter. As with SLE in general, its pulmonary manifestations are variable, yielding a heterogeneous clinical phenotype—from mild or essentially asymptomatic to severe and life-threatening. Although pulmonary disease is recognized as a leading cause of death and disability in SLE, over time, it has become increasingly clear that many patients with SLE have subclinical impairment in lung diffusing capacity and/or respiratory mechanics. The focus of this chapter will be on the clinical presentation, pathogenesis, pathology, management, and prognosis of SLE-associated lung conditions. Although lung cancer and pulmonary infections occur frequently in patients with SLE, they are not necessarily directly attributable to SLE disease activity and, therefore, will not be discussed here [2].

General

Before we begin the discussion of SLE-related pulmonary manifestations, we urge the reader to bear in mind that given the potential for subtle or subclinical pulmonary manifestations, the heterogeneity in clinical phenotype, and the potential for serious disease, clinicians must keep in mind a broad differential diagnosis anytime an SLE patient presents with chest or respiratory symptoms, and the etiology of those symptoms can be confidently identified and treated only through interdisciplinary dialogue/discussion. Because this chapter covers all the various ways SLE can affect the respiratory system, we begin the discussion with a brief overview of anatomy before moving to a general discussion of presenting symptoms. From there, we use a "compartments" approach to discuss how SLE may affect the vascular, parenchymal, pleural, or airways compartments of the respiratory system.

S. Mittoo, M.D., M.H.S., F.R.C.P.C. (✉)
Department of Medicine/Rheumatology,
Mount Sinai Hospital, 60 Murray Street, L2-003,
Toronto, ON, Canada M5T 3LP
e-mail: shikha.hopkins@gmail.com

J.J. Swigris, D.O., M.S.
Autoimmune Lung Center and Interstitial
Lung Disease Program, National Jewish Health,
1400 Jackson Street, Denver, CO 80206, USA
e-mail: swigrisj@njc.org

P.F. Dellaripa et al. (eds.), *Pulmonary Manifestations of Rheumatic Disease: A Comprehensive Guide*,
DOI 10.1007/978-1-4939-0770-0_6, © Springer Science+Business Media New York 2014

Table 6.1 Type, frequency, and clinical factors associated with specific pulmonary manifestations in systemic lupus erythematosus (SLE)

Type of pulmonary involvement	Estimated frequency/prevalence	Relevant clinical features associated with the specific type of pulmonary involvement
Pleural	30–50 % [56, 57, 69]	Positive antinuclear antibody in pleural fluid at a titer of ≥1:160, seropositivity for anti-ribonucleoprotein and anti-Sm antibodies, late-age (>50 years of age) onset of SLE, greater cumulative damage, and greater disease duration [57, 58]
Pulmonary hypertension	0.5–17.5 % [16]	Adult women, <40 years of age, within first 5 years of SLE disease onset, seropositivity for anticardiolipin and anti-ribonucleoprotein antibodies, Raynaud's phenomenon, rheumatoid factor [18, 21]
Shrinking lung syndrome	0.5–10 % [52, 53]	Greater disease duration, history of pleurisy, seropositivity for anti-ribonucleoprotein antibody [53]
Interstitial lung disease	1–15 % [38]	Older age at onset of SLE (>50 years old), greater disease duration (>10 years), sclerodactyly, abnormal nailfold capillaries, high levels of C-reactive protein, hypocomplementemia, serum cryoglobulins, lupus erythematosus cells in serum [38, 41–43]
Diffuse alveolar hemorrhage	Rare	Presence of nephritis, high disease activity, greater levels of anti-DS DNA antibody titers, low serum complement C3 levels [30, 70]
Larynx and airways disease	Rare, larynx [67, 68] Rare, airways [71]	Not known

Overview of Thoracic Cavity Anatomy

The pulmonary system, which includes the airways (trachea, bronchi and bronchioles, and alveoli), pleural, pulmonary vasculature, and parenchyma, is housed along with the esophagus, thymus, lymph nodes, heart, and its major blood vessels, in the thoracic cavity [3]. The thoracic cavity is surrounded by an osteocartilaginous complex (thoracic cage) comprised of thoracic vertebrae, ribs, sternum, and costal cartilage and is enveloped by intercostal muscles, nerves, and vessels; the thoracic cage is separated from the abdomen by the diaphragm [3]. Certain muscles that arise from the upper limb and neck (serratus anterior, pectoral muscles, latissimus dorsi, scalenes), and attach to the thoracic cage, can function as accessory muscles of respiration [3]. The larynx, which contains the vocal chords, is an extrathoracic structure, situated above the trachea, and comprised of small joints and cartilage. Vocal chord integrity, which can be threatened by direct involvement of the vocal chords or indirect damage/disease to structures within the larynx, is essential to voice quality and respiration. Any of these structures may be directly or indirectly affected by SLE.

Clinical Presentation and Mimicry of Pulmonary Disease in SLE

Cough, chest pain, and dyspnea are the most frequent respiratory system symptoms in SLE, and although they are suggestive, they are not specific for disease within the pulmonary system. In patients with SLE, cough may be caused by an airway or lung parenchymal problem, but as in the general population, it is more often a symptom of gastrointestinal reflux (GERD) or postnasal drip [4]. Like patients with other connective tissue diseases, those with SLE are at risk for esophageal disease, including GERD and dysmotility. They have been linked with the development and worsening of pulmonary complications including aspiration pneumonitis, aspiration pneumonia, and progression of interstitial lung disease [5–9]. Patients with SLE may present with SLE-related laryngeal involvement, such as paradoxical vocal fold motion, the symptoms of which may be difficult to distinguish from thoracic pathology. Patient with SLE can develop chest pain from musculoskeletal, cardiac, pulmonary, esophageal, or psychiatric causes. An SLE patient presenting with chest pain and/or dyspnea should be evaluated for a cardiovascular disease (accelerated atherosclerosis leading to coronary syndromes and/or congestive heart failure) given the high frequency and rate of cardiovascular mortality in this patient population [10, 11]. In this population, mimics of cardiovascular chest pain include pleural disease, esophageal spasm, costochondritis, or sternoclavicular arthritis (from SLE disease activity). The astute clinician will also be on the lookout for comorbid conditions commonly found in SLE, such as fibromyalgia or mood disorders (anxiety/ depression) [12–15].

Vascular Compartment

Pulmonary Hypertension

Epidemiology and Clinical Presentation
In various studies, the prevalence of pulmonary hypertension (PH) in SLE ranges from 0.5 to 17.5 %, depending on the case definition [16]. As in other CTDs, in SLE there are multiple potential reasons for PH to develop, so a number of causes must be carefully considered. Before a confident diagnosis of SLE-related PH (SLE-PH) is rendered (i.e., World Health Organization [WHO] Group 1 or pulmonary arterial hypertension [PAH]), the causes of WHO Groups 2–5 PH must be excluded [17]. Patients with SLE may develop WHO Group 2 PH, from either left ventricular dysfunction or left heart valvular abnormalities (related to SLE or not). SLE patients with significant interstitial lung disease (ILD) can develop PH from chronic hypoxia (WHO Group 3 PH), and those with antiphospholipid syndrome are at risk for developing WHO Group 4 PH (chronic thromboembolic PH or CTEPH). WHO Group 5 PH includes a number of disparate entities, including extrinsic compression of the pulmonary arteries, that are not particularly germane to SLE patients, but, as in other patients, these entities must be excluded in the evaluation of PH in the patient with SLE.

Typically, SLE patients develop PH within 5 years from SLE onset; there is no association between extrathoracic SLE disease activity and the development of PH. Most SLE patients with PH are adult women under the age of 40 years [18]. Although some patients with SLE-PH are asymptomatic, most present with one or more

symptoms, including chest pain, shortness of breath, or cough [19]. Approximately a third of SLE-PH patients will have pleural effusions, often associated with high right atrial pressure and right heart failure [16, 20]. Physical examination may reveal a prominent pulmonic component and/or fixed split of the second heart sound, murmurs of tricuspid or pulmonic regurgitation, a right ventricular heave, a palpable pulsation along the left sternal border, and, in advanced cases, overt signs of right heart failure. In a case-control study of 147 SLE patients, Raynaud's phenomenon and the presence of anticardiolipin and anti-U1 ribonucleoprotein (RNP) antibodies were predictive of PH, with odds ratios (ORs) of 3.2, 3.8, and 5.4, respectively [21]. In another study, investigators found that rheumatoid factor positivity was significantly more likely among SLE patients with PH compared to those without PH [19].

Pathophysiology
The main mechanisms driving the development of SLE-PH are believed to be organ-altering autoimmune effects directed at the pulmonary vasculature. Chronic inflammation, immune dysregulation, and vascular damage and remodeling are contributory. Rarely, vasculitis or pulmonary venoocclusive disease (PVOD) leads to SLE-PH [22]. With the exception of PVOD, the pathologic findings of SLE-PH include medial hypertrophy, intimal fibrosis, and, in severe cases, plexiform lesions.

Evaluation, Prognosis, and Management
Patients suspected to have SLE-PH may undergo screening evaluation with a transthoracic echocardiogram (TTE); however, TTE is notoriously inaccurate when the estimated right ventricular systolic pressure is not significantly elevated or other signs of right heart stress (e.g., dilation, impaired systolic function) are absent. Right heart catheterization (RHC) is needed to definitively diagnose PH. During RHC, the hemodynamic definition of PH is made when the mean pulmonary artery pressure is ≥25 mmHg in the face of a pulmonary capillary wedge pressure <15 mmHg [23]. As in patients without SLE, those with SLE-PH should undergo evaluation for other causes of PH. A thorough history looking for

current or past use of anorexigens or illicit drugs; testing that includes a screening polysomnogram to rule out obstructive sleep apnea, chest computed tomography (CT) angiogram and ventilation perfusion scan to evaluate for acute or chronic thromboembolic disease, and serologic testing for human immunodeficiency virus and chronic liver disease are suggested as part of the work-up for PH. If the history, physical exam, or lung function suggests the possibility of ILD, a high-resolution CT is indicated.

There are no consensus guidelines on the management of SLE-PH. In double-blind trials, in which only small numbers of patients ($n = 16$–35) were enrolled, PH-specific therapy (selective and nonselective endothelin receptor antagonists or phosphodiesterase-5 inhibitors) has demonstrated improvements in clinical and physiologic end points [16]. Data supporting the use of immunosuppressive medications, such as intravenous cyclophosphamide and glucocorticoids, for SLE-PH are limited. In certain retrospective series of small numbers of subjects, investigators have reported a modest physiologic benefit from the use of immunosuppression in combination with vasodilator therapy [24]. In a recent systematic review, elevated mean pulmonary artery pressure, Raynaud's phenomenon, thrombocytopenia, plexiform lesions, infection, thrombosis, pregnancy, pulmonary vasculitis, and anticardiolipin antibodies were associated with decreased survival among patients with SLE-PH [25]. Overall, SLE-PH has a 75 % 3-year survival [26].

Diffuse Alveolar Hemorrhage

Epidemiology and Clinical Presentation

Diffuse alveolar hemorrhage (DAH) is a rare and potentially catastrophic pulmonary manifestation of SLE. In SLE, DAH is the direct consequence of pulmonary capillaritis, defined pathologically by neutrophilic infiltration and destruction of vessel walls [27]. The clinical presentation is often dramatic: patients are often ill appearing with dyspnea and fever. Because hemoptysis occurs in only about 30 % of patients with DAH, its absence far from excludes the diagnosis. Chest imaging is notable for diffuse, bilateral consolidative or

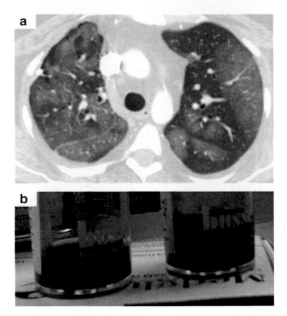

Fig. 6.1 (**a**) shows an axial slice from a chest computed tomography scan from the presented patient at the level of the azygous vein. The *image* shows bilateral, patchy ground glass opacities confirmed by bronchoalveolar lavage (**b**) to be due to diffuse alveolar hemorrhage

ground glass opacities (Fig. 6.1a). Depending on the amount of blood loss, patients may also present with falling hematocrit and/or overt anemia. Nephritis has been reported at the time of DAH presentation [28]. Notably, DAH can lead to pathologic changes in the lungs' terminal airways (alveoli) that are similar to renal involvement in SLE; immune complexes in addition to blood may be found in the alveolar wall in the setting of DAH [29]. At the time of DAH, high SLE disease activity, high titers of anti-DS DNA antibodies, and low complement C3 levels may be found [30].

Management and Prognosis

Catastrophic antiphospholipid antibody syndrome and overlap with primary vasculitides must be excluded, because their management differs from SLE-related DAH. All patients presenting with DAH should be screened for the presence of antiphospholipid, anti-glomerular basement membrane, and antineutrophil cytoplasmic antibodies in addition to serum complement C3, C4, ANA, and anti-DS DNA. Patients should also be evaluated for pulmonary infection as a cause of DAH. Pulse methylprednisolone, 1 g daily for

Case Vignette 1

Ms. J. is a 30-year-old African-American woman with long-standing SLE treated with hydroxychloroquine alone. She was found to have elevated antiphospholipid antibodies at the time of SLE diagnosis, but she has no history of arterial or venous thrombosis. She presents now to the emergency department (ED) with 2 days of dyspnea, cough, low-grade fever to 38 °C, and a vague "twinge" in her upper chest bilaterally.

A work-up in the ED shows her room air, resting, peripheral oxygen saturation to be 89 %, and her hematocrit is 30 %, down from 40 % 2 weeks ago. A chest computed tomography scan with contrast rules out acute or chronic pulmonary embolism but demonstrates bilateral, patchy ground glass opacities (Fig. 6.1a). Bronchoscopy with bronchoalveolar lavage (BAL) is performed; return from sequential BAL aliquots is progressively more bloody (Fig. 6.1b).

3 days and changed to 1–2 mg/kg/day oral prednisone over the next few days, is the initial treatment of DAH. Plasma exchange and cytotoxic agents may be used as well. Certain investigators have successfully treated SLE-related DAH with cyclophosphamide or rituximab [28, 31]. In DAH, poor prognostic markers include renal insufficiency, thrombocytopenia, and severity of clinical presentation (i.e., need for mechanical ventilation) [28]. Patients may experience recurrent episodes of DAH; thus, vigilant follow-up is required.

Pulmonary Embolism

Antiphospholipid antibodies (APLAs) are a heterogeneous group of autoantibodies that include anticardiolipin antibodies, lupus anticoagulant, and anti-glycoprotein-I antibodies. APLAs occur in around 1/3 of SLE patients [32]. When compared with SLE patients without a lupus anticoagulant or anticardiolipin antibodies, those with these antibodies are much more likely (six times

and 2.5 times) to develop deep venous thrombosis (DVT) or pulmonary embolism (PE) [33]. Moreover, lupus anticoagulant positivity is associated with a 50 % chance of DVT within 20 years of SLE diagnosis [34]. Interestingly, male gender is an independent predictor for thrombosis in SLE and, in addition to hypertension, is an important risk factor for thrombosis, even in the absence of APLAs [32].

As with the majority of pulmonary emboli, PE in SLE nearly always results from lower extremity DVT; intracardiac thrombi are a rare occurrence in SLE, even among those with APLA syndrome [35]. In SLE patients presenting with dyspnea and/or chest pain, particularly if they are seropositive for APLAs, PE must be part of the differential diagnosis. Bilateral lower extremity venous Doppler ultrasound, screen for APLAs, and CT angiogram should be considered for further work-up of PE.

Acute Reversible Hypoxemia

In this extremely rare entity, patients with SLE develop the abrupt onset of potentially profound hypoxemia. The cause is leuko-aggregation within pulmonary vessels [36, 37]. Substantially elevated blood levels of C3a suggest complement activation that plays a pivotal role. Treatment includes glucocorticoids and aspirin. Prognosis is believed to be favorable.

Parenchymal Compartment

Interstitial Lung Disease and Pneumonitis

Epidemiology
Clinically apparent ILD is far less common in SLE than in other connective tissue diseases, occurring in 1–15 % of SLE patients [38]. Although parenchymal abnormalities may occur in the setting of SLE, they are often not the direct consequence of the autoimmune aspect of the disease [39]. For example, an SLE patient presenting with radiographic opacities is much more likely to have infection than fibro/inflammatory parenchymal disease.

Clinical Presentation and Risk Factors

Patients with SLE-related ILD (SLE-ILD) typically present with exertional dyspnea and possibly a nonproductive cough. Because dyspnea is reported in nearly two-thirds of all-comers with SLE, it may be attributed to causes other than ILD, thus delaying the diagnosis of ILD until its later stages [40]. This may, in part, explain why two-thirds of patients with SLE-ILD have auscultatory crackles on chest examination upon presentation of ILD [41]. Clubbing and peripheral cyanosis, signs not infrequently observed in idiopathic pulmonary fibrosis, are rarely found in SLE-ILD [41]. Few predictors of SLE-ILD exist. Patients with long-standing disease (>10 years of disease duration), those with Raynaud's phenomenon, seropositivity for anti-(U1) RNP antibodies, sclerodactyly, and abnormal nailfold capillary loops are associated with radiographic evidence of ILD [41, 42]. Patients with an older age of SLE onset (>50 years of age) are significantly more likely than those with a younger age of onset to develop ILD [43]. Serologic abnormalities associated with SLE-ILD include a high levels of high-sensitivity C-reactive protein, cryoglobulins, hypocomplementemia, and serum lupus erythematosus cells [38].

Evaluation and Diagnosis

The diagnosis of SLE-ILD relies on a combination of clinical features, chest imaging, histopathology, and lung physiology. Before rending a diagnosis of SLE-ILD, it is important to exclude other causes of ILD including medication-related. Disease-modifying medications used in SLE such as methotrexate, leflunomide, imuran, tumor necrosis factor inhibitors, rituximab, cyclophosphamide, and sulfasalazine have been associated with the development of ILD. In addition, screening for environmental or occupational exposures must be undertaken (e.g., silica, asbestos, beryllium, dust, mold, bird feathers) [44]. It is also important to exclude overlapping disorders that may lead to ILD (sarcoidosis, other connective tissue disorders).

Although a surgical lung biopsy is the gold standard method to diagnose ILD, it is usually not performed. The most common histologic pattern of SLE-ILD is nonspecific interstitial pneumonia (NSIP); less common patterns include organizing pneumonia (OP), lymphoid interstitial pneumonia (LIP), usual interstitial pneumonia (UIP), desquamative interstitial pneumonia (DIP), and diffuse alveolar damage (DAD) [45]. In lieu of an invasive investigational approach, a high-resolution chest computed tomography (HRCT) scan in combination with restrictive physiology (a reduced forced vital capacity (FVC), total lung capacity, and/or diffusing capacity of carbon monoxide (DLCO) on pulmonary function tests (PFTs)) and/or compatible clinical features can clinch the diagnosis of ILD. However, clinicians must be vigilant to exclude ILD mimics such as DAH, drug toxicity congestive heart failure, uremia, or infection.

Management and Prognosis

Treatment for SLE-ILD is based largely on expert opinion. High-dose oral corticosteroids (1 mg/kg body weight of oral prednisone, up to 60 mg, or its equivalent) and a steroid-sparing agent, often cyclophosphamide (daily oral of 1–2 mg/kg depending on renal function and age of patient or intravenous equivalent), are initiated for severe ILD. Mild to moderate forms of ILD are sometimes treated initially with moderate doses of corticosteroids with either azathioprine or mycophenolate mofetil. Tapering of corticosteroid therapy is often guided by favorable clinical, physiologic, and/or radiographic response.

Case Vignette 2

Mrs. D. is a 58-year-old African-American female, never smoker, with SLE diagnosed 10 years ago. She has no other medical problems; she takes no medications associated with the development of pulmonary fibrosis; she owns no pets; she has no exposures, including feathers or dusts. Over the last 18 months, she has noticed gradually increasing exertional dyspnea and nonproductive cough. A slice from a chest computed tomography scan, shown in Fig. 6.2, confirms the presence of pulmonary fibrosis.

(continued)

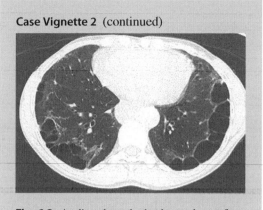

Case Vignette 2 (continued)

Fig. 6.2 A slice through the lower lungs from Mrs. D's chest computed tomography scan shows an interesting pattern of lower zone-, peripheral-, and subpleural-predominant fibrosis

Lupus Pneumonitis and Its Association with ILD

Lupus pneumonitis (LP) is probably best characterized as an acute interstitial pneumonia (AIP)-like reaction in a patient with SLE. It is a highly fatal syndrome characterized by acute onset of fever, pleuritic chest pain, and tachypnea; up to 50 % mortality rate is seen with this rare condition. It is often accompanied with auscultatory crackles, and hemoptysis may rarely occur. Chest imaging usually reveals bilateral opacities [46]. If alveolar hemorrhage is found, we prefer the term DAH and reserve the term LP for cases in which an AIP-like reaction is the cause of the patient's acute decompensation. Pneumonitis may be a precursor to chronic ILD in a subset of patients [46]. In one case series, 3 of 12 patients with pneumonitis progressed to chronic ILD, despite treatment with high-dose corticosteroids. In both LP and SLE-ILD, immune complexes, lymphocytic aggregates, and vascular pathology are common [46].

Physiology Impairment: Restrictive Lung Disease and Shrinking Lung Syndrome

Restrictive Lung Disease
Epidemiology

PFT abnormalities in SLE are very common and can occur in patients who are not suspected to have lung involvement [47, 48]. In a study of 43 SLE patients, 88 % had pulmonary dysfunction with the most common abnormality being a reduction in DLCO (72 %), followed by restrictive (49 %) or obstructive (9 %) patterns on PFT [48]. In a study of 70 non-smoking SLE patients, the majority of whom were asymptomatic with a normal chest radiograph, 67 % had an isolated reduction in DLCO, and 6 % had a restrictive pattern [49]. In another study of 110 Japanese SLE patients, an abnormal DLCO and restrictive changes were found in 47 % and 8 % of patients, respectively; only 13 % of patients with PFT abnormalities had other clinical and/or radiographic evidence for lung involvement [50].

Shrinking Lung Syndrome
Clinical Presentation

Dyspnea and physiologic restriction, in the absence of parenchymal disease on chest imaging, are major features of shrinking lung syndrome (SLS). In the original report of SLS by Hoffbrand and colleagues, SLS was characterized by unexplained dyspnea, small lung volumes, and restrictive lung physiology, with or without diaphragmatic elevation, in the absence of interstitial, alveolar, or vascular pulmonary disease [51].

Epidemiology and Risk Factors

SLS is often considered a rare manifestation of SLE, occurring in 0.5 % of patients [52]. In a recent study of 110 consecutively enrolled SLE patients systematically evaluated for the presence of pulmonary involvement, a surprising 10 % of patients met the definition of SLS [53]. The higher frequency of SLS compared with prior reports may in part be due to the fact that in that study SLE patients were screened with PFTs and chest imaging for the presence of parenchymal lung involvement. In this study, greater disease duration, seropositivity for anti-RNP antibodies, and a history of pleuritis were independently associated with SLS in a multivariate analysis [53]. The exact cause of SLS remains unclear, but some data suggest progressive impairment in diaphragmatic excursion from weakness is the main contributing factor [54].

Management

There is limited information on the management and prognosis of SLS. Corticosteroids (moderate to high doses), cytotoxic agents, biologic therapies (rituximab), theophylline, and high-dose beta-agonists have all been used to successfully treat this condition [54].

Case Vignette 3

Ms. P. is a 40-year-old white female with several years of malar rash, photosensitivity, Raynaud's phenomenon, and oral ulcers who was diagnosed with SLE 2 years ago when recalcitrant cough brought her to medical attention. Over the last 2 years, she has noticed gradually increasing exertional dyspnea.

A posteroanterior chest radiograph showed small lung volumes characteristic for SLS (Fig. 6.3). A chest computed tomography scan showed no parenchymal or pleural abnormalities. Seated, her FVC is 1.7 L, which is 45 % of the predicted value based on her age, height, and weight. Supine, her FVC is 1.2 L, which represents a 29 % decline from seated. Her maximal inspiratory pressure (MIP) is only 30 % of the predicted value. Results from a maximal cardiopulmonary exercise test are in Table 6.2. Note the failure in her ability to recruit tidal volume (Vt) as the test progresses; minute ventilation increases throughout exercise only because her respiratory rate climbs excessively. The constellation of findings supports a diagnosis of SLS.

Table 6.2 Results from maximal cardiopulmonary exercise test showing inability to recruit (i.e., increase) tidal volume (Vt) as test progresses

Time	Work (W)	VE (L/min)	Vt (mL)	RR (breaths/min)
1:00	0	10.6	493	22
2:00	0	8.4	542	16
3:00	0	8.8	459	19
Start exercise				
4:00	5	19.9	634	31
5:00	10	21.3	590	36
6:00	15	17.2	509	34
7:00	20	23.2	504	46
8:00	25	23.9	519	46
9:00	30	30.0	528	57

This is a hallmark of restrictive pulmonary physiology, but can be most profound in cases of respiratory muscle weakness

VE minute ventilation, *L/min* liters per minute, *mL* milliliters, *RR* respiratory rate

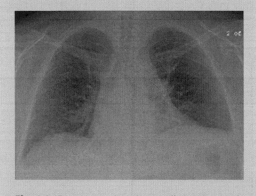

Fig. 6.3 Posteroanterior chest radiograph reveals small lung volumes

Pleural Compartment

Epidemiology and Clinical Presentation

Pleuritis (with or without pleural effusion) is the most common SLE-related pulmonary manifestation and part of the classification criteria for SLE [55]. In large observational cohorts from Europe and Canada, nearly a third of prospectively followed SLE patients developed clinically identifiable pleuritis, whereas up to 2/3 will have involvement at autopsy [24, 56, 57]. Disease duration, late age of diagnosis of SLE (after age 50 years), greater cumulative damage, and concomitant seropositivity for anti-RNP and anti-Sm antibodies are factors that increased the risk of pleuritis by nearly twofold [57, 58]. Pleuritic chest pain is the most common symptom, but patients may also report cough, dyspnea, and fever.

Evaluation, Prognosis, and Management

A pleural rub may be heard on physical examination, and chest imaging may reveal pleural effusion(s). Pleural effusions are often bilateral and small; rarely, effusions from SLE disease activity involve more than 2/3 of the lung fields [24]. Before diagnosing SLE-related pleuritis, other causes of a pleural effusion in SLE, such as cardiac or renal failure, must be excluded [59]. A thoracentesis and/or pleural biopsy is not necessary to diagnose an effusion and are rarely performed. These procedures may be performed when there is a concern for infection, blood in the pleural space, or malignancy.

The majority of SLE-related pleural effusions are not life-threatening and respond favorably to treatment with nonsteroidal anti-inflammatory drugs, for mild or asymptomatic effusions, and/or oral corticosteroids at a dose of 20–40 mg daily, for moderate to severe effusions [60]. Treatment can be discontinued in 3–4 weeks depending on clinical response. Pleurodesis may be considered in refractory, treatment-resistant cases [61].

Airways Compartment and Larynx

Large and/or small airways may be affected by SLE. Bronchiectasis can be seen in SLE, but is often an incidental finding on chest imaging; its clinical significance in this population is not known [62]. Inflammatory (e.g., lymphocytic) bronchiolitis may occur. Obliterative bronchiolitis (OB) is an uncommon manifestation of SLE that presents with cough and dyspnea. It is associated with severe, often progressive, airways obstruction (a reduced ratio of forced expiratory volume in 1 s to FVC), air trapping (that is often nicely accentuated on expiratory imaging), but usually a normal DLCO on PFT [63, 64]. Although various agents have been tried, no regimen has been proved effective [65, 66]. Borrowing from the lung transplantation literature, clinicians often prescribe OB patients macrolide antibiotics, because of their putative anti-inflammatory and perhaps antifibrotic effects.

Laryngeal involvement is an uncommon manifestation of SLE, often presenting with hoarseness and dyspnea. In a review of 97 SLE patients with laryngeal involvement, there were various pathologic changes found, from mild ulcerations to subglottic stenosis, but laryngeal edema and vocal chord paralysis were more frequently observed, at a rate of 28 % and 11 %, respectively [67]. It results from varying levels of upper airway mucosal inflammation and is responsive to treatment with oral corticosteroids. In rare circumstances, mucosal inflammation is accompanied by edema and can lead to airway obstruction [68].

How to Approach the Evaluation of a Patient with SLE Who Presents with Dyspnea

In any patient with SLE who presents with a respiratory complaint, particularly dyspnea, infection must be excluded. The concern for infection is heightened further in the dyspneic patient who is receiving chronic immunomodulatory therapy. It should be recognized that patients on glucocorticoids alone, or in combination with an immunomodulatory agent, may not manifest classic symptoms of infection, so a high index of suspicion for infection by typical (bacteria) and atypical (Mycobacteria, fungi, Pneumocystis) agents must be maintained. Bronchoscopy should be considered in any patient on immune-suppressing drugs who is found to have opacities on chest imaging. Besides confirming or ruling out pulmonary infection, as demonstrated in the representative case discussed, findings at bronchoscopy may prove useful for identifying the true cause of a patient's symptoms (e.g., DAH). If infection is confidently ruled out, consideration is given to other potential etiologies for dyspnea; top on the list, particularly in an SLE patient with risk factors for thromboembolism (e.g., hypercoagulable state or history of thromboembolism), is PE. In the appropriate scenario, a CT angiogram, with or without a lower extremity venous duplex with Doppler ultrasound, can be useful for confirming or ruling out thromboembolic disease.

The added benefit to performing CT angiogram is that it shows the lung parenchyma as well as the vasculature. However, because of the intravenous contrast given and the technique-mandated lower lung volumes used for a CT angiogram, the lung parenchyma will be more radiodense than on a high-resolution CT scan; this can make discerning whether ground glass opacities are present or not quite challenging. Depending on the acuity of symptoms, PFTs and an assessment of peripheral oxygen saturation (SpO_2) during exertion may add important information that can be used to help direct the evaluation. The DLCO may be elevated in DAH and reduced in the setting of interstitial lung disease or PH. Pulmonary vascular disease should be considered—and its presence assessed—in any patient with otherwise unexplained dyspnea or exertion-induced oxygen desaturation (SpO_2 decline ≥ 4 from resting value, even if nadir during exertion remains >90 %).

The SLE Patient Without Respiratory Complaints and the One with Known SLE-Related Pulmonary Complications

There are no data to guide the practitioner on whether and how to evaluate an SLE patient who has no respiratory complaints. Mild abnormalities on spirometry and/or diffusion capacity testing are common in asymptomatic SLE patients; most often, these abnormalities remain stable over time. It is our practice to use imaging and other testing as appropriate for the clinical scenario and not to "screen" asymptomatic SLE patients. However, patients should have a chest radiograph before the start of a disease-modifying medication, particularly before methotrexate is initiated, to rule out any underlying preexisting parenchymal disease. Our approach to following the patient with known SLE-related pulmonary complications varies depending on the particular complication present. For example, we routinely evaluate patients with SLE-ILD every 3–4 months in clinic with spirometry, DLCO, and an assessment of their functional status and exertion-related oxygen requirements.

Concluding Remarks

Pulmonary involvement is common during the disease course of SLE and can involve any part of the respiratory tract. It is important to identify the underlying etiology when pulmonary involvement occurs; clinicians need to particularly be vigilant in excluding other etiologies, such as infections, before attributing the manifestation to SLE. Being mindful of the clinical context, including the serologic profile of the patient, may help support the diagnosis of specific SLE-related pulmonary manifestations. Management of pulmonary manifestations is based largely on clinical experience and case series; studies in large cohorts and/or clinical trials are needed to establish effective therapies for pulmonary disease in SLE.

References

1. Pines A, et al. Pleuro-pulmonary manifestations of systemic lupus erythematosus: clinical features of its subgroups. Prognostic and therapeutic implications. Chest. 1985;88(1):129–35.
2. Bernatsky S, et al. Mortality in systemic lupus erythematosus. Arthritis Rheum. 2006;54(8):2550–7.
3. Moore KL, Agur A, Dalley AF. Essential Clinical Anatomy. 4th ed. Philadelphia: Lippincott Williams & Wilkins; 2010.
4. Azad AK, et al. Cough in systemic lupus erythematosus. Mymensingh Med J. 2013;22(2):300–7.
5. Zhang XJ, et al. Association of gastroesophageal factors and worsening of forced vital capacity in systemic sclerosis. J Rheumatol. 2013;40(6):850–8.
6. Marie I, et al. Esophageal involvement and pulmonary manifestations in systemic sclerosis. Arthritis Rheum. 2001;45(4):346–54.
7. Marie I, et al. Polymyositis and dermatomyositis: short term and longterm outcome, and predictive factors of prognosis. J Rheumatol. 2001;28(10):2230–7.
8. Savarino E, et al. [Possible connection between gastroesophageal reflux and interstitial pulmonary fibrosis in patients with systemic sclerosis]. Recenti Prog Med. 2009;100(11):512–6.
9. Fagundes MN, et al. Esophageal involvement and interstitial lung disease in mixed connective tissue disease. Respir Med. 2009;103(6):854–60.
10. Symmons DP, Gabriel SE. Epidemiology of CVD in rheumatic disease, with a focus on RA and SLE. Nat Rev Rheumatol. 2011;7(7):399–408.
11. Sinicato NA, da Silva Cardoso PA, Appenzeller S. Risk factors in cardiovascular disease in systemic lupus erythematosus. Curr Cardiol Rev. 2013;9(1):15–9.

12. Wolfe F, et al. Fibromyalgia, systemic lupus erythematosus (SLE), and evaluation of SLE activity. J Rheumatol. 2009;36(1):82–8.

13. Palagini L, et al. Depression and systemic lupus erythematosus: a systematic review. Lupus. 2013;22(5): 409–16.

14. Donmez S, et al. Autoimmune rheumatic disease associated symptoms in fibromyalgia patients and their influence on anxiety, depression and somatisation: a comparative study. Clin Exp Rheumatol. 2012;30(6 Suppl 74):65–9.

15. Peppercorn MA, Docken WP, Rosenberg S. Esophageal motor dysfunction in systemic lupus erythematosus. Two cases with unusual features. JAMA. 1979;242(17):1895–6.

16. Dhala A. Pulmonary arterial hypertension in systemic lupus erythematosus: current status and future direction. Clin Dev Immunol. 2012;2012:854941.

17. Simonneau G, et al. Updated clinical classification of pulmonary hypertension. J Am Coll Cardiol. 2009; 54(1 Suppl):S43–54.

18. Badesch DB, et al. Medical therapy for pulmonary arterial hypertension: ACCP evidence-based clinical practice guidelines. Chest. 2004;126(1 Suppl):35S–62.

19. Kamel SR, et al. Asymptomatic pulmonary hypertension in systemic lupus erythematosus. Clin Med Insights Arthritis Musculoskelet Disord. 2011;4:77–86.

20. Luo YF, et al. Frequency of pleural effusions in patients with pulmonary arterial hypertension associated with connective tissue diseases. Chest. 2011; 140(1):42–7.

21. Lian F, et al. Clinical features and independent predictors of pulmonary arterial hypertension in systemic lupus erythematosus. Rheumatol Int. 2012;32(6):1727–31.

22. Kishida Y, et al. Pulmonary venoocclusive disease in a patient with systemic lupus erythematosus. J Rheumatol. 1993;20(12):2161–2.

23. Galie N, et al. Guidelines for the diagnosis and treatment of pulmonary hypertension: the Task Force for the Diagnosis and Treatment of Pulmonary Hypertension of the European Society of Cardiology (ESC) and the European Respiratory Society (ERS), endorsed by the International Society of Heart and Lung Transplantation (ISHLT). Eur Heart J. 2009; 30(20):2493–537.

24. Swigris JJ, et al. Pulmonary and thrombotic manifestations of systemic lupus erythematosus. Chest. 2008;133(1):271–80.

25. Chow SL, et al. Prognostic factors for survival in systemic lupus erythematosus associated pulmonary hypertension. Lupus. 2012;21(4):353–64.

26. Condliffe R, et al. Connective tissue disease-associated pulmonary arterial hypertension in the modern treatment era. Am J Respir Crit Care Med. 2009;179(2):151–7.

27. Fishbein GA, Fishbein MC. Lung vasculitis and alveolar hemorrhage: pathology. Semin Respir Crit Care Med. 2011;32(3):254–63.

28. Martinez-Martinez MU, Abud-Mendoza C. Predictors of mortality in diffuse alveolar haemorrhage associated with systemic lupus erythematosus. Lupus. 2011;20(6):568–74.

29. Hughson MD, et al. Alveolar hemorrhage and renal microangiopathy in systemic lupus erythematosus. Arch Pathol Lab Med. 2001;125(4):475–83.

30. Chen GX, Dong Y, Ju ZB. [A clinical analysis of 32 patients with diffuse alveolar hemorrhage in diffuse connective tissue diseases]. Zhonghua Nei Ke Za Zhi. 2008;47(5):362–5.

31. Narshi CB, et al. Rituximab as early therapy for pulmonary haemorrhage in systemic lupus erythematosus. Rheumatology (Oxford). 2010;49(2):392–4.

32. Tektonidou MG, et al. Risk factors for thrombosis and primary thrombosis prevention in patients with systemic lupus erythematosus with or without antiphospholipid antibodies. Arthritis Rheum. 2009;61(1): 29–36.

33. Wahl DG, et al. Risk for venous thrombosis related to antiphospholipid antibodies in systemic lupus erythematosus—a meta-analysis. Lupus. 1997;6(5):467–73.

34. Somers E, Magder LS, Petri M. Antiphospholipid antibodies and incidence of venous thrombosis in a cohort of patients with systemic lupus erythematosus. J Rheumatol. 2002;29(12):2531–6.

35. Pardos-Gea J, et al. Cardiac manifestations other than valvulopathy in antiphospholipid syndrome: long-time echocardiography follow-up study. Int J Rheum Dis 2013 Oct 17. doi:10.1111/1756-185X.12191 [Epub ahead of print].

36. Martinez-Taboada VM, et al. Acute reversible hypoxemia in systemic lupus erythematosus: a new syndrome or an index of disease activity? Lupus. 1995;4(4):259–62.

37. Abramson SB, et al. Acute reversible hypoxemia in systemic lupus erythematosus. Ann Intern Med. 1991;114(11):941–7.

38. Mittoo S, Fischer A, Strand V, Meehan R, Swigris JJ. Systemic lupus erythematosus-related interstitial lung disease. Curr Rheumatol Rev. 2010;6(2):99–107.

39. Quadrelli SA, et al. Pulmonary involvement of systemic lupus erythematosus: analysis of 90 necropsies. Lupus. 2009;18(12):1053–60.

40. Hellman DB, et al. Dyspnea in ambulatory patients with SLE: prevalence, severity, and correlation with incremental exercise testing. J Rheumatol. 1995;22(3): 455–61.

41. Eisenberg H, et al. Diffuse interstitial lung disease in systemic lupus erythematosus. Ann Intern Med. 1973;79(1):37–45.

42. ter Borg EJ, et al. Clinical associations of antiribonucleoprotein antibodies in patients with systemic lupus erythematosus. Semin Arthritis Rheum. 1990;20(3): 164–73.

43. Ward MM, Polisson RP. A meta-analysis of the clinical manifestations of older-onset systemic lupus erythematosus. Arthritis Rheum. 1989;32(10):1226–32.

44. Schwaiblmair M, et al. Drug induced interstitial lung disease. Open Respir Med J. 2012;6:63–74.

45. Galie N, et al. Guidelines on diagnosis and treatment of pulmonary arterial hypertension. Rev Esp Cardiol. 2005;58(5):523–66.

46. Matthay RA, et al. Pulmonary manifestations of systemic lupus erythematosus: review of twelve cases of acute lupus pneumonitis. Medicine (Baltimore). 1975;54(5):397–409.

47. Groen H, et al. Pulmonary function in systemic lupus erythematosus is related to distinct clinical, serologic, and nailfold capillary patterns. Am J Med. 1992;93(6):619–27.

48. Silberstein SL, et al. Pulmonary dysfunction in systemic lupus erythematosus: prevalence classification and correlation with other organ involvement. J Rheumatol. 1980;7(2):187–95.

49. Andonopoulos AP, et al. Pulmonary function of nonsmoking patients with systemic lupus erythematosus. Chest. 1988;94(2):312–5.

50. Nakano M, et al. Pulmonary diffusion capacity in patients with systemic lupus erythematosus. Respirology. 2002;7(1):45–9.

51. Hoffbrand BI, Beck ER. "Unexplained" dyspnoea and shrinking lungs in systemic lupus erythematosus. Br Med J. 1965;1(5445):1273–7.

52. Bertoli AM, Vila LM, Apte M, Fessler BJ, Bastian HM, Reveille JD, Alarcon GS. Systemic lupus erythematosus in a multiethnic US Cohort LUMINA XLVIII: factors predictive of pulmonary damage. Lupus. 2007;16(6):410–7.

53. Allen D, et al. Evaluating systemic lupus erythematosus patients for lung involvement. Lupus. 2012; 21(12):1316–25.

54. Carmier D, Diot E, Diot P. Shrinking lung syndrome: recognition, pathophysiology and therapeutic strategy. Expert Rev Respir Med. 2011;5(1):33–9.

55. Tan EM, Cohen AS, Fries JF, Masi AT, McShane DJ, Rothfield NF, Schaller JG, Talal N, Winchester RJ. The 1982 revised criteria for the classification of systemic lupus erythematosus. Arthritis Rheum. 1982;25(11):1271–7.

56. Cervera R, et al. Systemic lupus erythematosus in Europe at the change of the millennium: lessons from the "Euro-Lupus Project". Autoimmun Rev. 2006; 5(3):180–6.

57. Mittoo S, et al. Clinical and serologic factors associated with lupus pleuritis. J Rheumatol. 2010;37(4): 747–53.

58. Boddaert J, et al. Late-onset systemic lupus erythematosus: a personal series of 47 patients and pooled analysis of 714 cases in the literature. Medicine (Baltimore). 2004;83(6):348–59.

59. Badui E, et al. Cardiovascular manifestations in systemic lupus erythematosus. Prospective study of 100 patients. Angiology. 1985;36(7):431–41.

60. Winslow WA, Ploss LN, Loitman B. Pleuritis in systemic lupus erythematosus: its importance as an early manifestation in diagnosis. Ann Intern Med. 1958;49(1):70–88.

61. Glazer M, et al. Successful talc slurry pleurodesis in patients with nonmalignant pleural effusion. Chest. 2000;117(5):1404–9.

62. Fenlon HM, et al. High-resolution chest CT in systemic lupus erythematosus. AJR Am J Roentgenol. 1996;166(2):301–7.

63. Weber F, et al. Cyclophosphamide therapy is effective for bronchiolitis obliterans occurring as a late manifestation of lupus erythematosus. Br J Dermatol. 2000;143(2):453–5.

64. Porter DR. Bronchiolitis obliterans in systemic lupus erythematosus. Ann Rheum Dis. 1992;51(7):927.

65. Kawahata K, et al. Severe airflow limitation in two patients with systemic lupus erythematosus: effect of inhalation of anticholinergics. Mod Rheumatol. 2008;18(1):52–6.

66. Godeau B, Cormier C, Menkes CJ. Bronchiolitis obliterans in systemic lupus erythematosus: beneficial effect of intravenous cyclophosphamide. Ann Rheum Dis. 1991;50(12):956–8.

67. Teitel AD, et al. Laryngeal involvement in systemic lupus erythematosus. Semin Arthritis Rheum. 1992;22(3):203–14.

68. Karim A, et al. Severe upper airway obstruction from cricoarytenoiditis as the sole presenting manifestation of a systemic lupus erythematosus flare. Chest. 2002; 121(3):990–3.

69. Cervera R, et al. Systemic lupus erythematosus: clinical and immunologic patterns of disease expression in a cohort of 1,000 patients. The European Working Party on Systemic Lupus Erythematosus. Medicine (Baltimore). 1993;72(2):113–24.

70. Martinez-Martinez MU, Abud-Mendoza C. Recurrent diffuse alveolar haemorrhage in a patient with systemic lupus erythematosus: long-term benefit of rituximab. Lupus. 2012;21(10):1124–7.

71. Hariri LP, et al. Acute fibrinous and organizing pneumonia in systemic lupus erythematosus: a case report and review of the literature. Pathol Int. 2010;60(11): 755–9.

Pulmonary Manifestations in Mixed Connective Tissue Disease

7

Kristin B. Highland and Richard M. Silver

Abbreviations

DM	Dermatomyositis
FEV1	Forced expiratory volume in 1 second
HRCT	High-resolution chest computed tomography
ILD	Interstitial lung disease
MCTD	Mixed connective tissue disease
PAH	Pulmonary arterial hypertension
PFT	Pulmonary function testing
PH	Pulmonary hypertension
PM	Polymyositis
PVOD	Pulmonary veno-occlusive disease
RA	Rheumatoid arthritis
SLE	Systemic lupus erythematosus
SSc	Systemic sclerosis, scleroderma
TLC	Total lung capacity

K.B. Highland, M.D., M.S.C.R. (✉)
Respiratory Institute, Cleveland Clinic, Desk A90,
9500 Euclid Avenue, Cleveland, OH 44195, USA
e-mail: highlak@ccf.org

R.M. Silver, M.D.
Division of Rheumatology and Immunology,
Medical University of South Carolina, 96 Jonathan
Lucas Street, Suite 816, Charleston, SC 29425, USA
e-mail: silver@musc.edu

Introduction

Mixed connective tissue disease (MCTD) is defined by the combined presence of U1 ribonucleoprotein autoantibodies and clinical features including Raynaud's phenomenon, "puffy" hands, sclerodactyly, arthralgias/arthritis, pleuritis, pericarditis, myositis, esophageal dysmotility, renal disease, pulmonary hypertension, and interstitial lung disease (ILD) [1]. The most common clinical manifestations at disease onset are Raynaud's phenomenon, arthralgias, swollen hands, sausage-like appearance of the fingers, and muscle weakness. They appear in 90 % of patients and usually develop insidiously [2]. This disease has been reported in children and in adults over the age of 80 years, although it is more common in women in the third decade of life [3]. The prevalence of MCTD is unknown, but most studies suggest an overall prevalence of approximately 3–10/100,000, with juvenile-onset presentations accounting for nearly a quarter of these cases [4–6].

Controversy persists on whether this disease is actually a distinct disorder or represents an overlap between systemic sclerosis (scleroderma, SSc), polymyositis/dermatomyositis (PM/DM), rheumatoid arthritis (RA), and systemic lupus erythematosus (SLE). This is due to the difficulty in distinguishing MCTD patients from SLE, SSc, PM/DM, and RA and because many patients who have anti-U1 RNP antibodies often eventually

P.F. Dellaripa et al. (eds.), *Pulmonary Manifestations of Rheumatic Disease: A Comprehensive Guide*,
DOI 10.1007/978-1-4939-0770-0_7, © Springer Science+Business Media New York 2014

Table 7.1 Pleuropulmonary manifestations associated with mixed connective tissue disease (MCTD)

- Aspiration pneumonia/pneumonitis
- Diaphragmatic dysfunction
- Diffuse alveolar hemorrhage
- Interstitial lung disease (ILD)
  - Nonspecific interstitial pneumonia
  - Organizing pneumonia
  - Usual interstitial pneumonia
- Malignancy
- Obstructive airways disease
  - Bronchiolitis
  - Bronchiectasis
- Pleural effusion
- Pleurisy
- Pneumothorax
- Pulmonary arterial hypertension (PAH)
- Pulmonary edema
- Pulmonary infections
- Pulmonary vasculitis
- Respiratory muscle weakness
- Thromboembolic disease

satisfy the criteria for SLE, SSc, PM/DM, and/or RA during their clinical course [7, 8].

Respiratory complications of MCTD are now accepted as a major feature of MCTD (Table 7.1) and are associated with the highest morbidity and mortality in MCTD. Pulmonary features are an integral part of two of the four proposed classification criteria for MCTD (Table 7.2) [9–12] and have a reported prevalence as high as 90 % [3, 13–15]. The two most prevalent pulmonary complications in MCTD are pulmonary hypertension (PH) and ILD.

Interstitial Lung Disease

Although ILD can be found in most adult MCTD patients depending upon methods used for detection, the majority of patients are asymptomatic. Nevertheless, the presence of dyspnea, cough, tachycardia, and bibasilar crackles is often associated with active ILD [16].

Although ILD also occurs in patients with juvenile-onset MCTD, it is usually less common and less severe. In a study of 24 patients with juvenile-onset MCTD, ILD was identified in only 25 % and the median extent of ILD in

the parenchyma was only 2.0 %. Radiographic findings did not seem to be associated with PFT results or disease duration. In this study, patients tended to have fine fibrosis and had an absence of a honeycomb pattern. There was also no evidence of airways disease and only minor pleural disease noted by HRCT scan [4].

In studies of adult patients from tertiary referral centers, abnormal PFTs showing predominantly a restrictive pattern have been reported in up to 90 % of patients with MCTD [2, 3, 5, 17]. The most common PFT abnormality is a reduction in the carbon monoxide diffusing capacity (DLCO), followed by a reduction of FEV1 and TLC (total lung capacity). A reduction in DLCO has been shown to be the most sensitive test for predicting the presence of ILD on HRCT. However, the overall correlation of pulmonary function with radiographic appearance is poor [16].

The most common chest imaging abnormality in MCTD is an interstitial pattern [18, 19]. On HRCT, the reported frequencies of abnormalities consistent with pulmonary fibrosis range from 0 to 20 %, while the frequency of ground-glass attenuation varies between 12 and 100 % [16, 19, 20]. Abnormalities on HRCT in patients with MCTD-ILD have been primarily characterized by the presence of ground-glass attenuation, interlobular septal and nonseptal linear opacities, and subpleural micronodules, all with a peripheral and lower lobe predominance [16, 19–21] (Fig. 7.1). The pattern on HRCT is most consistent with NSIP similar to that found in patients with SSc or PM/DM [6]. In a small retrospective study [19] that compared MCTD patients with other CTD patients, the frequency of ground-glass opacity in MCTD was significantly lower; the frequency of honeycombing was lower than in SSc, but higher than in PM/DM.

There is little published regarding the histology of ILD in MCTD, although it is believed that the major lung injury patterns include nonspecific interstitial pneumonia and usual interstitial pneumonia [20, 22–24]. Alveolar septal infiltration by lymphocytes and plasma cells, as well as the deposition of type III collagen, has been described [25, 26].

Table 7.2 Proposed criteria for mixed connective tissue diagnosis

	Major criteria	Minor criteria	Requirement for diagnosis

Sharp [11]	1. Myositis
	2. Pulmonary involvement
	  a. DLCO<70 %
	  b. PH
	  c. PAH on biopsy
	3. Raynaud's phenomenon
	4. Esophageal hypomotility
	5. Swollen hands
	6. Anti-ENA >1:10,000
	  with (+) anti-U1 RNP
	  and (−) anti-Smith
		1. Alopecia
		2. Leukopenia
		3. Anemia
		4. Pleuritis
		5. Pericarditis
		6. Arthritis
		7. Trigeminal neuropathy
		8. Malar rash
		9. Thrombocytopenia
		10. Mild myositis
		11. History of swollen hands
			Inclusion:
			1. Four major criteria+anti-U1 RNP≥1:4,000 *or*
			2. Two major criteria from criteria 1 and 2 and 3+2 minor criteria+anti-U1 RNP titer of at least 1:1,000
			Exclusion:
			+Anti-Smith antibody

Alarcón-Segovia [12]	Anti-RNP titer >1:1,600	1. Edema in hands 2. Synovitis 3. Myositis 4. Raynaud's phenomenon 5. Acrosclerosis	Major criteria+at least three minor criteria (one of which must be either synovitis or myositis)

Kasukawa [10]	1. Raynaud's phenomenon
	2. Swollen fingers or hands
	3. Anti-RNP (+)
		1. SLE-like symptoms
		  a. Polyarthritis
		  b. Lymphadenopathy
		  c. Facial erythema
		  d. Pericarditis or pleuritis
		  e. Leuko-thrombocytopenia
		2. SSc-like findings
		  a. Sclerodactyly
		  b. Pulmonary fibrosis, restrictive PFTs, or decreased DLCO
		  c. Esophageal hypomotility or dilatation
		3. PM-like findings
		  a. Muscle weakness
		  b. Elevated muscle enzymes
		  c. Myogenic pattern on EMG
			(+) Anti-U1 RNP+1 other major criteria+1 more of the minor criteria in at least two of the three disease categories

Kahn [9]	1. High-titer anti-U1 RNP corresponding to speckled ANA titer ≥1:2,000 2. Raynaud's phenomenon	1. Synovitis 2. Myositis 3. Swollen fingers	Both major criteria and at least two of the three minor criteria

Case Vignette

A 57-year-old white female presented with 3 years of nonproductive cough and progressive shortness of breath and dyspnea on exertion with activities of daily living. Her exercise tolerance is also limited by a concomitant myopathy. She had 10 years of Raynaud's phenomenon that has been complicated by digital ulcers. She also described recent episodes of near-syncope. She has had no overt syncope. She denied any chest pain. She had occasional palpitations. She denied PND, orthopnea, or lower extremity edema. Her past medical history is significant for severe gastroesophageal reflux disease and review of systems was also notable for significant sicca symptoms.

Pertinent physical examination findings included a heart rate of 97 beats per minute, respiratory rate 20 breaths per minute, blood pressure 101/60 mmHg, and oxygen saturation 88 % on room air. She had dry mucous membranes. She had elevated jugular venous distention. There were bilateral crackles on chest auscultation. Cardiac examination revealed a grade II/VI systolic murmur consistent with

(continued)

Case Vignette (continued)

tricuspid regurgitation and an increased P2. Extremities were notable for sclerodactyly with visible Raynaud's phenomenon at ambient temperature and the presence of digital pitted scars. She also had mild lower extremity edema. Musculoskeletal examination was unremarkable. She had grade 4-/5 proximal muscle strength.

Laboratory evaluation revealed an ANA >1:2,560 (speckled); ENA panel was notable for RNP >8.0 AI and SSA 3.1 AI. CPK was 547 and aldolase was 10.7. PM-1 (PM-Scl) antibody was positive. Her NT-BNP was 723 pg/mL.

Pulmonary function testing (PFT) was notable for FVC, 1.53 L (43 % predicted); forced expiratory volume in 1 second (FEV1), 1.36 L (49 % predicted); FEV1/FVC, 89 %; and diffusion, 26 % predicted consistent with severe restriction. FVC% predicted/DLCO% predicted was 1.6. She walked 332 m (59 % predicted) in 6 min. Her lowest oxygen saturation was 90 % despite 2 L of oxygen. She had an abnormal cardiovascular response to exercise with drop in diastolic blood pressure from 73 to 58 mmHg.

High-resolution chest computed tomography (HRCT) revealed bilateral ground-glass opacities, intralobular interstitial thickening, and traction bronchiectasis in an NSIP pattern. She also had significant esophageal dilatation (Fig. 7.1). Echocardiogram (Fig. 7.2) revealed a pericardial effusion as well as evidence of a pressure-overloaded right ventricle. The right atrium and right ventricle were dilated, and the peak right ventricular systolic pressure was estimated at 100 mmHg. Right heart catheterization revealed an RA 17 mmHg, mean PAP 54 mmHg, pulmonary capillary wedge pressure (PCWP) 13 mmHg, CI 1.9 L/min/m², and PVR 12 Wood units.

The patient was diagnosed with MCTD, fulfilling all four proposed criteria (Table 7.2), as well as ILD and severe pulmonary hypertension felt to be "out of proportion" to her ILD and likely due to pulmonary arterial hypertension (PAH). Severe gastroesophageal reflux was also felt to be a significant contributor to her pulmonary complaints, and treatment of GERD was optimized with twice daily PPI

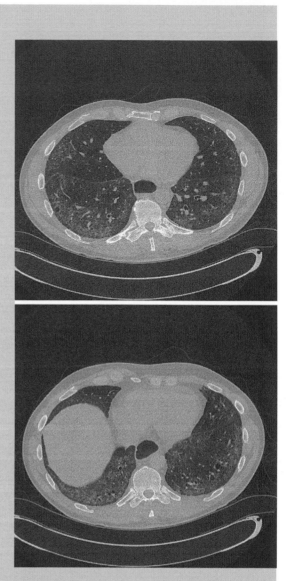

Fig. 7.1 High-resolution CT images of patient with MCTD and ILD. Note massive esophageal dilatation, basilar and peripheral predominance of reticulation, and ground-glass opacification with an absence of honeycombing. There is also the presence of traction bronchiectasis

and bedtime H2 blocker. She was also treated with corticosteroids and oral cyclophosphamide for ILD, as well as with combination therapy with a PDE5 inhibitor, ERA, and inhaled prostanoids for severe PAH. This therapeutic regimen resulted in a modest improvement in her pulmonary function, exercise tolerance, and hemodynamics over the course of the following year.

(continued)

Case Vignette (continued)

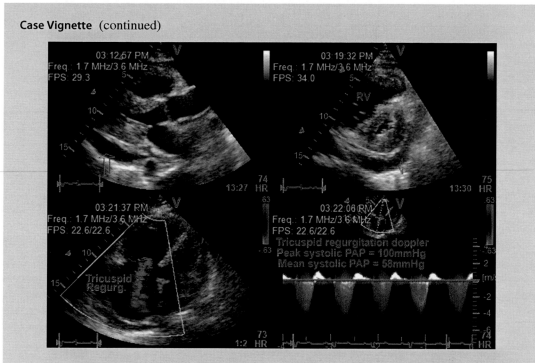

Fig. 7.2 Echocardiographic images of an MCTD patient with severe PAH. *Upper left* is a parasternal long axis and *upper right* is a parasternal short axis. Both views show evidence of a pericardial effusion (*arrows*) as well as evidence of a pressure-overloaded right ventricle; note septal flattening with a D-shaped left ventricle on the parasternal axis view. *Lower left corner* is an apical four-chamber view revealing a dilated right atrium and ventricle with Doppler evidence of tricuspid regurgitation. *Lower right* is the conventional Doppler of the tricuspid regurgitant jet, which was measured to reveal a peak right ventricular systolic pulmonary artery pressure of 100 mmHg and an estimated mean systolic pulmonary artery pressure of 58 mmHg

The pathologic mechanisms that trigger ILD in MCTD remain unknown. It is likely that alveolar macrophages and CD8-positive T cells play a major role. Bronchoalveolar lavage studies in patients with MCTD-ILD have consistently shown a neutrophilic predominance [27, 28]. Total cell counts and CD8-positive lymphocyte counts have also been shown to correlate negatively with DLCO [27]. Elevated eosinophils and CD4-positive lymphocytes and low CD71-positive alveolar macrophages have also been reported [27, 28].

Although a causal relationship between esophageal and pulmonary involvement remains unproven, there is a strong association between esophageal dysfunction and ILD in patients with MCTD. In a study of 50 consecutive patients with MCTD esophageal dilatation, gastroesophageal reflux and esophageal motor impairment were each found to be highly prevalent; moreover, the presence of interstitial changes on HRCT was

Table 7.3 Risk factors for severe fibrosis/ILD

- Advanced age
- Early disease
- Esophageal dilatation
- Esophageal motor dysfunction
- Fulfillment of all four MCTD criteria sets
- Worse baseline functional status
- Worse baseline lung function

significantly higher among patients with esophageal dilatation (Fig. 7.1) and among patients with severe esophageal motor dysfunction [21].

Severe lung fibrosis is common in MCTD, has an impact on pulmonary function and overall physical capacity, and is associated with increased mortality. Risk factors for severe fibrosis (Table 7.3) include advanced age, presence of ILD early in disease, worse baseline lung function/functional status, and esophageal dysfunction.

Patients with severe ILD also were more likely to fulfill all MCTD criteria sets [6, 21].

Outcomes in MCTD-ILD are not always predictable, although more than 20 % of patients will go on to become hypoxemic [3], 30 % will develop significant fibrosis despite therapy [16], and the presence of ILD increases the risk of death [6]. In a Norwegian cohort of 126 MCTD patients, the overall mortality was 7.9 % for ILD patients compared with 3.3 % mortality in patients who had a normal HRCT over a mean follow-up period of 4.2 years. Patients with severe fibrosis had a 20.8 % mortality and the death rate for patients with baseline HRCT abnormalities was 12.3 % [6].

There are also no prospective randomized controlled trials in MCTD-ILD. Retrospective reports and small case series suggest improvement with corticosteroids, alone or with the addition of cyclophosphamide or mycophenolate mofetil, with reported resolution (in some patients) of symptoms, crackles, radiographic, and PFT abnormalities. In a case series that included 96 patients with MCTD-ILD patients [16], 46.9 % of patients responded well to 2 mg/kg/day corticosteroids, whereas 53.1 % of patients required combination of corticosteroids and cyclophosphamide. However, 30 % of patients went on to develop mild pulmonary fibrosis with one patient eventually developing subpleural honeycomb changes.

Pulmonary Hypertension

Pulmonary hypertension in the setting of MCTD may be due to a number of causes (Table 7.4) including obliteration of the pulmonary arterioles as seen in PAH, pulmonary veno-occlusive disease (PVOD), recurrent thromboembolic disease, pulmonary vasculitis, parenchymal lung disease (ILD), left ventricular dysfunction, valvular heart disease, or myocarditis; often, it is multifactorial. PH is considered to be the most serious, often fatal, complication of MCTD [5, 29–32].

PAH defined as a mean pulmonary arterial pressure greater than 25 mmHg in the absence of elevation of the pulmonary capillary wedge pressure (PCWP ≤ 15 mmHg) is a significant cause of

Table 7.4 Causes of pulmonary hypertension in MCTD

- Chronic thromboembolism
- Diaphragmatic dysfunction
- ILD
- Left ventricular diastolic dysfunction
- Left ventricular systolic dysfunction
- Myocarditis
- PAH
- Pulmonary vasculitis
- Pulmonary veno-occlusive disease
- Valvular heart disease (Libman-Sacks endocarditis)

morbidity and is responsible for ~50 % of deaths among patients with MCTD [3, 33].

It has been suggested that the more pronounced inflammation, endothelial dysfunction, and dysregulated angiogenesis seen in patients with MCTD-PAH may partially explain the worse prognosis as compared to patients with idiopathic pulmonary arterial hypertension (IPAH). From a histological standpoint, the pulmonary vascular lesions in PAH complicating MCTD demonstrate intimal hyperplasia, smooth muscle cell hypertrophy medial thickening, plexogenic lesions, and in situ thrombosis [25], which is nearly indistinguishable from those present in IPAH. These lesions result in increased pulmonary vascular resistance that ultimately leads to right ventricular failure and eventually to death.

Estimates of the prevalence of PAH in MCTD have varied widely based on the definition of pulmonary hypertension and the method of diagnosis and have been reported to range from 25 to 75 % [3, 34].

Risk factors for the development of PAH in MCTD (Table 7.5) include long disease duration; more severe inflammation as evidenced by high serum levels of IL-6; severe overall organ involvement; Raynaud's phenomenon; progressive decline in diffusion capacity; the presence of high-titer anti-U1RNP, anti-β2-glycoprotein I antibodies, anti-cardiolipin antibodies, anti-endothelial cell antibodies, and von Willebrand factor antigen; and high serum levels of thrombomodulin [30, 33, 35, 36].

The symptoms of PAH are often nonspecific and physical findings may be absent in early disease. Using Doppler echocardiography as a

Table 7.5 Risk factors for PAH in MCTD

- Anti-cardiolipin antibodies
- Anti-endothelial antibodies
- Anti-$\beta 2$ glycoprotein I antibodies
- Elevated B-type natriuretic peptide
- High serum IL-6 levels
- High serum thrombomodulin levels
- High serum von Willebrand factor antigen levels
- High-titer anti-U1 RNP
- Long-standing disease
- More severe overall organ involvement
- Progressive decline in diffusion capacity
- Raynaud's phenomenon

screening tool, investigators found a significant number (13.3 %) of scleroderma and MCTD patients with an elevated estimated right ventricular systolic pressure consistent with undiagnosed PAH. Many of these patients had Doppler echocardiographic evidence of RV dysfunction, an abnormally low DLCO, and decreased exercise tolerance suggestive of advanced disease. These data support the use of Doppler echocardiographic evaluation of MCTD patients irrespective of symptoms in order to detect patients who may need further evaluation, close surveillance, and/or treatment for underlying PAH [37].

In a large international registry, it was found that MCTD patients with PAH had better hemodynamic and more favorable echocardiographic findings compared to IPAH patients, but a higher prevalence of pericardial effusion (Fig. 7.2). They also were found to have higher levels of B-type natriuretic peptide and a lower DLCO. One-year survival and discharge from hospitalization were lower in patients with MCTD and PAH when compared to patients with SLE, SSc, or RA with PAH [38].

There have been no trials specifically addressing the therapy of MCTD-associated PAH. Approach to therapy for MCTD-associated PAH includes the use of anticoagulation, oxygen, diuretics, and pulmonary vasodilators including the phosphodiesterase type 5 inhibitors, endothelin receptor antagonists, and prostanoids. Treatment strategies are largely extrapolated from studies of scleroderma spectrum disease patients and IPAH patients as only small numbers

of MCTD patients have been enrolled in pivotal trials [39, 40]. Two caveats are that vasodilator therapy with high-dose calcium channel blockers may not be effective as patients with MCTD are unlikely to demonstrate an acute vasodilator response during hemodynamic testing [41], and anticoagulation is controversial due to the possibility of increased risk of bleeding in patients who may have gastrointestinal sources of hemorrhage, e.g., mucosal telangiectasias.

There are also no randomized controlled trials evaluating the efficacy of immunosuppressive therapy for the treatment of MCTD-PAH. Nevertheless, there are reports of some patients with MCTD who have demonstrated a positive response to immunosuppressive therapy, further suggesting that inflammation and autoimmunity may play major roles in the pathogenesis of MCTD-PAH [42, 43]. The immunosuppressive regimen and duration of therapy varies significantly between reported cases; patients who were responsive to immunotherapy tended to have a less advanced functional class (New York Heart Association I or II) and less severe hemodynamic impairment (cardiac index >3.1 L/min/m^2) [43].

In the modern PAH treatment era, the 1- and 3-year survival rates for MCTD-PAH are 83 % and 66 %, respectively [44], whereas historically the median survival from the onset of PAH was 4.4 years [31]. This suggests that patients with MCTD-PAH may be less responsive to modern PAH therapies when compared with IPAH patients. This is likely due to the systemic nature of MCTD with multiple comorbidities and a heightened inflammatory state contributing to the pathogenesis of PAH in these patients. Age, sex, mixed venous oxygen saturation, cardiac index, and WHO functional class have each been identified as independent prognostic factors in patients with MCTD-PAH and may be useful in making treatment decisions [43, 44].

Pleural Manifestations

Pleural manifestations of MCTD are common. The overall incidence of pleural effusion and pleuritic chest pain in MCTD has been estimated

Table 7.6 Recommended cardiopulmonary screening in MCTD

Test	MCTD population and frequency
Echocardiogram	• Baseline and annual in all MCTD patients
Spirometry	• Baseline and annual in all MCTD patients
	• Every 3–4 months in symptomatic patients or those at high risk for severe fibrosis (Table 7.3)
Lung volumes	• Baseline and annual in all MCTD patients
Diffusion capacity	• Baseline and annual in all MCTD patients
	• Every 3–4 months in symptomatic patients or those at high risk for severe fibrosis (Table 7.3)
MVV, MIP/MEP, sitting and supine spirometry	• Baseline in patients with restriction and myositis
HRCT	• Baseline in all MCTD patients
	• Repeat as needed for worsening symptoms/pulmonary function
Right heart catheterization	• PRVSP on echocardiogram >40 mmHg or evidence of right ventricular pressure/volume overload or dysfunction
	• FVC%/DLCO% >1.6
	• Isolated diffusion <40 %
	• Symptomatic and at high risk for pulmonary hypertension (Table 7.5)
Ventilation/perfusion scan	• Pulmonary hypertension demonstrated by right heart catheterization
Six-minute walk test (with oximetry)	• Baseline and annual in all MCTD patients
	• Every 3–4 months in patients with PAH or ILD
BNP or NT-BNP	• Pulmonary hypertension demonstrated by right heart catheterization

to be as high as 50 % and 40 %, respectively, and can occasionally be the presenting symptom of MCTD [3, 45]. Pleural effusions are frequently exudative in nature and often are self-limited.

Alveolar Hemorrhage

There are case reports of patients who have MCTD presenting with alveolar hemorrhage [46, 47]. The etiology of alveolar hemorrhage in MCTD is unclear, although it is presumably similar in etiology to that seen in SLE and may involve immune complex deposition and be responsive to aggressive immunosuppressive therapy with or without plasma exchange.

Conclusions

Pleuropulmonary manifestations are major features of MCTD, particularly PAH and ILD, which contribute significantly to morbidity and mortality. Our recommended pulmonary screening in MCTD patients is outlined in Table 7.6. Unfortunately there is a paucity of data in regard

to epidemiology, pathogenesis, and treatment, and inferences must be made from other forms of CTD, primarily SSc. The pleuropulmonary manifestations of MCTD should be the focus of future research.

References

1. Sharp GC, Irvin WS, Tan EM, Gould RG, Holman HR. Mixed connective tissue disease—an apparently distinct rheumatic disease syndrome associated with a specific antibody to an extractable nuclear antigen (ENA). Am J Med. 1972;52:148–59.
2. Bennett RM, O'Connell DJ. Mixed connective tissue disease: a clinicopathologic study of 20 cases. Semin Arthritis Rheum. 1980;10:25–51.
3. Sullivan WD, Hurst DJ, Harmon CE, Esther JH, Agia GA, Maltby JD, et al. A prospective evaluation emphasizing pulmonary involvement in patients with mixed connective tissue disease. Medicine (Baltimore). 1984;63:92–107.
4. Aaløkken TM, Lilleby V, Søyseth V, Mynarek G, Pripp AH, Johansen B, et al. Chest abnormalities in juvenile-onset mixed connective tissue disease: assessment with high-resolution computed tomography and pulmonary function tests. Acta Radiol. 2009;4:430–6.
5. Burdt MA, Hoffman RW, Deutscher SL, Wang GS, Johnson JC, Sharp GC. Long-term outcome in

mixed connective tissue disease: longitudinal clinical and serologic findings. Arthritis Rheum. 1999;42: 899–909.

6. Gunnarsson R, Aaløkken TM, Molberg Ø, Lund MB, Mynarek GK, Lexberg ÅS, et al. Prevalence and severity of interstitial lung disease in mixed connective tissue disease: a nationwide, cross-sectional study. Ann Rheum Dis. 2012;71:1966–72.

7. Zimmerman C, Steiner G, Skriner K, Hassfeld W, Petera P, Smolen JS. The concurrence of rheumatoid arthritis and limited systemic sclerosis: clinical and serological characteristics of an overlap syndrome. Arthritis Rheum. 1998;41:1938–45.

8. Ortega-Hernandez O-D, Shoenfeld Y. Mixed connective tissue disease: an overview of clinical manifestations, diagnosis and treatment. Best Pract Res Clin Rheumatol. 2012;26:61–72.

9. Kahn MF, Appelboom T. Syndrome de Sharp. In: Kahn MF, Peltier AP, Meyer O, Piette JC, editors. Les maladies systemiques. 3rd ed. Paris: Flammarion; 1991. p. 454–6.

10. Kasukawa R, Tojo T, Miyawaki S. Preliminary diagnostic criteria for classification of mixed connective tissue disease. In: Kasukawa R, Sharp G, editors. Mixed connective tissue disease and antinuclear antibodies. Amsterdam: Elsevier; 1987. p. 41–7.

11. Sharp GC. Diagnostic criteria for classification of MCTD. In: Kasukawa R, Sharp GC, editors. Mixed connective tissue diseases and antinuclear antibodies. Amsterdam: Elsevier; 1987. p. 23–32.

12. Alarcón-Segovia D, Villareal M. Classification and diagnostic criteria for mixed connective tissue disease. In: Kasukawa R, Sharp GC, editors. Mixed connective tissue disease and antinuclear antibodies. Amsterdam: Elsevier; 1987. p. 33–40.

13. O'Connell DJ, Bennett RM. Mixed connective tissue disease: clinical and radiological aspects of 20 cases. Br J Radiol. 1977;50:620–5.

14. Wiener-Kronish JP, Solinger AM, Warnock ML, Churg A, Ordonez N, Golden JA. Severe pulmonary involvement in mixed connective tissue disease. Am Rev Respir Dis. 1981;124:499–503.

15. Derderian SS, Tellis CJ, Abbbrecht PH, Welton RC, Rajagopal KR. Pulmonary involvement in mixed connective tissue disease. Chest. 1985;88:45–8.

16. Bodolay E, Szekanecz Z, Dévényl K, Galuska L, Csípő I, Veègh J, et al. Evaluation of interstitial lung disease in mixed connective tissue disease (DMTC). Rheumatology. 2005;44:656–81.

17. Alpert MA, Goldberg SH, Singsen BH, Durham JB, Sharp GC, Ahmad M, et al. Cardiovascular manifestations of mixed connective tissue disease in adults. Circulation. 1983;68:1182–93.

18. Prakash UB. Lungs in mixed connective tissue disease. J Thorac Imaging. 1992;7:55–61.

19. Saito Y, Terada M, Takada T, Ishida T, Moriyama H, Ooi H, et al. Pulmonary involvement in mixed connective tissue disease: comparison with other collagen vascular disease using high resolution CT. J Comput Assist Tomogr. 2002;36:349–57.

20. Kozuka T, Johkoh T, Honda O, Mihara N, Koyama M, Tomiyama N, et al. Pulmonary involvement in mixed connective tissue disease: high resolution CT findings in 41 patients. J Thorac Imaging. 2001;16:94–8.

21. Fagundes MN, Caleiro MTC, Navarro-Rodriguez T, Baldi BG, Kavakama J, Salge JM, et al. Esophageal involvement and interstitial lung disease in mixed connective tissue disease. Respir Med. 2009;103: 854–60.

22. American Thoracic Society/European Respiratory Society International Multidisciplinary Consensus Classification of the Idiopathic Interstitial Pneumonias. This Joint Statement of the American Thoracic Society (ATS) and the European Respiratory Society (ERS) was adopted by the ATS Board of Directors, June 2001, and The ERS Executive Committee, June 2001. Am J Respir Crit Care Med. 2002;165:277–304.

23. Bull TM, Fagan KA, Badesch DB. Pulmonary vascular manifestations of mixed connective tissue disease. Rheum Dis Clin North Am. 2005;31:451–64.

24. Kim EA, Lee KS, Johkoh T, Kim TS, Suh GY, Kwon OJ, Han J. Interstitial lung diseases associated with collagen vascular diseases: radiologic and histopathologic findings. Radiographics. 2002;22:15S–65.

25. Hosada T. Review of pathology of mixed connective tissue disease. In: Kasukawa R, Sharp GC, editors. Mixed connective tissue disease and anti-nuclear antibodies. Amsterdam: Excerpta Medica; 1987. p. 281–90.

26. Hurst DJ, Baker WM, Gilbert G. Lung collagen synthesis and type analysis in patients with mixed connective tissue disease (MCTD). Arthritis Rheum. 1980;19:801–4.

27. Enomoto K, Takada T, Suzuki E, Ishida T, Moriyama H, Ooi H, et al. Bronchoalveolar lavage fluid cells in mixed connective tissue disease. Respirology. 2003;8:149–56.

28. Nagai N. The value of BALF cell findings for differentiation of idiopathic UIP, BOOP, and interstitial pneumonia associated with collagen vascular disease. In: Harasawa M, Fukuchi Y, Morinari H, editors. Interstitial pneumonia of unknown etiology. Tokyo: University of Tokyo Press; 1989. p. 27.

29. Jensen GG. Reversible pulmonary hypertension in a woman with connective tissue disease. Ugeskr Laeger. 1992;154:3065–6.

30. Ueda N, Mimura K, Maeda H, Sugiyama T, Kado T, Kobayashi K, Fukuzaki H. Mixed connective tissue disease with fatal pulmonary hypertension and a review of literature. Virchows Arch A Pathol Anat Histopathol. 1984;404:335–40.

31. Nishimaki T, Aotuka S, Kondo H, Yamamoto K, Takasaki Y, Sumiya M, Yokohari R. Immunological analysis of pulmonary hypertension in connective tissue diseases. J Rheumatol. 1999;26:2357–62.

32. Grant KD, Adams LE, Hess EV. Mixed connective tissue disease—a subset with sequential clinical and laboratory features. J Rheumatol. 1981;8:587–98.

33. Miyata M, Suzuki K, Sakuma F, Miyata M, Watanabe H, Kaise S, Nishimaki T, Kasukawa R. Anticardiolipin antibodies are associated with pulmonary hypertension in patients with mixed connective tissue disease

or systemic lupus erythematosus. Int Arch Allergy Immunol. 1993;100:351–4.

34. Simonson JS, Schiller NB, Petri M, Hellmannn DB. Pulmonary hypertension in systemic lupus erythematosus. J Rheumatol. 1989;16:918–25.

35. Hasegawa EM, Caleiro MTC, Fuller R, Carvalho JF. The frequency of anti-β2-glycoprotein I antibodies is low and these antibodies are associated with pulmonary hypertension in mixed connective tissue disease. Lupus. 2009;18:618–21.

36. Vegh J, Szodoray P, Kappelmayer J, Csipo I, Udvardy M, Lakos G, et al. Clinical and immunoserological characteristics of mixed connective tissue disease associated with pulmonary arterial hypertension. Scand J Immunol. 2006;64:69–76.

37. Wigley FM, Lima JA, Mayes M, McLain D, Chapin JL, Ward-Able C. The prevalence of undiagnosed pulmonary arterial hypertension in subjects with connective tissue disease at the secondary health care level of community-based rheumatologists (the UNCOVER study). Arthritis Rheum. 2005;53:2125–32.

38. Chung L, Liu J, Parsons L, McGoon M, Badesch DB, Miller DP, et al. Characterization of connective tissue disease-associated pulmonary arterial hypertension from REVEAL: identifying systemic sclerosis as a unique phenotype. Chest. 2010;138:1383–94.

39. Fagan KA, Badesch DB. Pulmonary hypertension associated with connective tissue disease. Prog Cardiovasc Dis. 2002;45(3):225–34.

40. Hassoun PM. Pulmonary arterial hypertension complicating connective tissue diseases. Semin Respir Crit Care Med. 2009;30:429–39.

41. Humbert M, Sitbon O, Chaouat A, Bertocchi M, Habib G, Gressin V, et al. Pulmonary arterial hypertension in France: results from a national registry. Am J Respir Crit Care Med. 2006;173:1023–30.

42. Sanchez O, Sitbon O, Jaïs X, Simonneau G, Humbert M. Immunosuppressive therapy in connective tissue diseases-associated pulmonary arterial hypertension. Chest. 2006;130:182–9.

43. Jaïs X, Launay D, Yaici A, Le Pavec J, Tchérakian C, Sitbon O, et al. Immunosuppressive therapy in lupus- and mixed connective tissue disease-associated pulmonary arterial hypertension: a retrospective analysis of twenty-three cases. Arthritis Rheum. 2008;58: 521–31.

44. Condliffe R, Kiely DG, Peacock AJ, Corris PA, Gibbs JS, Vrapi F, et al. Connective tissue disease-associated pulmonary arterial hypertension in the modern treatment era. Am J Respir Crit Care Med. 2009;179: 151–7.

45. Hoogsteden HC, van Dongen JJ, van der Kwast TH, Hooijkaas H, Hilvering C. Bilateral exudative pleuritis, an unusual pulmonary onset of mixed connective tissue disease. Respiration (Herrlisheim). 1985;48: 164–7.

46. Germain MJ, Davidman M. Pulmonary hemorrhage and acute renal failure in a patient with mixed connective tissue disease. Am J Kidney Dis. 1984;3:420–4.

47. Schwarz MI, Zamora MR, Hodges TN, Chan ED, Bowler RP, Tuder RM, et al. Isolated pulmonary capillaritis and diffuse alveolar hemorrhage in rheumatoid arthritis and mixed connective tissue disease. Chest. 1998;113:1609–15.

Pulmonary Manifestations of Primary Sjögren's Syndrome

8

Tracy R. Luckhardt and Barri J. Fessler

Introduction

Sjögren's syndrome (SS) is a chronic systemic inflammatory syndrome whose hallmark is exocrine gland dysfunction due to lymphocytic infiltration. Its etiology is unknown. Although the most common symptoms are dryness of the eyes and mouth, any organ in the body may be affected during the disease course [1, 2]. When it occurs by itself, it is called primary Sjögren's syndrome (pSS); if it occurs in association with another systemic autoimmune disease (e.g., rheumatoid arthritis, systemic lupus erythematosus, or systemic sclerosis) it is called secondary Sjögren's syndrome. The name of the syndrome honors a Swedish ophthalmologist, Henrik Sjögren, who wrote his doctoral thesis on keratoconjunctivitis sicca in 1933 although Johann Mikulicz described parotid and lacrimal gland hypertrophy with inflammatory cell infiltrates in 1888 and Henri Gougerot, a French dermatologist, described three cases of salivary gland atrophy associated with dryness of the eyes, mouth, and vagina in 1925 [3].

Epidemiology

The prevalence of SS worldwide ranges from 0.1 to 4.8 % depending on the location and the classification criteria used [4]. It affects women more commonly than men (9:1). Disease onset is predominantly in middle age with approximately 15 % developing prior to age 35 and 15 % after age 70 [1]. pSS in the pediatric population is uncommon and tends to be mild [5].

Classification Criteria

Over the past 50 years, more than ten different classification or diagnostic criteria for SS have been published. The American and European Consensus group (AECG) criteria published in 2002 (Table 8.1) are used frequently in clinical trials and epidemiologic studies but have both strengths and limitations (reviewed in [6]). The newest classification criteria published in 2012 (Table 8.2) were proposed by expert consensus by the American College of Rheumatology (ACR) Sjögren's International Collaborative Clinical Alliance (SICCA) which are based on objective criteria and have a sensitivity of 93 % and specificity of 95 % [7].

T.R. Luckhardt, M.D., M.S. (✉)
Department of Pulmonary, Allergy and Critical Care Medicine, University of Alabama Birmingham, 1900 University Boulevard, THT 433A, Birmingham, AL, USA
e-mail: tluck@uab.edu

B.J. Fessler, M.D., M.S.P.H.
Division of Clinical Immunology and Rheumatology, University of Alabama at Birmingham, 510 20th Street South, Faculty Office Tower 844, Birmingham, AL 35294, USA
e-mail: bjf@uab.edu

P.F. Dellaripa et al. (eds.), *Pulmonary Manifestations of Rheumatic Disease: A Comprehensive Guide*,
DOI 10.1007/978-1-4939-0770-0_8, © Springer Science+Business Media New York 2014

Table 8.1 2002 American-European Consensus Group (AECG) criteria, revised international classification criteria for Sjögren's syndrome

1. Ocular symptoms: a positive response to at least one of the following questions:
   (a) Have you had daily, persistent, troublesome dry eyes for more than 3 months?
   (b) Do you have a recurrent sensation of sand or gravel in the eyes?
   (c) Do you use tear substitutes more than three times a day?
2. Oral symptoms: a positive response to at least one of the following questions:
   (a) Have you had a daily feeling of dry mouth for more than 3 months?
   (b) Have you had recurrently or persistently swollen salivary glands as an adult?
   (c) Do you frequently drink liquids to aid in swallowing dry food?
3. Ocular signs: that is, objective evidence of ocular involvement defined as a positive result for at least one of the following two tests:
   (a) Schirmer test performed without anesthesia (<5 mm wetting in 5 min)
   (b) Rose Bengal score or other ocular dye score (>4 according to van Bijsterveld's scoring system)
4. Histopathology: In minor salivary glands (obtained through normal-appearing mucosa) focal lymphocytic sialoadenitis, evaluated by an expert histopathologist, with a focus score >1, defined as a number of lymphocytic foci (which are adjacent to normal-appearing mucous acini and contain more than 50 lymphocytes) per 4 mm² of glandular tissue
5. Salivary gland involvement: objective evidence of salivary gland involvement defined by a positive result for at least one of the following diagnostic tests:
   (a) Unstimulated whole salivary flow (<1.5 mL in 15 min)
   (b) Parotid sialography showing the presence of diffuse sialectasias (punctuate, cavitary, or destructive pattern), without evidence of obstruction in the major ducts
   (c) Salivary scintigraphy showing delayed uptake, reduced concentration, and/or delayed excretion of tracer
6. Autoantibodies: the presence in the serum of the following autoantibodies:
   (a) Antibodies to Ro (SSA) or La (SSB) antigens or both

Revised rules for classification

For primary SS

In patients without any potentially associated disease, primary SS may be defined as follows:
   (a) The presence of any four of the six items is indicative of primary SS, as long as either item IV or VI is positive
   (b) The presence of any three of the four objective criteria items (that is, items III, IV, V, VI)

For secondary SS

In patients with a potentially associated disease (for instance, another well-defined connective tissue disease), the presence of item I or item II plus any two from among items III, IV, and V may be considered as indicative of secondary SS.

Exclusion criteria: Past head and neck radiation treatment, hepatitis C infection, acquired immunodeficiency disease syndrome (AIDS), preexisting lymphoma, sarcoidosis, graft versus host disease, use of anticholinergic drugs.

Used with permission from Vitali C, Bombardieri S, Jonsson R, Moutsopoulos HM, Alexander EL, Carsons SE, Daniels TE, Fox PC, Fox RI, Kassan SS, Pillemer SR, Talal N, Weisman MH; European Study Group on Classification Criteria for Sjögren's Syndrome. Classification criteria for Sjögren's syndrome: a revised version of the European criteria proposed by the American-European Consensus Group. Ann Rheum Dis. 2002 Jun;61(6):554–8

Table 8.2 2012 classification criteria from the Sjögren's International Collaborative Clinical Alliance (SICCA)[a]

1. Positive serum anti-SSA/Ro and/or anti-SSB/La or (positive rheumatoid factor and ANA titer ≥1:320)
2. Labial salivary gland biopsy exhibiting focal lymphocytic sialadenitis with a focus score ≥1 focus/4 mm²
3. Keratoconjunctivitis sicca with ocular staining ≥3 (assuming that individual is not currently using daily eye drops for glaucoma and has not had corneal surgery or cosmetic eyelid surgery in the last 5 years)

Prior diagnosis of any of the following conditions would exclude participation in SS studies or therapeutic trials because of overlapping clinical features or interference with criteria tests: history of head and neck radiation treatment, hepatitis C infection, AIDS, sarcoidosis, amyloidosis, graft versus host disease, and IgG4-related disease
Used with permission from Shiboski SC et al. American College of Rheumatology Classification Criteria for Sjögren's syndrome: a data-driven, expert consensus approach in the Sjögren's International Collaborative Clinical Alliance Cohort. Arthritis Care Research 2012; 64:475-487
[a]Patient is considered to have SS if at least two of the three objective features are met

Clinical Manifestations

Glandular Manifestations

The characteristic symptoms of SS are dry eyes (keratoconjunctivitis sicca) and dry mouth (xerostomia) related to progressive lymphocytic infiltration in exocrine glands seen in up to 93 %

and 87 % of patients, respectively [2, 8]. Approximately 30 % of patients have disease limited to sicca symptoms with the remainder developing extraglandular manifestations [1]. Ocular symptoms include a foreign body sensation, grittiness, or irritation in the eyes. There is an increased incidence of dental caries, gingivitis, and oral candidiasis. The parotid or other salivary glands may swell up. Symptoms of dryness may also affect the skin, oropharynx, and other mucosal membranes such as the vagina resulting in dyspareunia.

Non-visceral Manifestations

Constitutional symptoms including chronic fatigue, low grade fever, and myalgias are common. Joint complaints, which may precede the onset of sicca symptoms, are seen in 50–75 % of patients [9]. Arthralgias are most frequent, but polyarticular symmetric synovitis which is nonerosive may also be seen. Fibromyalgia and chronic pain commonly accompany Sjögren's syndrome. Depression is present in 50 % of patients and is one of the key predictors of poor function, along with pain [10].

Skin manifestations include dry scaly skin, flat purpura associated with hypergammaglobulinemia and palpable purpura associated with cryoglobulinemia, and cutaneous vasculitis [11]. Raynaud's phenomenon may be seen in 15–50 % of patients and is typically not associated with digital ulcerations [9]. Vasculitis may manifest as localized cutaneous vasculitis or as a systemic necrotizing vasculitis involving small- and medium-sized arteries affecting major organs. Patients with vasculitis are more likely to have joint involvement, Raynaud's phenomenon, peripheral neuropathy, renal involvement, and Sjögren's-associated autoantibodies [11].

Hematologic manifestations including leukopenia, autoimmune hemolytic anemia, and thrombocytopenia may be observed in SS and may develop prior to sicca symptoms [12].

Visceral Manifestations (Non-pulmonary)

Renal disease in pSS manifests primarily with interstitial nephritis with or without renal tubular acidosis; distal tubular acidosis is most commonly observed [13, 14]. Untreated renal tubular acidosis may lead to nephrolithiasis, nephrocalcinosis, and compromised renal function. Glomerulonephritis is less commonly seen and is associated with a decreased C4 [13]. Interstitial cystitis has been described.

Neurologic manifestations of SS may affect the central, peripheral, and/or autonomic nervous system [15]. Sensory, sensorimotor, and small fiber neuropathies are most commonly observed. Cranial neuropathies affecting the trigeminal, optic, and cochlear nerves may also be seen. Mononeuritis multiplex is rare [16]. A wide variety of central nervous system manifestations have been described including focal motor or sensory deficits, aphasia, seizures, encephalopathy, aseptic meningitis, cognitive dysfunction, transverse myelitis, and multiple sclerosis-like disease [17].

Gastrointestinal manifestations include dysphagia from dryness of the pharynx and esophageal dysmotility and reflux. Chronic atrophic gastritis and lymphocytic infiltration may be seen on gastric biopsies. Acute or chronic pancreatitis is rare. There is an increased incidence of autoimmune liver diseases including primary biliary cirrhosis and autoimmune hepatitis in patients with pSS [18].

Acute pericarditis is uncommon, but echocardiography may show evidence of thickened pericardium indicative of asymptomatic involvement as well as valvular regurgitation [19]. Pulmonary hypertension may be observed but is also rare [20]. Impaired autonomic response to orthostasis and sympathetic failure is seen in patients with pSS [21].

Patients with SS have an increased occurrence of organ-specific autoimmune diseases including autoimmune thyroid disease (e.g., Hashimoto's thyroiditis and Graves disease), celiac disease, primary biliary cirrhosis, and autoimmune liver disease [22].

Diagnostic Tests

No single blood test or test of oral or ocular involvement is sufficiently sensitive and specific enough to definitively establish a diagnosis of SS. A combination of symptoms, objective signs, and laboratory tests is needed. The differential diagnosis of SS is shown in Table 8.3.

Ocular testing includes the Schirmer tear test, Rose Bengal staining of the corneal epithelium, and tear film breakup time. The Schirmer test evaluates tear secretion by the lacrimal gland. The end of a piece of filter paper 30 mm in length is placed under the lower lid with the remainder of the paper hanging below. After 5 min the wetting length of the paper is measured; if there is <5 mm wetting after 5 min, this is indicative of decreased tear production. This is not a specific test as many conditions may decrease tear production. Rose Bengal staining consists of a slit lamp examination of the cornea following topical administration of the stain demonstrating damaged epithelium, punctuate, or filamentary keratitis. Finally, a drop of fluorescein is placed in the eye and the time from the last blink to the development of non-fluorescent areas in the tear film is measured [23].

There are numerous measures of salivary involvement. Sialometry measures salivary flow rate but is nonspecific. Sialography is a radiographic method of assessing the anatomic changes in the salivary duct system. Scintigraphy allows functional assessment of salivary glands following injection of technetium 99 pertechnetate; while it is sensitive, it is not specific [23].

Table 8.3 Differential diagnosis of Sjögren's syndrome

Sarcoidosis
Lipoproteinemias (type II, IV, V)
Hypertriglyceridemia
Diabetes mellitus
Amyloidosis
Chronic graft versus host disease
Viral infections: HIV, HTLV-1, hepatitis C

Finally, minor salivary gland biopsy is the cornerstone for diagnosis. In a recent systematic review, the sensitivity ranged from 64 to 94 % and specificity from 61 to 100 % [24]. Minor salivary gland biopsy has been used to help establish the underlying disease process in asymptomatic patients presenting with interstitial lung disease (ILD) suggesting that Sjögren's may be subclinical in some patients [25].

The most common autoantibodies seen in patients with pSS are anti-SSA and anti-SSB antibodies occurring in 40–75 % and 25–50 %, respectively. These antibodies are associated with earlier disease onset, longer disease duration, and female gender. Other autoantibodies observed in SS include antinuclear antibodies (usually speckled pattern on immunofluorescence) and rheumatoid factor. Cryoglobulins are found in 10–15 % of patients with SS and have been associated with more severe disease, an increased risk of developing non-Hodgkin's lymphoma (NHL), and higher risk for SS-related death. The number of antibodies correlates with the total number of extraglandular manifestations, with anti-SSA being the strongest predictor of extraglandular manifestations. In contrast, 10–20 % of patients may be seronegative, usually experiencing milder clinical disease [26]. Hypocomplementemia may be observed and is closely associated with systemic expression and adverse outcomes [27].

Anti-centromere antibodies identify a small unique subset of SS patients characterized by high prevalence of Raynaud's phenomenon, and dysphagia with lower prevalence of dry eyes and anti-SSA and anti-SSB antibodies. This subset has a high risk of NHL [28]. Anti-mitochondrial antibodies can be seen in a subset of patients with SS who are at increased risk for primary biliary cirrhosis. In addition, anti-smooth muscle and anti-liver kidney microsomal antibodies characterize a subset of SS patients prone to developing autoimmune hepatitis. Finally, antibodies directed against carbonic anhydrase have been associated with renal manifestations in SS, particularly renal tubular acidosis [29].

Pulmonary Manifestations

In patients with pSS, there is a wide variety of possible pulmonary complications. These range from airway diseases, to ILD and malignancies. The true prevalence of pulmonary disease in pSS patients is unclear. Studies have reported a prevalence of 11–80 %; the large variability is due to how the pulmonary disease was defined, location of the study, and criteria for SS used [1, 8, 30–37]. Kelly et al. evaluated 100 pSS patients in England and demonstrated that within 6 months of diagnosis 43 % of pSS patients had pulmonary symptoms with 24 % having abnormalities in pulmonary function [33, 34]. These patients were followed longitudinally and at 34 months 9 % had developed pleuropulmonary disease [6] and at 10 years there were no new cases of pulmonary fibrosis [2].

Several different factors have been identified as possible risk factors for developing pulmonary disease in pSS. Consistently, disease duration, increasing age, and male gender have been shown to predispose to developing lung disease [1, 35]. Yazisiz et al. showed that male gender, smokers, Raynaud's phenomenon, and multiple serologic markers including positive ANA, rheumatoid factor, anti-La, anti-Ro, and hypergammaglobulinemia correlated with an increased risk of pulmonary disease [37].

Interstitial Lung Disease

ILD is the most common pulmonary manifestation of pSS [38, 39], with up to 61 % of patients with lung disease having evidence for ILD. The most common CT findings in pSS patients with ILD are cysts, ground-glass opacities, interlobular septal and interstitial thickening, and honeycomb change [39, 40]. Pulmonary function tests (PFTs) generally show a restrictive pattern with decreased forced vital capacity (FVC) and total lung capacity (TLC), and impairment in gas exchange as evidenced by a low diffusion capacity for carbon monoxide (DLCO). Varying

histological patterns of interstitial pneumonia have been described in pSS patients including nonspecific interstitial pneumonia (NSIP), organizing pneumonia with and without bronchiolitis obliterans, usual interstitial pneumonia (UIP), lymphocytic interstitial pneumonitis (LIP), and diffuse amyloidosis [41].

NSIP appears to be the most common pattern associated with pSS. Ito et al. reported that 61 % of pSS patients with lung disease had evidence of NSIP with most of those being the fibrosing form (95 %) as opposed to the cellular form [38]. A CT pattern consistent with NSIP (although how this was determined was not described in the manuscript) had a 94 % positive predictive value for a pathologic diagnosis of NSIP [38].

LIP, although not as common as NSIP, is an ILD that is unique to SS patients. CT findings include ground-glass opacities, interlobular septal thickening, and thin-walled cysts [42]. On histology there is interstitial infiltration of small polyclonal lymphocytes, as well as plasma cells and reactive follicles [42, 43]. It has been hypothesized that LIP can transform to lymphoma; however, in the one large case series in the literature, there was no evidence for this [44].

In pSS patients with ILD, the prognosis is usually good. Most patients improve with treatment or remain stable over several years. The 5-year survival rate for NSIP in pSS patients has been reported at 83 % [38], although other reports have been less favorable [41]. report a mortality rate of 39 % in pSS patients with ILD [38] with nearly half of the deaths being from ILD. Evidence of fibrosis either with an increased fibrotic score [45] or by evidence of microscopic honeycomb change [38] increases the mortality associated with pSS-ILD.

Airways Disease and Nodular Pulmonary Amyloidosis

Airway Disease

Airways disease in pSS can occur in isolation or in combination with ILD [46]. It is thought that airway disease is due to dessication or "sicca"

Case Vignette 1

Forty-seven-year-old Caucasian male presents with dyspnea and dry cough in the setting of a 7-year history of pSS manifested by sicca symptoms, diffuse arthralgias, and anti-Ro antibodies. He had an initial high-resolution CT scan (HRCT) which demonstrated diffuse ground-glass opacities, consolidations, interlobular septal thickening, and traction bronchiectasis (Fig. 8.1a). Surgical lung biopsy demonstrated patchy organizing pneumonia, desquamated intra-alveolar cells, and mild fibrotic changes with early microscopic honeycomb change. He was treated with prednisone and azathioprine for 5 years and then switched to hydroxychloroquine. His pulmonary symptoms and pulmonary function remained stable over time. Repeat imaging 8 years later demonstrated a decrease in ground-glass opacities and consolidation, with a mild increase in fibrotic changes and traction bronchiectasis (Fig. 8.1b).

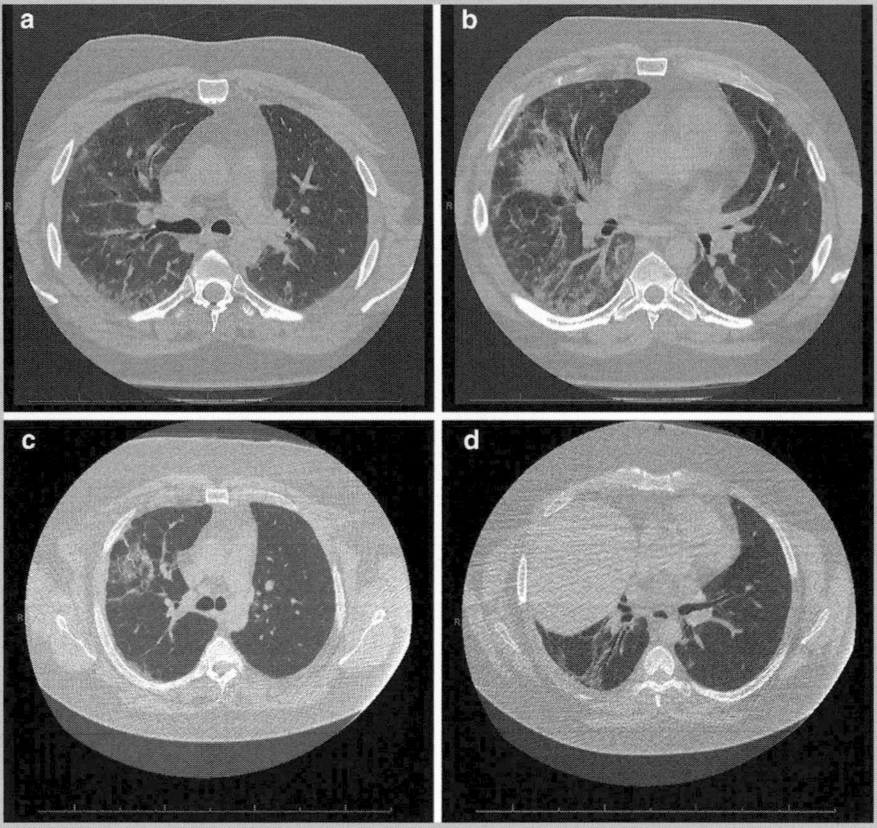

Fig. 8.1 (**a, b**) Initial HRCT demonstrating diffuse ground-glass opacities, consolidations, interlobular septal thickening, and traction bronchiectasis. (**c, d**) HRCT 8 years later demonstrating marked improvement in ground-glass opacities, with increased fibrotic changes and traction bronchiectasis

symptoms of the main airways, as well as a peri-bronchiolar lymphoid infiltrate and follicular bronchiolitis [47–50]. Most patients present with a dry cough [50]; however, rarely some patients will develop severe airway disease characterized by chronic bronchorrhea, recurrent sinusitis, and respiratory failure [48]. Obstructive lung disease in pSS patients appears to be more common in current and former smokers than in patients who have never smoked [51].

The most common findings on pulmonary function testing are reductions in the mid-expiratory flow rates (MEF25 and MEF50) [52], and a reduction in forced expiratory volume in 1 second (FEV$_1$). Papiris et al. demonstrated that in a group of 61 pSS patients, the FEV$_1$ was lower than a control group [50]. In an 11-year follow-up study in Sweden, pSS patients demonstrated an increase in vital capacity (VC) and TLC over time, with a concomitant decrease in FEV$_1$, FEV$_1$ to VC ratio, and DLCO [51]. Indices of hyperinflation, mainly elevation in the residual volume to TLC ratio, have also been demonstrated [53]. Up to 60 % of pSS patients will have bronchial hyperreactivity in response to methacholine challenge [54, 55]; however, the obstructive lung disease often does not respond to bronchodilator challenge [50].

Abnormal chest radiographs (CXR) are seen in 78 % of pSS patients [50] and Taouli et al. found that 54 % of pSS patients had evidence of large and/or small airway abnormalities on CT scan [56]. The most common findings on CT scan are bronchial wall thickening, bronchiectasis, centrilobular nodules, mosaic perfusion, air trapping, and bullae [48, 50, 51, 56]. Mandl et al. in their longitudinal analysis did not see any correlation between CT scan findings and lung function [51]. Histopathology in pSS patients with obstructive lung disease usually demonstrates a peribronchiolar lymphocytic infiltrate, lymphocytic bronchiolitis, or follicular bronchiolitis [48–50].

Nodular Pulmonary Amyloidosis

A rare pulmonary finding in pSS is nodular pulmonary amyloidosis. In most case reports and series, it presents as multiple nodules, often as an incidental finding [57, 58]. There is one case report of a solitary nodule in a pSS patient being amyloidosis [59]. This is usually limited to the lung with no other systemic findings of amyloidosis [57, 58]. In a case series of five patients in Korea, the most common findings on CT scan are multiple nodules, 3–24 mm in size with irregular borders and often with calcifications. The nodules are often accompanied by thin-walled cysts [60]. The nodules can show intense uptake on F-18 fluorodeoxyglucose positron emission

tomography (FDG-PET) [61]. No specific therapy has been shown to be needed with nodular amyloidosis, and no progression or complications have been reported in the literature.

Malignancy

In a recent meta-analysis, pSS has been shown to carry an overall increased risk of malignancy of 53 %, and in particular NHL and thyroid cancer [62]. In the lung, pSS can be associated with

> **Case Vignette 2**
> Sixty-four-year-old woman with a 20-year history of anti-SSA-positive pSS presents with years of progressive dyspnea, dry cough, and wheezing. She is a former smoker. PFTs reveal an obstructive pattern with an FVC of 2.44 L (81 % of predicted), FEV$_1$ of 1.48 L (67 % of predicted), an FEV$_1$/FVC of 61 %, TLC 4.62 L (95 % of predicted), residual volume 2.13 L (114 % of predicted), and a DLCO of 10.6 mL/mmHg/min (59 % of predicted). HRCT shows mild centrilobular nodules, bronchiectasis, and air trapping on expiratory images (Fig. 8.2). She was treated with bronchodilators, oral prednisone, and hydroxychloroquine with improvement in her symptoms and radiology.

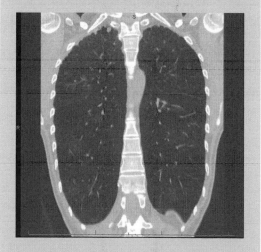

Fig. 8.2 HRCT demonstrating very mild changes with centrilobular nodules and bronchiectasis

extranodal marginal zone B-cell lymphoma of the mucosa-associated (MALT) or bronchus-associated lymphoid tissue (BALT) type. These can have a very nonspecific pattern on radiology with nodular, peribronchovascular, alveolar, or interstitial changes. These pulmonary lymphomas can often mimic ILD on radiology, which suggests that there should be a lower threshold of surgical biopsy in patients with pSS and chest radiographic abnormalities [63–65]. These are often treated with chemotherapy or rituximab [64]. Other forms of lung cancer such as adenocarcinoma [66] and small cell lung carcinoma [67] have been reported in pSS patients, but are not as common as lymphoma.

Treatment

Oral dryness is treated symptomatically using sugar-free lemon candies, frequent sips of water, and saliva substitute sprays. Frequent follow-up with a dentist is recommended to address dental caries and periodontal disease. Oral cholinergic agonists (e.g., pilocarpine and cevimeline) may be used to increase saliva production. Ocular dryness is initially treated with preservative-free teardrops and ocular lubricating ointments. Cyclosporin eye drops are used for more severe symptoms [68]. Nonsteroidal anti-inflammatory drugs may help alleviate mild musculoskeletal symptoms. Hydroxychloroquine is used to treat oral dryness, arthralgias, myalgias, and fatigue [69] although small clinical trials have shown little benefit [68].

For major organ involvement, corticosteroids and immunosuppressive medications are used although evidence-based recommendations are lacking. For peripheral neuropathies, antidepressants and gabapentin are frequently used followed by intravenous immunoglobulins in refractory cases. For central nervous system involvement and vasculitis, corticosteroids and cyclophosphamide have been used. Rituximab appears to be a promising new treatment for cryoglobulinemia and vasculitis.

Treatment of ILD is typically with corticosteroids and/or other immunosuppressants including

Case Vignette 3

Sixty-seven-year-old Caucasian female presents with a 3-year history of progressive dyspnea, dry cough, and recurrent pneumonias. She has had sicca symptoms and Raynaud's phenomenon for 30 years. She had been diagnosed with Sjögren's syndrome by her dentist 30 years earlier but had never sought treatment. PFTs revealed a restrictive pattern with a TLC of 3.43 L (61 % of predicted) and severe impairment in gas exchange with a DLCO of 36 % of predicted. HRCT revealed multi-lobar consolidations and ground-glass opacities with a few thin-walled cysts (Fig. 8.3). Because of the 30-year history of suspected Sjögren's syndrome and concern for possible pulmonary lymphoma, the patient underwent surgical lung biopsy which revealed adenocarcinoma in situ with evidence of invasion. After surgery, the patient had progressive respiratory failure and passed away without treatment.

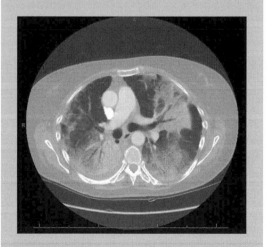

Fig. 8.3 HRCT revealing multi-lobar consolidations and ground-glass opacities with a thin-walled cyst

azathioprine and cyclophosphamide [45]. There are no clinical trials of treatment in pSS-associated ILD. In our pSS-ILD population, patients with clinically significant disease or evidence of progressive disease are usually treated with azathioprine or mycophenolate mofetil either alone or in combination with corticosteroids. Organizing pneumonia and LIP are often more responsive to corticosteroids alone [43, 44, 70]. There are recent reports of successful treatment of ILD associated with pSS with rituximab [71, 72].

The mainstay of treatment of airways disease is to treat the underlying pSS. Inhaled bronchodilators and corticosteroids have not been studied in this group of patients, but may be useful. Follicular bronchiolitis usually responds well to steroids and other immunosuppressive agents such as azathioprine [48, 73]. There are also case reports of successful treatment with macrolide therapy [48, 74] and rituximab [75].

Conclusion

SS is a chronic systemic autoimmune disease of unknown etiology with a wide spectrum of clinical manifestations. A diagnosis is established based on a combination of signs, symptoms, and autoantibodies. Pulmonary involvement is common and may present prior to development of sicca symptoms or autoantibodies. Studies of novel therapeutic agents are needed.

References

1. Ramos-Casals M, Solans R, Rosas J, Camps MT, Gil A, Del Pino-Montes J, Calvo-Alen J, Jimenez-Alonso J, Mico ML, Beltran J, Belenguer R, Pallares L. Primary Sjogren syndrome in Spain: clinical and immunologic expression in 1010 patients. Medicine (Baltimore). 2008;87:210–9.
2. Malladi AS, Sack KE, Shiboski S, et al. Primary Sjögren's syndrome as a systemic disease: a study of participants enrolled in an international Sjögren's syndrome registry. Arthritis Care Res (Hoboken). 2012;64:911–8.
3. Blatt IM. On sialectasis and benign lymphosialdenopathy (the pyogenic parotitis, Gougerot-Sjoegren's syndrome, Mikulicz's disease complex). A ten year study. Laryngoscope. 1964;74:1684–746.
4. Mavragani CP, Moutsopoulos HM. The geoepidemiology of Sjögren's syndrome. Autoimmun Rev. 2010; 9:A305–10.
5. Cimaz R, Casadei A, Rose C, Bartunkova J, Sediva A, Falcini F, Picco P, Taglietti M, Zulian F, Ten Cate R, Sztajnbok FR, Voulgari PV, Drosos AA, et al. Primary Sjogren syndrome in the paediatric age; a multicentric survey. Eur J Pediatr. 2003;162:661–5.
6. Baldini C, Talarico R, Tzioufas AG, Bombardieri S. Classification criteria for Sjögren's syndrome: a critical review. J Autoimmun. 2012;39(1–2):9–14.
7. Shiboski SC, Shiboski CH, Criswell L, Baer A, Challacombe S, Lanfranchi H, Schiødt M, Umehara H, Vivino F, Zhao Y, Dong Y, Greenspan D, Heidenreich AM, Helin P, Kirkham B, Kitagawa K, Larkin G, Li M, Lietman T, Lindegaard J, McNamara N, Sack K, Shirlaw P, Sugai S, Vollenweider C, Whitcher J, Wu A, Zhang S, Zhang W, Greenspan J, Daniels T, Sjögren's International Collaborative Clinical Alliance (SICCA) Research Groups. American College of Rheumatology Classification Criteria for Sjögren's syndrome: a data-driven, expert consensus approach in the Sjögren's International Collaborative Clinical Alliance Cohort. Arthritis Care Res. 2012;64:475–87.
8. Lin DF, Yan SM, Zhao Y, Zhang W, Li MT, Zeng XF, Zhang FC, Dong Y. Clinical and prognostic characteristics of 573 cases of primary Sjögren's syndrome. Chin Med J (Engl). 2010;123:3252–7.
9. Skopouli FN, Dafni U, Ioannidis JP, Moutsopoulos HM. Clinical evolution, and morbidity and mortality of primary Sjögren's syndrome. Semin Arthritis Rheum. 2000;29:296–304.
10. Lendrem D, Mitchell S, McMeekin P, Bowman S, Price E, Pease CT, Emery P, Andrews J, Lanyon P, Hunter J, Gupta M, Bombardieri M, Sutcliffe N, Pitzalis C, McLaren J, Cooper A, Regan M, Giles I, Isenberg D, Vadivelu S, Coady D, Dasgupta B, McHugh N, Young-Min S, Moots R, Gendi N, Akil M, Griffiths B, Ng WF; on behalf of the UK primary Sjögren's Syndrome Registry. Health-related utility values of patients with primary Sjögren's syndrome and its predictors. Ann Rheum Dis. 2013 Jun 12. [Epub ahead of print].
11. Ramos-Casals M, Anaya JM, García-Carrasco M, Rosas J, Bové A, Claver G, Diaz LA, Herrero C, Font J. Cutaneous vasculitis in primary Sjögren syndrome: classification and clinical significance of 52 patients. Medicine (Baltimore). 2004;83:96–106.
12. Baimpa E, Dahabreh IJ, Voulgarelis M, Moutsopoulos HM. Hematologic manifestations and predictors of lymphoma development in primary Sjögren syndrome: clinical and pathophysiologic aspects. Medicine (Baltimore). 2009;88(5):284–93.
13. Ren H, Wang WM, Chen XN, Zhang W, Pan XX, Wang XL, Lin Y, Zhang S, Chen N. Renal involvement and followup of 130 patients with primary Sjögren's syndrome. J Rheumatol. 2008;35(2):278–84.
14. Maripuri S, Grande JP, Osborn TG, Fervenza FC, Matteson EL, Donadio JV, Hogan MC. Renal involvement in primary Sjögren's syndrome: a clinicopathologic study. Clin J Am Soc Nephrol. 2009;4(9): 1423–31.
15. Fauchais AL, Magy L, Vidal E. Central and peripheral neurological complications of primary Sjögren's syndrome. Presse Med. 2012;41(9 Pt 2):e485–93.

16. Pavlakis PP, Alexopoulos H, Kosmidis ML, Mamali I, Moutsopoulos HM, Tzioufas AG, Dalakas MC. Peripheral neuropathies in Sjögren's syndrome: a critical update on clinical features and pathogenetic mechanisms. J Autoimmun. 2012;39(1–2):27–33.

17. Massara A, Bonazza S, Castellino G, Caniatti L, Trotta F, Borrelli M, Feggi L, Govoni M. Central nervous system involvement in Sjögren's syndrome: unusual, but not unremarkable—clinical, serological characteristics and outcomes in a large cohort of Italian patients. Rheumatology (Oxford). 2010;49(8):1540–9.

18. Ebert EC. Gastrointestinal and hepatic manifestations of Sjogren syndrome. J Clin Gastroenterol. 2012;46(1):25–30.

19. Vassiliou VA, Moyssakis I, Boki KA, Moutsopoulos HM. Is the heart affected in primary Sjögren's syndrome? An echocardiographic study. Clin Exp Rheumatol. 2008;26(1):109–12.

20. Launay D, Hachulla E, Hatron PY, Jais X, Simonneau G, Humbert M. Pulmonary arterial hypertension: a rare complication of primary Sjögren syndrome: report of 9 new cases and review of the literature. Medicine (Baltimore). 2007;86(5):299–315.

21. Ng WF, Stangroom AJ, Davidson A, Wilton K, Mitchell S, Newton JL. Primary Sjögren's syndrome is associated with impaired autonomic response to orthostasis and sympathetic failure. QJM. 2012; 105(12):1191–9.

22. Lazarus MN, Isenberg DA. Development of additional autoimmune diseases in a population of patients with primary Sjögren's syndrome. Ann Rheum Dis. 2005;64(7):1062–4.

23. Tzioufas AG, Mitsias DI, Moutsopoulos HM. Sjögren syndrome. In: Harris ED, Budd RC, Firestein GS, Genovese MC, Sergent JS, Ruddy S, Sledge CB, editors. St Clair EW. Sjogren's syndrome. In: Firestein GS, Budd RC, Gabriel SE, McInnes IB, O'Dell JR, editors. Kelley's textbook of rheumatology. 9th ed. Philadelphia: Elsevier; 2013. p. 1184–85.

24. Guellec D, Cornec D, Jousse-Joulin S, Marhadour T, Marcorelles P, Pers JO, Saraux A, Devauchelle-Pensec V. Diagnostic value of labial minor salivary gland biopsy for Sjögren's syndrome: a systematic review. Autoimmun Rev. 2013;12(3):416–20.

25. Fischer A, Swigris JJ, du Bois RM, Groshong SD, Cool CD, Sahin H, Lynch DA, Gillis JZ, Cohen MD, Meehan RT, Brown KK. Minor salivary gland biopsy to detect primary Sjogren syndrome in patients with interstitial lung disease. Chest. 2009;136(4):1072–8.

26. ter Borg EJ, Risselada AP, Kelder JC. Relation of systemic autoantibodies to the number of extraglandular manifestations in primary Sjögren's syndrome: a retrospective analysis of 65 patients in the Netherlands. Semin Arthritis Rheum. 2011;40(6):547–51.

27. Ramos-Casals M, Brito-Zerón P, Yagüe J, et al. Hypocomplementemia as an immunological marker of morbidity and mortality in patients with primary Sjögren's syndrome. Rheumatology (Oxford). 2005; 44:89–94.

28. Baldini C, Mosca M, Della Rossa A, Pepe P, Notarstefano C, Ferro F, Luciano N, Talarico R, Tani C, Tavoni AG, Bombardieri S. Overlap of ACA-positive systemic sclerosis and Sjögren's syndrome: a distinct clinical entity with mild organ involvement but at high risk of lymphoma. Clin Exp Rheumatol. 2013;31(2):272–80.

29. Bournia VK, Vlachoyiannopoulos PG. Subgroups of Sjögren syndrome patients according to serological profiles. J Autoimmun. 2012;39(1–2):15–26.

30. Constantopoulos SH, Papadimitriou CS, Moutsopoulos HM. Respiratory manifestations in primary Sjögren's syndrome. A clinical, functional, and histologic study. Chest. 1985;88:226–9.

31. Davidson BK, Kelly CA, Griffiths ID. Ten year follow up of pulmonary function in patients with primary Sjögren's syndrome. Ann Rheum Dis. 2000;59:709–12.

32. Franquet T, Gimenez A, Monill JM, Diaz C, Geli C. Primary Sjögren's syndrome and associated lung disease: CT findings in 50 patients. AJR Am J Roentgenol. 1997;169:655–8.

33. Kelly CA, Foster H, Pal B, Gardiner P, Malcolm AJ, Charles P, Blair GS, Howe J, Dick WC, Griffiths ID. Primary Sjögren's syndrome in north east England—a longitudinal study. Br J Rheumatol. 1991;30:437–42.

34. Kelly C, Gardiner P, Pal B, Griffiths I. Lung function in primary Sjögren's syndrome: a cross sectional and longitudinal study. Thorax. 1991;46:180–3.

35. Palm O, Garen T, Berge Enger T, Jensen JL, Lund MB, Aalokken TM, Gran JT. Clinical pulmonary involvement in primary Sjögren's syndrome: prevalence, quality of life and mortality—a retrospective study based on registry data. Rheumatology (Oxford). 2013;52:173–9.

36. Uffmann M, Kiener HP, Bankier AA, Baldt MM, Zontsich T, Herold CJ. Lung manifestation in asymptomatic patients with primary Sjogren syndrome: assessment with high resolution CT and pulmonary function tests. J Thorac Imaging. 2001;16:282–9.

37. Yazisiz V, Arslan G, Ozbudak IH, Turker S, Erbasan F, Avci AB, Ozbudak O, Terzioglu E. Lung involvement in patients with primary Sjögren's syndrome: what are the predictors? Rheumatol Int. 2010;30:1317–24.

38. Ito I, Nagai S, Kitaichi M, Nicholson AG, Johkoh T, Noma S, Kim DS, Handa T, Izumi T, Mishima M. Pulmonary manifestations of primary Sjögren's syndrome: a clinical, radiologic, and pathologic study. Am J Respir Crit Care Med. 2005;171:632–8.

39. Matsuyama N, Ashizawa K, Okimoto T, Kadota J, Amano H, Hayashi K. Pulmonary lesions associated with Sjögren's syndrome: radiographic and CT findings. Br J Radiol. 2003;76:880–4.

40. Lohrmann C, Uhl M, Warnatz K, Ghanem N, Kotter E, Schaefer O, Langer M. High-resolution CT imaging of the lung for patients with primary Sjögren's syndrome. Eur J Radiol. 2004;52:137–43.

41. Parambil JG, Myers JL, Lindell RM, Matteson EL, Ryu JH. Interstitial lung disease in primary Sjogren syndrome. Chest. 2006;130:1489–95.

42. Dalvi V, Gonzalez EB, Lovett L. Lymphocytic interstitial pneumonitis (lip) in Sjögren's syndrome: a case report and a review of the literature. Clin Rheumatol. 2007;26:1339–43.

43. Elzbieta R, Elzbieta W, Dariusz G, Langfort R, Ptak J. [Lymphocytic interstitial pneumonia in primary Sjogren syndrome]. Pneumonol Alergol Pol. 2005;73: 277–80.

44. Cha SI, Fessler MB, Cool CD, Schwarz MI, Brown KK. Lymphoid interstitial pneumonia: clinical features, associations and prognosis. Eur Respir J. 2006; 28:364–9.

45. Kocheril SV, Appleton BE, Somers EC, Kazerooni EA, Flaherty KR, Martinez FJ, Gross BH, Crofford LJ. Comparison of disease progression and mortality of connective tissue disease-related interstitial lung disease and idiopathic interstitial pneumonia. Arthritis Rheum. 2005;53:549–57.

46. Shi JH, Liu HR, Xu WB, Feng RE, Zhang ZH, Tian XL, Zhu YJ. Pulmonary manifestations of Sjögren's syndrome. Respiration. 2009;78:377–86.

47. Bellido-Casado J, Plaza V, Diaz C, Geli C, Dominguez J, Margarit G, Torrejon M, Giner J. Bronchial inflammation, respiratory symptoms and lung function in primary Sjögren's syndrome. Arch Bronconeumol. 2011;47:330–4.

48. Borie R, Schneider S, Debray MP, Adle-Biasssette H, Danel C, Bergeron A, Mariette X, Aubier M, Papo T, Crestani B. Severe chronic bronchiolitis as the presenting feature of primary Sjögren's syndrome. Respir Med. 2011;105:130–6.

49. Papiris SA, Saetta M, Turato G, La Corte R, Trevisani L, Mapp CE, Maestrelli P, Fabbri LM, Potena A. Cd4-positive t-lymphocytes infiltrate the bronchial mucosa of patients with Sjögren's syndrome. Am J Respir Crit Care Med. 1997;156:637–41.

50. Papiris SA, Maniati M, Constantopoulos SH, Roussos C, Moutsopoulos HM, Skopouli FN. Lung involvement in primary Sjögren's syndrome is mainly related to the small airway disease. Ann Rheum Dis. 1999;58:61–4.

51. Mandl T, Diaz S, Ekberg O, Hesselstrand R, Piitulainen E, Wollmer P, Theander E. Frequent development of chronic obstructive pulmonary disease in primary SS—results of a longitudinal follow-up. Rheumatology (Oxford). 2012;51:941–6.

52. Nakanishi M, Fukuoka J, Tanaka T, Demura Y, Umeda Y, Ameshima S, Nishikawa S, Kitaichi M, Itoh H, Ishizaki T. Small airway disease associated with Sjögren's syndrome: clinico-pathological correlations. Respir Med. 2011;105:1931–8.

53. Lahdensuo A, Korpela M. Pulmonary findings in patients with primary Sjögren's syndrome. Chest. 1995;108:316–9.

54. Gudbjornsson B, Hedenstrom H, Stalenheim G, Hallgren R. Bronchial hyperresponsiveness to methacholine in patients with primary Sjögren's syndrome. Ann Rheum Dis. 1991;50:36–40.

55. Ludviksdottir D, Janson C, Bjornsson E, Stalenheim G, Boman G, Hedenstrom H, Venge P, Gudbjornsson B, Valtysdottir S. Different airway responsiveness profiles in atopic asthma, nonatopic asthma, and Sjögren's syndrome. BHR study group. Bronchial hyperresponsiveness. Allergy. 2000;55:259–65.

56. Taouli B, Brauner MW, Mourey I, Lemouchi D, Grenier PA. Thin-section chest CT findings of primary Sjögren's syndrome: correlation with pulmonary function. Eur Radiol. 2002;12:1504–11.

57. Sakai T, Tsushima T, Kimura D, Fukuda I, Kamata Y, Hatanaka R, Yamada Y. [Multiple nodular pulmonary amyloidosis complicated with Sjogren syndrome]. Kyobu Geka. 2010;63:818–21.

58. Miyagawa T, Mochizuki Y, Nakahara Y, Kawamura T, Sasaki S, Kobashi Y. A case of Sjogren syndrome with pulmonary nodular amyloidosis and pulmonary multiple cysts. Nihon Kokyuki Gakkai Zasshi. 2009; 47:737–41.

59. Sakai K, Ohtsuki Y, Hirasawa Y, Hashimoto A, Nakamura K. Sjögren's syndrome with solitary nodular pulmonary amyloidosis. Nihon Kokyuki Gakkai Zasshi. 2004;42:330–5.

60. Jeong YJ, Lee KS, Chung MP, Han J, Chung MJ, Kim KI, Seo JB, Franquet T. Amyloidosis and lymphoproliferative disease in Sjogren syndrome: thin-section computed tomography findings and histopathologic comparisons. J Comput Assist Tomogr. 2004; 28:776–81.

61. Umeda Y, Demura Y, Takeda N, Morikawa M, Uesaka D, Nakanishi M, Mizuno S, Ameshima S, Sasaki M, Itoh H, Ishizaki T. [FDG-PET findings of nodular pulmonary amyloidosis with a long-term observation]. Nihon Kokyuki Gakkai Zasshi. 2007;45:424–9.

62. Liang Y, Yang Z, Qin B, Zhong R. Primary Sjögren's syndrome and malignancy risk: a systematic review and meta-analysis. Ann Rheum Dis. 2014:73(6): 1151–6.

63. Watanabe Y, Koyama S, Miwa C, Okuda S, Kanai Y, Tetsuka K, Nokubi M, Dobashi Y, Kawabata Y, Kanda Y, Endo S. Pulmonary mucosa-associated lymphoid tissue (MALT) lymphoma in Sjögren's syndrome showing only the lip pattern radiologically. Intern Med. 2012;51:491–5.

64. Papiris SA, Kalomenidis I, Malagari K, Kapotsis GE, Harhalakis N, Manali ED, Rontogianni D, Roussos C, Moutsopoulos HM. Extranodal marginal zone b-cell lymphoma of the lung in Sjögren's syndrome patients: reappraisal of clinical, radiological, and pathology findings. Respir Med. 2007;101:84–92.

65. Ingegnoli F, Sciascera A, Galbiati V, Corbelli V, D'Ingianna E, Fantini F. Bronchus-associated lymphoid tissue lymphoma in a patient with primary Sjögren's syndrome. Rheumatol Int. 2008;29:207–9.

66. Takabatake N, Sayama T, Shida K, Matsuda M, Nakamura H, Tomoike H. Lung adenocarcinoma in lymphocytic interstitial pneumonitis associated with primary Sjögren's syndrome. Respirology. 1999;4: 181–4.

67. Nishimura T, Tasaka S, Yamada W, Hasegawa N, Soejima K, Sayama K, Asano K, Ishizaka A. [Small cell lung cancer with Sjögren's syndrome and Lambert-Eaton myasthenic syndrome]. Nihon Kokyuki Gakkai Zasshi. 2006;44:775–8.

68. Ramos-Casals M, Tzioufas AG, Stone JH, Sisó A, Bosch X. Treatment of primary Sjögren syndrome: a systematic review. JAMA. 2010;304(4):452–60.

69. Fox RI, Dixon R, Guarrasi V, Krubel S. Treatment of primary Sjögren's syndrome with hydroxychloroquine: a retrospective, open-label study. Lupus. 1996;5 Suppl 1:S31–6.

70. Hayashi R, Yamashita N, Sugiyama E, Maruyama M, Matsui S, Yoshida Y, Arai N, Kobayashi M. [A case of primary Sjögren's syndrome with interstitial pneumonia showing bronchiolitis obliterans organizing pneumonia pattern and lymphofollicular formation]. Nihon Kokyuki Gakkai Zasshi. 2000;38:880–4.

71. Gottenberg JE, Cinquetti G, Larroche C, Combe B, Hachulla E, Meyer O, Pertuiset E, Kaplanski G, Chiche L, Berthelot JM, Gombert B, Goupille P, Marcelli C, Feuillet S, Leone J, Sibilia J, Zarnitsky C, Carli P, Rist S, Gaudin P, Salliot C, Piperno M, Deplas A, Breban M, Lequerre T, Richette P, Ghiringhelli C, Hamidou M, Ravaud P, Mariette X. Efficacy of rituximab in systemic manifestations of primary Sjogren's syndrome: results in 78 patients of the autoimmune and rituximab registry. Ann Rheum Dis. 2013;72: 1026–31.

72. Swartz MA, Vivino FB. Dramatic reversal of lymphocytic interstitial pneumonitis in Sjögren's syndrome with rituximab. J Clin Rheumatol. 2011;17:454.

73. Romero S, Barroso E, Gil J, Aranda I, Alonso S, Garcia-Pachon E. Follicular bronchiolitis: clinical and pathologic findings in six patients. Lung. 2003;181: 309–19.

74. Kobayashi H, Kanoh S, Motoyoshi K, Aida S. Tracheo-broncho-bronchiolar lesions in Sjögren's syndrome. Respirology. 2008;13:159–61.

75. Saraux A, Devauchelle V, Jousse S, Youinou P. Rituximab in rheumatic diseases. Joint Bone Spine. 2007;74:4–6.

Pulmonary Manifestations of Sarcoidosis

Kristin B. Highland and Daniel A. Culver

Introduction

Sarcoidosis is a systemic disease of unknown etiology with protean clinical manifestations. Because of the systemic nature of the disease, the wide range of symptoms and manifestations, and the need for immunosuppression, rheumatologists are frequently central in the diagnosis, assessment, and management of individuals with sarcoidosis.

The diagnosis of sarcoidosis generally requires clinicoradiological findings that are supported by the demonstration of noncaseating granulomas on histopathology and the exclusion of other disorders known to cause granulomatous disease [1, 2]. However, granulomatous inflammation is a nonspecific immune reaction that can be triggered by a wide range of causes. Therefore, the evaluation and management of sarcoidosis requires a healthy dose of skepticism about the accuracy of the diagnosis.

The clinical course of sarcoidosis is markedly heterogeneous; those with acute or asymptomatic presentations have a high likelihood of spontaneous resolution, whereas individuals with indolent presentations are more likely to have persistent disease. Other strong predictors of the long-term outcome include the pattern of organ involvement, need for treatment, and race/ethnicity.

For example, multiple studies suggest that sarcoidosis is more common and more severe in blacks [3–10]. The overall mortality from sarcoidosis ranges from 1 to 5 % [2], most commonly due to respiratory failure [8, 11]. Although any organ can be affected by sarcoidosis, the respiratory system is affected in more than 90 % of cases and will be the focus of this chapter [10].

Epidemiology

Sarcoidosis occurs throughout the world, affecting all ethnic and racial groups [2]. The true prevalence and incidence of sarcoidosis are probably underestimated since asymptomatic individuals may not be included in epidemiologic studies, or true sarcoidosis cases may be misclassified in countries where there is a high prevalence of mycobacterial diseases. In countries with historical population-based mass chest radiographic screening programs, approximately 50 % of the diagnosed sarcoidosis cases were made in asymptomatic individuals [12]. An autopsy study in Northeast Ohio suggested that prevalence of sarcoidosis may be underestimated by up to tenfold [13]. Therefore, the majority of published incidence and prevalence estimates account only for sarcoidosis that is clinically overt, not all possible sarcoidosis.

Sarcoidosis is most commonly diagnosed before the age of 50 with a peak incidence in the third decade of life; it is slightly more common in females [2, 14]. Sarcoidosis in females can also

K.B. Highland, M.D., M.S.C.R. • D.A. Culver, D.O. (✉)
Respiratory Institute, Cleveland Clinic, Desk A90,
9500 Euclid Avenue, Cleveland, OH 44195, USA
e-mail: culverd@ccf.org

P.F. Dellaripa et al. (eds.), *Pulmonary Manifestations of Rheumatic Disease: A Comprehensive Guide*,
DOI 10.1007/978-1-4939-0770-0_9, © Springer Science+Business Media New York 2014

occur frequently after the age of 50 [14–16]. The annual incidence of sarcoidosis in the Black Women's Health Study, a prospective cohort comprising 59,000 black females in the United States, was 71/100,000 with a peak of 92/100,000 in women ages 40–49 [17]. In a survey from a health maintenance organization in the Detroit, Michigan area, the age-adjusted incidence rates were 10.9/100,000 in whites and 35.5/100,000 in blacks, based on diagnosis during usual health care [7]. Worldwide prevalence estimates range from less than 1/100,000 population in the United Kingdom to 102/100,000 in Sweden [18]. Besides susceptibility, race and ethnicity also influence disease phenotype, with blacks far more likely to exhibit chronic disease, multiple organ involvement, and higher morbidity [2, 18].

Pathophysiology

The exact cause of sarcoidosis is unknown. It most likely develops when a genetically susceptible host is exposed to an exogenous (likely inhaled) agent. Evidence for the importance of environmental factors comes from epidemiologic studies of disease incidence patterns, reports of case clusters in small populations, transmission by organ transplantation, and the worldwide reproducibility of intradermal granulomatous reactions only in sarcoidosis subjects following injection of sarcoidosis lymph node homogenate (the Kveim–Siltzbach test) [19]. There may also be exposures that modify the risk of developing sarcoidosis but do not directly trigger the disease [20, 21]. Examples of positive risk modifiers include woodsmoke, rural residence, photocopier toner, pesticides, and bioaerosols [22–25]. A strong negative risk modifier is a history of smoking (odds ratio 0.65) [23].

As reviewed previously, the epidemiologic data are consistent with the possibility that sarcoidosis could be caused by an infectious agent. Despite those data, multiple attempts to culture an organism that might cause sarcoidosis have failed. Using molecular techniques, there is now mounting evidence that immune responses to mycobacteria may trigger sarcoidosis [26, 27].

For example, cellular immune responses to the mycobacterial catalase antigen (KatG) are found in most sarcoidosis patients, and the responses are dependent on HLA type, similar to human disease [28]. KatG protein may be found in granulomas from sarcoidosis patients, but not those with other inflammatory diseases [26]. In support of the hypothesis that viable (poorly pathogenic) nontuberculous mycobacteria are the agents causing sarcoidosis, two small open-label studies suggested that treatment with concomitant levofloxacin, ethambutol, azithromycin, and rifampin for 8 weeks was substantially effective for refractory cutaneous and pulmonary sarcoidosis [29, 30]. An alternative hypothesis holds that sarcoidosis is triggered by persistence of certain mycobacterial antigens in the context of heightened innate immune responses mediated by serum amyloid A protein [31].

Propionibacteria species have also been promulgated as a possible etiologic agent, based on culture of the organism from sarcoidosis granulomas and its ability to trigger granuloma formation in an animal model of sarcoidosis [32]. However, there are also data suggesting that Propionibacterium is not capable of inducing cellular immune responses, at least in American sarcoidosis patients [33]. It is possible that there may be more than one etiologic agent that causes sarcoidosis, depending on geographic location, host immunity, and genetic background [34]. Regardless of the specific etiology, it seems likely that development of a sarcoidosis reaction to a triggering antigen depends on a combination of genetic polymorphisms, the status of the host immune system, and the exposure itself.

Besides a relevant exposure, genetic polymorphisms modulate both susceptibility and phenotype of sarcoidosis [35]. A registry-based study of 210 affected twin pairs in Denmark and Finland documented an 80-fold increased susceptibility risk for monozygotic twins versus population controls, compared to only a sevenfold increased chance in dizygotic pairs [36]. Heritable risk for sarcoidosis has also been demonstrated in other populations [37, 38]. HLA genes governing the expression of the type II major histocompatibility complex (MHC) on antigen-presenting cells are the most consistently documented genetic risk factors [35, 39]. A review of the genetic loci associated with sarcoidosis is beyond the scope of this chapter but has been discussed recently [40].

Diagnosis

The diagnosis of sarcoidosis requires careful assessment of all the relevant data—there is no single test that "rules in" or "rules out" sarcoidosis [34, 41]. Since there are many causes of granulomatous inflammation, the diagnosis is never certain. Instead, labeling a patient's syndrome as "sarcoidosis" implies that the likelihood of finding an alternate diagnosis is so low that further testing is not warranted [42]. Thus, diagnosis inherently involves the use of clinical judgment. Factors that are inconsistent or unusual for sarcoidosis should be weighed carefully. Sometimes, an individual patient must be managed as "provisional sarcoidosis" to allow time to help define the diagnosis more clearly.

Presentation

The presenting symptoms depend on the organs involved. In acute presentations, which are more common in Caucasian populations [2], the most common complaints include periarticular inflammation or arthritis of the ankles, fevers, weight loss, and fatigue; fewer than half of patients have concomitant erythema nodosum, which tends to be more frequent in women [43]. Frequently, patients with acute presentations may recall an antecedent event, such as a viral syndrome or a noxious exposure.

When sarcoidosis presentations are more indolent, the symptoms are dominated by the pattern of organ involvement. Nonproductive cough, exertional dyspnea, wheezing, and chest discomfort are all common in pulmonary sarcoidosis. The cough in sarcoidosis is commonly exacerbated by exposure to dusts, cold air, or other irritants, making differentiation from asthma difficult at times. The chest discomfort is usually described as a non-remitting mid-sternal dull ache or pressure that is not associated with exertion. It is not related to the size of thoracic lymph nodes [44]. When the presentation is dominated by pulmonary symptoms, the diagnosis required an average of five physician visits in one epidemiologic survey, probably since the symptoms were misattributed to asthma or other causes [45]. Arthralgias involving multiple joints are also frequently present, though true polyarthritis is very unusual [46].

When sarcoidosis is suspected, the history should probe for unexplained past medical events that may have been due to sarcoidosis. The most common of these include renal lithiasis, Bell's palsy, unexplained uveitis, and lymphocytic (viral) meningitis. Occasionally, patients may carry prior diagnoses of inflammatory bowel disease, multiple sclerosis, fibromyalgia, or inflammatory arthritis that actually represent prior manifestations of sarcoidosis if the clinical scenario and pathology are carefully examined.

Examination

The physical exam is useful to identify potential biopsy sites and characterize organ involvement. Peripheral lymphadenopathy is present in up to 15–33 % of patients [2, 47]; epitrochlear and supraclavicular lymph nodes may be easily accessible biopsy targets [47]. The lymph nodes in sarcoidosis are not typically tender, hard, or ulcerating.

Cutaneous sarcoidosis is present in approximately 20 % of patients [10]. The granulomas of cutaneous sarcoidosis have a predilection to involve tattoos, scars, and needle tracks. Subcutaneous nodules, sometimes painful, can frequently be found along tendon sheaths in the upper and lower extremities. Other physical examination findings that may be sought include lacrimal or parotid enlargement, organomegaly, upper airways mucosal involvement (Fig. 9.1), and auscultatory features of cardiopulmonary disease. Digital clubbing and/or rales are extremely rare in sarcoidosis—alternative diagnoses should be aggressively sought if they are present.

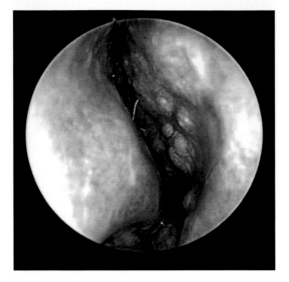

Fig. 9.1 Nasal sarcoidosis with pearl-colored mucosal nodules. Erythema, friability, and crusting are also frequently seen

Table 9.1 Selected features influencing the likelihood of sarcoidosis

More likely	Less likely
• African-American or Northern European	• Age <18
	• Age >50 in males
	• Smoking
• Female	• Exposure to metal dusts, bioaerosols, organic antigens
• Symmetric bilateral hilar adenopathy	• History of exposure to tuberculosis
• Asymptomatic presentation	
• Peripheral blood lymphopenia	• History of recurrent infections
	• Hypogammaglobulinemia
• BAL lymphocytes >15 % and/or BAL CD4/CD8 ratio >3.5	• Systemic disease capable of inducing granulomatous reactions
• Multisystem involvement	Malignancy
	Inflammatory bowel disease
• Elevated serum ACE	Immunodeficiency

BAL bronchoalveolar lavage, *ACE* angiotensin-converting enzyme
Adapted with permission from Judson MA. The diagnosis of sarcoidosis. Clin Chest Med. 2008; 29:415–427, viii

Clinical and Laboratory Features

The likelihood of sarcoidosis is influenced by a variety of clinical features (Table 9.1) [48]. The items listed on the right side of the table are unexpected or rare—when present, the diagnostician should be cautious about conferring a label of sarcoidosis. In particular, a careful exposure history is important to exclude sarcoidosis mimics such as chronic beryllium disease or hypersensitivity pneumonitis [49].

There is no currently available blood test that is either sensitive or specific enough to diagnose sarcoidosis. Angiotensin-converting enzyme (ACE), which is released by epithelioid histiocytes in granulomas and by pulmonary endothelial cells, loosely reflects the overall total granuloma burden in the body [50]. Previously, ACE was proposed as a useful diagnostic tool, but it may be elevated in a number of other conditions, including certain infections, alcoholic liver disease, and other conditions [51, 52]. In a series of 1,941 patients with sarcoidosis, 1,575 healthy controls, and 1,355 patients with other diseases, the diagnostic sensitivity of an elevated serum ACE was 57 %, the specificity 90 %, and positive predictive value 90 %, but negative predictive

value was only 60 % [50]. In a second study of 128 sarcoidosis patients and 208 control subjects, the sensitivity of ACE for sarcoidosis was only 58 %, and specificity was 84 %, but these increased significantly if only patients with clinically active sarcoidosis were evaluated [53]. A common genetic polymorphism also modulates ACE level and function, further confounding the interpretation of the test [54]. Elevations more than twofold the upper limits of normal are thought to be more specific. Nonetheless, ACE is currently viewed as only supportive evidence for sarcoidosis, but cannot be used in isolation to confirm the diagnosis.

Other blood tests, such as erythrocyte sedimentation rate (ESR), C-reactive protein (CRP), soluble interleukin 2 receptor, chitotriosidase, lysozyme, and a variety of cytokines may be abnormally elevated in sarcoidosis [55–57]. However, none of these markers is sufficiently sensitive or specific for confident diagnostic distinction between sarcoidosis and other inflammatory diseases. As a management tool, ESR and CRP are simultaneously so insensitive and nonspecific that their measurement is just as likely to lead to confusion as to be helpful. On the other hand, hypergammaglobulinemia and peripheral lymphopenia occur more than 50 % of the time [58, 59].

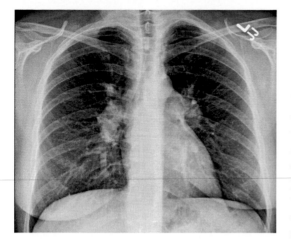

Fig. 9.2 Chest radiograph demonstrating classic bilateral hilar lymph node enlargement

Diagnostic Strategy

In most cases, a biopsy is required to confirm the diagnosis. However, in a few situations, a confident diagnosis can be reached on clinical grounds only, provided there are no evident alternative explanations for the findings. These situations include:

- Löfgren's syndrome (bilateral hilar lymphadenopathy, erythema nodosum, usually periarticular ankle inflammation, and usually constitutional symptoms)
- Isolated bilateral hilar lymphadenopathy in an asymptomatic patient
- Heerfordt's syndrome (uveoparotid fever—uveitis, parotid swelling, usually constitutional symptoms, often facial nerve palsy)
- Gallium uptake in the panda (parotid, lacrimal glands)-lambda (right paratracheal and bihilar lymph node) pattern

A common scenario is isolated bilateral lymph node enlargement seen on chest X-ray (CXR) in an asymptomatic or minimally symptomatic patient (Fig. 9.2). Many of these individuals will also have had chest computed tomography (CT), which often uncovers other abnormalities, such as mediastinal lymph node enlargement or parenchymal lesions. However, for diagnostic decision-making, the CXR alone can be used to make a confident diagnosis. In a seminal study,

Winterbauer et al. reviewed the chest radiograph in 99 patients with sarcoidosis, 212 patients with lymphoma, 500 patients with lung cancer, and 1,201 patients with extrathoracic malignancies [60]. Among the patients with isolated bilateral hilar lymphadenopathy, all patients had sarcoidosis except those who had either obvious extrathoracic tumor on physical exam or significant symptoms due to undiagnosed malignancy. One calculation suggested that approximately 1,833 patients with isolated bilateral hilar adenopathy would require mediastinoscopy to uncover each single patient with an alternative (non-sarcoidosis) diagnosis [61].

For most patients, a biopsy site should be identified after a complete physical exam and basic laboratory testing. In general, a reasonable biopsy target can be identified without resorting to advanced imaging techniques such as 18-fluorodeoxyglucose positron emission tomography (FDG-PET). In difficult cases, however, FDG-PET can identify unsuspected foci of inflammation. In a retrospective review of FDG-PET scans in 137 patients, biopsy sites were identified only by FDG-PET scan in 15 % of patients [62]. Frequently, the FDG-avid lymph nodes are barely discernible by standard CT scanning and may be deemed not to be technically enlarged. PET scan appears to be a more sensitive tool than 67-gallium imaging [63].

Since the lungs and intrathoracic lymph nodes are most commonly involved, most diagnoses of sarcoidosis are made by sampling within the chest. In A Case Control Etiologic Study of Sarcoidosis (ACCESS), a multicenter epidemiologic study of 736 incident sarcoidosis cases in the United States, an intrathoracic location was the site of the biopsy in 74 % of the subjects [64]. Two-thirds of the biopsies were bronchoscopic, and the remaining 1/3 were obtained by mediastinoscopy. More recently, however, endobronchial ultrasound-guided transbronchial needle aspiration (EBUS-TBNA) has emerged as a sensitive tool to diagnose sarcoidosis and can replace mediastinoscopy in many cases. A recent meta-analysis estimated the accuracy of EBUS-TBNA in patients suspected of sarcoidosis to be 79 %, with a minimal complication rate [65].

The sensitivity of EBUS-TBNA to confirm sarcoidosis ranges from 83 to 93 %, with 100 % specificity [66, 67]. EBUS-TBNA is more convenient and, in some settings, more cost-effective than mediastinoscopy.

Other bronchoscopic techniques are also useful, including transbronchial forceps biopsy (approximately 70 % sensitive) [67], blind transbronchial needle aspirate of the lymph nodes (sensitivity approximately 70 %) [68], and endobronchial mucosal biopsy (sensitivity 30–50 %) [69]. Combining multiple sampling modalities increases the diagnostic yield by 20–30 % [70, 71]. Bronchoalveolar lavage (BAL) with examination of lymphocyte populations (CD4/CD8 ratio) may be useful to support the diagnosis. Differential cell count of the leukocytes in the BAL demonstrating more than 15 % lymphocytes is 90 % sensitive for the diagnosis of sarcoidosis, although the specificity is low [72]. Specificity is improved with higher proportions of lymphocytes or when the CD4/CD8 ratio is more than >3.5 [72]. The American Thoracic Society recommends routine assessment of cell count and targeted assessment of CD4/CD8 ratio in patients with interstitial lung disease who have bronchoscopy [73].

Sarcoidosis granulomas are comprised of well-formed clusters of epithelioid histiocytes, often harboring multinucleate giant cells that are surrounded by an outer rim of T lymphocytes (Fig. 9.3). Collagen and some fibroblasts may surround the granuloma, and a few B lymphocytes may be found in the granuloma. Pathologic evaluation should include stains and cultures for mycobacteria and fungi, which can occasionally cause non-necrotizing granulomas. Sarcoidosis granulomas frequently exhibit focal necrosis [74], but it is rarely widespread or suppurative. Pathologic features that may be useful in the diagnosis are listed in Table 9.2. Sarcoidal granulomas may contain a variety of inclusion bodies, all of which are nonspecific. These include calcium bodies (Schaumann bodies, which are made up of calcium carbonate but may contain birefringent calcium oxalate crystals), asteroid bodies within multinucleate giant cells, and Hamazaki-Wesenberg bodies (which may resemble fungal yeast forms).

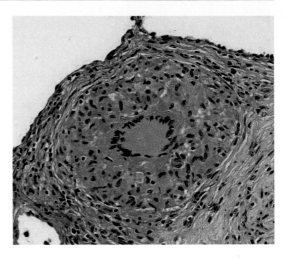

Fig. 9.3 Well-formed granuloma typically seen in sarcoidosis. The granuloma is comprised of a core of epithelioid histiocytes and multinucleated giant cells surrounded by a few lymphocytes. There is little inflammation in the adjacent lung. (Courtesy of Carol Farver, M.D.)

Table 9.2 Pathologic features of sarcoidosis granulomas

Favor sarcoidosis	Favor alternate diagnosis
Morphologic descriptors	
Well formed or compact	Loosely formed
Non-necrotizing, or minimal central necrosis	Widespread necrosis
Naked granulomas (<25 % of granuloma diameter comprised of inflammatory cells other than histiocytes)[a]	Polarizable material[b] Palisading architectural arrangement of histiocytes Substantial granulocytes (polymorphonuclear cells or eosinophils)
Perigranuloma features	
Circumferential hyalinization	Fibromyxoid plugs in the alveolar ducts (organizing pneumonia reaction)
Granuloma confluence	Substantial non-granulomatous inflammatory cell infiltrates (i.e., alveolitis or bronchitis) Nearby granuloma trigger (tumor, foreign body)
Granuloma distribution	
Lungs: perilymphatic (bronchocentric, intralobular septae, pleural)	Lungs: bronchocentric only, random, intraparenchymal only
Lymph nodes: confluent and widespread	Lymph nodes: scattered or few

[a]May be seen in nontuberculous mycobacterial infections
[b]Excluding calcium bodies (e.g., Schaumann bodies—see text)

Extrapulmonary sarcoidosis may be diagnosed either by biopsy of the affected organ or by inferring its involvement when the diagnosis of sarcoidosis is already well established. Inferential diagnosis of other organ involvement entails documenting consistent imaging or other testing findings in the affected organ and some "reasonably aggressive" exclusion of other causes for the observed abnormalities. This approach, in turn, implies a crucial role for clinical judgment about how much testing is needed to exclude other causes for symptoms or organ dysfunction. For example, cardiac sarcoidosis is inferred when imaging features are consistent with granulomatous myocarditis (e.g., patchy mid-myocardial delayed enhancement in a patient without coronary artery disease), and the diagnosis of extracardiac sarcoidosis was previously established. In some situations, bronchoscopy with BAL may be useful, even in patients with relatively unremarkable CXRs. For example, in a study of 61 Japanese patients with uveitis suspicious for sarcoidosis but no CXR abnormality, the yield of bronchoscopy was 62 % [75].

When possible, it has been suggested to establish involvement of a second organ in all patients with suspected sarcoidosis in order to improve specificity of the diagnosis [2, 34]. For example, a liver biopsy demonstrating granulomatous hepatitis could represent sarcoidosis, but the process may be confined to the liver—in that case, it would be consistent with idiopathic granulomatous hepatitis, a relatively benign condition with a good prognosis [76]. In the skin, it is not uncommon to have isolated granulomatous reactions to foreign bodies or debris, which cannot be labeled as sarcoidosis unless a second organ is also involved. From a practical standpoint, biopsying a second organ is rarely necessary; imaging or examination is usually sufficient.

A common scenario is isolated pulmonary sarcoidosis, since there are no non-pulmonary organs affected by sarcoidosis in more than one-quarter of patients. In the ACCESS cohort, approximately 50 % of the patients had only pulmonary involvement at the time of diagnosis, implying that establishing the diagnosis by documenting two-organ involvement is not always

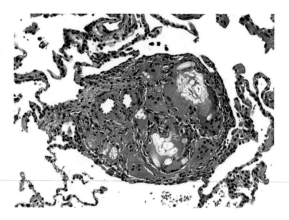

Fig. 9.4 Granuloma due to a foreign body reaction. In this case, silicone from leaking breast implants entered the lung, causing a pulmonary granulomatous reaction. (Courtesy of Andrea Arrossi, M.D.)

necessary or even possible [10]. However, when diagnosing isolated pulmonary sarcoidosis, a variety of alternative causes for granulomatous inflammation should be carefully considered. Salient masqueraders include:
- Granulomatous infections (especially endemic fungi)
- Hypersensitivity pneumonitis
- Chronic beryllium disease
- Granulomatous reactions (foreign bodies, particulates, tumors) (Fig. 9.4)

Systemic granulomatous reactions can occur in several diseases that may be confused with sarcoidosis. For example, patients with dysregulated immune responses such as common variable immune deficiency (CVID) may exhibit multiorgan granulomatous inflammation [77]. The granulomas in CVID tend to be less compact than in sarcoidosis (Fig. 9.5), and there are often also nonspecific inflammatory cell infiltrates in affected tissues. Some patients, but not all, have a history of recurring infections. Other clues to the diagnosis are a history of (multiple) autoimmune syndromes and the presence of splenomegaly. Since hypergammaglobulinemia is expected in sarcoidosis, any low serum immunoglobulin level or absent serological response to immunizations may confirm the diagnosis. Controlling the inflammation may require immunosuppressive medication in combination with immune globulin replacement therapy.

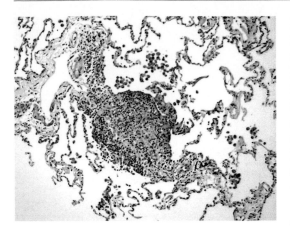

Fig. 9.5 Poorly formed (loose) granuloma in a patient with chronic variable immune deficiency. Besides the granuloma, the alveolar septae are widened by chronic inflammatory cells, mainly lymphocytes. (Courtesy of Carol Farver, M.D.)

Another second multisystem granulomatous disorder is an extremely rare entity known as granulomatous lesions of undetermined significance (GLUS), a syndrome characterized by fever; granulomas in the liver, bone marrow, spleen, and peripheral lymph nodes; and a tendency not to cause end-stage organ failure [78]. It is thought to differ from usual sarcoidosis because (1) the lung is never involved; (2) the serum ACE level is normal; (3) when done, the Kveim–Siltzbach test is negative; and (4) it does not cause hypercalcemia [79]. A third multisystem granulomatous disorder is Blau syndrome, a very rare disorder caused by autosomal dominant mutations in the CARD15/NOD2 gene [80]. Characteristically, Blau syndrome causes uveitis, symmetric polyarticular arthritis, and granulomatous dermatitis.

Sarcoidosis Effects on the Respiratory System

Parenchymal Lung Disease

Pulmonary involvement is seen in 90–95 % of patients at the time of diagnosis; symptoms are present in approximately half of individuals with radiographic evidence of pulmonary involvement

[2, 10]. Even when extrapulmonary manifestations dominate the clinical presentation, the lungs are usually involved on at least a histologic level [75, 81]. When present, infiltrates have a predilection for the mid- and upper lung zones. The most common parenchymal findings are reticulonodular infiltrates, but alveolar infiltrates, consolidation, perihilar conglomerate masses, and larger nodules may also be seen. The degree of reticulonodular infiltrates correlates most closely with the response to treatment [82].

Chest CT scanning can show more specific signs of sarcoidosis and can identify enlarged lymph nodes more readily, but it is not always necessary for the diagnosis of uncomplicated pulmonary sarcoidosis. For example, CT scanning in a patient with typical bihilar lymphadenopathy on CXR or a presentation consistent with Löfgren's syndrome will be extremely unlikely to identify an alternate diagnosis. For routine follow-up of pulmonary sarcoidosis, chest CT scanning is widely overused—the main indication for chest CT scanning in established pulmonary sarcoidosis is when a superimposed complication or coexistent alternate diagnosis is suspected. Complications of sarcoidosis, such as pulmonary fibrosis, bullae, mycetomas, bronchiectasis, and architectural distortion, are seen more readily on CT than CXR [83].

Characteristic features on chest CT include mediastinal or hilar adenopathy, micronodular infiltrates, and bronchial wall thickening (Fig. 9.6). Less common CT features include reticulations, peribronchial or subpleural ground-glass opacities, consolidation, macronodules, and pleural effusions. Rarely, honeycombing may occur. It should be noted that the Scadding system for prognostication (Table 9.3) refers to the posterior-anterior chest radiograph, not to whatever can be seen on chest CT [84].

Pulmonary function tests (PFTs) are recommended at the time of diagnosis to establish a baseline, even in individuals without pulmonary symptoms [2]. Forced viral capacity (FVC) is the most reproducible test, but the single-breath diffusing capacity for carbon monoxide (DLCO) provides additional complementary clinical information [85]. Abnormal PFTs are found in

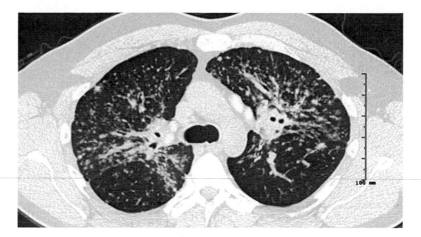

Fig. 9.6 Classic computed tomography (CT) findings in pulmonary sarcoidosis. There are innumerable small poorly circumscribed nodules found predominantly in the mid- and upper lung zones. The nodules are typically found in a lymphatic distribution, along the bronchovascular bundles and the pleural surfaces

Table 9.3 Scadding chest radiograph staging system

Stage	Description	Frequency (%)	Likelihood of CXR remission at 5-year after diagnosis (%)
I	Bilateral hilar lymphadenopathy with or without right paratracheal lymphadenopathy	40–67	80–90
II	Lymphadenopathy + parenchymal infiltrates	20–40	50–65
III	Parenchymal infiltrates alone	10–20	20–30
IV	Pulmonary fibrosis	0–10	0

approximately 20 % of patients with Scadding stage I radiographs, whereas 40–80 % of those with more advanced radiographic stages have abnormal values [86]. Although restrictive physiology is widely assumed to be typical for sarcoidosis, obstructive lung disease is seen as often. At the time of diagnosis, it is present in up to 63 % of patients [87, 88]. Similarly, bronchial hyperresponsiveness documented by bronchoprovocation testing is present in 21–58 % of subjects, regardless of chronicity or radiographic stage [89, 90]. Other tests of pulmonary physiology, such as the 6-min walk test, total body plethysmography, cardiopulmonary exercise testing, or measurements of respiratory muscle strength, can be considered in the appropriate clinical context [91].

The minimal clinically important difference for PFTs in sarcoidosis is unknown. In general, most patients with worsening sarcoidosis will not demonstrate conventionally defined deterioration of >10–15 % of FVC prior to seeking treatment, so that a consistent decline of 5–10 %, along with worsening symptoms or radiographic changes, may be sufficient to escalate treatment [85]. It is also important to carefully identify what mechanism is causing symptoms determining treatment. For example, muscle weakness, as assessed by quadriceps peak torque, hamstrings peak torque, peak inspiratory force, or hand grip, is prevalent in sarcoidosis patients [92]. The reductions of muscle strength correlate with lower 6-min walk distances, more dyspnea, and worse quality of life [93]. These may in turn be effects of obesity or myopathy related to corticosteroid administration. In one study, the dose of steroids was inversely correlated with the quadriceps peak torque, suggesting that subclinical steroid myopathy is a contributor to the symptoms [93].

Upper Respiratory Tract Sarcoidosis

Sarcoidosis of the upper respiratory tract (SURT) is an underappreciated manifestation of sarcoidosis and may be present in the nose, sinuses, larynx, oral cavity, or ear. The estimated incidence of sinonasal involvement is between 1 and 6.8 % [10, 94–96], with laryngeal involvement in less than 1 % [97]. SURT appears to be more common in African-American and female patients and those with lupus pernio [95]. It can be a presenting manifestation of sarcoidosis, although there is often a substantial delay in the diagnosis of SURT. Nasal congestion is the most common symptom, but crusting, anosmia, and hoarseness may also occur. Erythematous nodules can often be identified on the turbinates and septum (Fig. 9.1). Destruction of the nasal sinuses, saddle nose deformity, and septal perforation are features of more chronic disease.

Because laryngeal involvement could be potentially life-threatening, clinicians should consider fiber-optic laryngoscopy for significant laryngeal symptoms [98, 99]. Some patients may respond to topical or intralesional corticosteroids [99], although the majority of patients require more aggressive systemic corticosteroids or immunosuppressive medications to control the disease [94, 95]. Sinus surgery should be reserved as a procedure of last resort for severe SURT that has failed aggressive medical management, as there is increased risk of nasal septal perforation and recurrence of disease after surgical intervention [100, 101]. Patients with SURT have a lower likelihood of remission compared to sarcoidosis patients without upper respiratory tract involvement [95, 102].

Endobronchial Sarcoidosis

As mentioned previously, sarcoidosis granulomas tend to cluster along the bronchovascular bundle and in the vicinity of the airways. When the granulomatous airways inflammation is clinically overt, it is associated with increased respiratory symptoms and higher mortality [103]. Endobronchial disease typically manifests as an obstructive ventilatory defect, although pulmonary function testing may also be normal [104, 105].

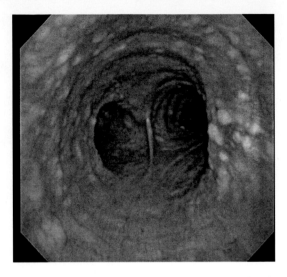

Fig. 9.7 Airways mucosal involvement from sarcoidosis in the trachea. This appearance has been termed "pebbly mural" or "cobblestoning"

Bronchiolar involvement from sarcoidosis can occasionally occur in early sarcoidosis without pulmonary parenchymal involvement, leading to radiologic and physiologic air trapping that correlates with evidence of small airways disease and airways hyperreactivity on pulmonary function testing [106]. However, airways obstruction is far more common in patients with advanced parenchymal disease, probably due to the overall granuloma burden, as well as the presence of architectural airways distortion from peribronchiolar fibrosis [107, 108]. Significant endoluminal narrowing from bronchostenosis is rare, occurring in fewer than 1 % of patients [104].

The most common endobronchial abnormalities include erythema and/or mucosal thickening. As the airways disease progresses, the mucosa may demonstrate waxy yellow mucosa nodules, cobblestoning, and friability (Fig. 9.7). Although diffuse airways narrowing can lead to near total obstruction of the airways, greater than two-thirds of patients have multiple stenotic sites [104]. The most common clinical features are cough and airways hyperreactivity [89]. Wheezing, squeaks, and stridor are less common and, when focal, should prompt bronchoscopic examination or dedicated airways imaging to evaluate whether there is a mechanical obstruction that can be treated with interventional bronchoscopic modalities.

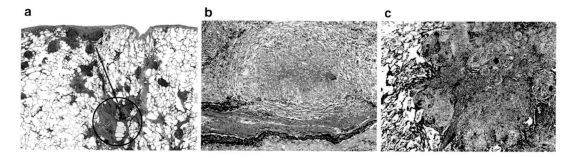

Fig. 9.8 (**a–c**) Sarcoidosis can cause pulmonary hypertension through a variety of mechanisms, but it tends to be more common than in idiopathic pulmonary fibrosis due to the distribution of the granulomas in the bronchovascular bundle where the pulmonary arteries are located (**a**, *circle*) as well as adjacent to the veins, which run through the intralobular septae (**a**, *line*). The sarcoidosis granulomas may cause a destructive arteriopathy (**b**), eroding through the vascular wall. When the granuloma burden is high, there is often direct physical occlusion of the vasculature (**c**), where the pulmonary vein is compressed

Pulmonary Hypertension

The prevalence of sarcoidosis-associated pulmonary hypertension (SAPH) ranges from 1 to 28 %, depending on how pulmonary hypertension is defined, the technique used for detection, and the population studied [109–111]. It may be as high as 75 % in patients awaiting lung transplantation [112]. Generally, the mean pulmonary artery pressure is modestly elevated, but severe pulmonary hypertension with cor pulmonale and systemic level PA pressures may also occur [111, 113]. Right heart catheterization is necessary to confirm suspected SAPH, since elevated pulmonary pressures are frequently due to pulmonary venous hypertension from cardiac sarcoidosis or other causes of elevated left heart filling pressures such as hypertensive heart disease [114]. The presence of SAPH is a predictor of significant morbidity and lower survival, particularly when the right atrial pressure is elevated (>15 mmHg) [114, 115]. Therefore, under the current organ allocation system for lung transplantation, added priority has been given to those patients with sarcoidosis who suffer from pulmonary hypertension.

The mechanism of SAPH is multifactorial, leading to its inclusion in World Health Organization Group 5 (miscellaneous causes). A key factor responsible for the high prevalence of SAPH in sarcoidosis is that the anatomic location of sarcoidosis granulomas tends to favor a perivascular distribution, leading to direct as well as indirect effects on the pulmonary arterioles and veins (Fig. 9.8a–c) [116]. Many patients also develop pulmonary hypertension from hypoxemic vasoconstriction and progressive loss of the vascular bed in patients with severe fibrosis [116, 117]. However, the lung parenchyma is normal in a small subset (10 %) of patients [117]. Other mechanisms may include obstructive sleep apnea, which is common in patients with sarcoidosis, occlusion of the pulmonary vasculature by granulomatous vasculitis, pulmonary veno-occlusive disease, and external compression from lymphadenopathy [116]. Patients with sarcoidosis are also at increased risk for thromboembolism [118], which can occasionally lead to chronic thromboembolic pulmonary hypertension. Rarely, portopulmonary hypertension can occur in individuals with sarcoidosis-associated cirrhosis.

A high index of suspicion is necessary to identify patients with sarcoidosis who have pulmonary hypertension. Patients with SAPH are more likely to have advanced radiographic disease and more impaired lung volumes, although patients with preserved lung function and no pulmonary fibrosis have also been reported [119]. Patients with a diffusion capacity <60 % predicted, those requiring supplemental oxygen, and those with oxygen desaturation <90 % on 6-min walk testing have a relatively high likelihood of having pulmonary hypertension [112, 119].

Although there are reports of successful reversal of SAPH with corticosteroids, most patients do not respond to immunosuppressive therapies [112, 120]. The usefulness of specific pulmonary hypertension therapies in SAPH is relatively understudied. A single randomized, double-blind placebo-controlled trial showed improvements in pulmonary hemodynamics but not in 6-min walk distance at 16 weeks for those treated with bosentan but not placebo [121]. Other small case series and uncontrolled trials have reported variably positive results [111, 122, 123].

Pleural Sarcoidosis

The major forms of pleural involvement in sarcoidosis are pleural effusions, pneumothorax, and pleural thickening, although pleural nodules, hydropneumothorax, trapped lung, pleural calcification, hemothorax, and chylothorax have also been described [124–127]. The reported incidence of pleural effusions ranges from 0.7 to 10 %, with most studies supporting a prevalence of 1–2 % [124, 128–130]. The effusion is typically a paucicellular, lymphocyte-predominant exudate, with a pleural/serum protein ratio more consistently in the exudative range than the serum: pleural fluid lactate dehydrogenase (LDH) criteria. The more predominant protein elevation suggests that the pathogenesis of sarcoid-related pleural effusions is more likely to be a consequence of increased capillary permeability rather than of pleural space inflammation [130]. Pleural effusions are more likely to occur in CXR stage 2 disease but the majority resolve spontaneously in 1–3 months [124, 130]. With the progression of parenchymal disease, the prevalence of pleural effusions decreases, while the prevalence of pleural thickening and pneumothorax increases [124].

Mycetoma

Advanced fibrocystic pulmonary sarcoidosis is the main risk factor for the development of mycetomas (typically aspergillomas). The true prevalence of mycetomas in sarcoidosis is unknown, but has ranged from 2.7 % in unselected cohorts

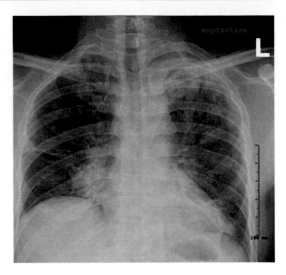

Fig. 9.9 Monod's (crescent) sign due to a mycetoma in the left upper lobe in a patient with fibrobullous sarcoidosis

to a high of 44 % in groups with advanced lung disease [131–133].

Mycetomas most commonly occur in the upper lobes, can affect both lungs equally, and can present as single or multiple lesions [134]. The classic radiographic appearance is that of a round, mobile mass topped by a clear crescent which separates the mass from the wall of the cavity (crescent sign—Fig. 9.9). In the presence of a crescent sign and a positive serum precipitin test, the diagnosis of aspergilloma can be confidently made without resorting to cultures or invasive testing [135]. Invasive fungal infection or dissemination of the infection, even in the setting of immune modulating therapy, is very rare [136, 137].

Most patients are asymptomatic. In a minority of individuals, hemoptysis may occur, ranging from scanty blood-streaked sputum to massive hemoptysis that results in variable amounts of hemoptysis with risk for mortality from asphyxiation. The risk for hemoptysis does not correlate with the size of the mycetoma [134]; however, once bleeding starts, the mortality rate from the episode ranges from 5 to 26 % [132, 134, 138]. Surgical resection is the only known definitive therapy but it is associated with high perioperative morbidity and mortality [134]. Bronchial artery embolization may be a temporizing measure. Pharmacologic treatment options are limited. Direct, CT-guided, intracavitary instillation of antifungal agents has been studied and shown to be effective in small case series [134, 139–141].

Other Considerations

Pulmonary Embolism

Epidemiologic surveys in the United States and in England have suggested that the risk of pulmonary embolism (PE) in patients with sarcoidosis is more than twofold greater than the risk of PE in the general population, regardless of gender, race, or age [118, 142]. One potential explanation for a heightened risk of thrombosis may be due to increased procoagulant activity that has been demonstrated in the BAL fluid of patients [143]. Other effects of chronic inflammation, or decreased mobility due to complications of severe sarcoidosis, may also account for the elevated thrombotic risk. In sarcoidosis patients with worsening respiratory status, PE should be considered as a potential explanation.

Sleep Apnea

Patients with sarcoidosis are at increased risk for sleep apnea, possibly due to factors such as steroid use, neurosarcoidosis, or upper airways obstruction. In a single-center prospective study, sleep apnea was identified in 17 % of patients when screening consisted solely of the Epworth Sleepiness Scale, followed by polysomnography in those with a high screening score [144]. In that cohort, the only independent risk factor for the presence of sleep apnea was lupus pernio [144]. Similar to the general population, obstructive sleep apnea occurs more commonly in males, but in the sarcoidosis population, it is relatively frequent in females as well [144]. Excessive daytime sleepiness and fatigue are very common in sarcoidosis cohorts, but are only partially explained by the presence of sleep apnea [145, 146].

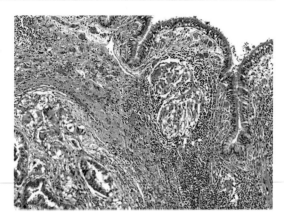

Fig. 9.10 Bronchogenic malignancy (adenocarcinoma) causing a local granulomatous reaction in the overlying airways mucosa that was initially mistaken for sarcoidosis when only granulomas were identified on a superficial (endobronchial) biopsy

Malignancy

Sarcoidosis has been reported to occur in patients preceding, concurrent with, or after the diagnosis of cancer. Whether the incidence of sarcoidosis after a diagnosis of cancer is truly elevated above the population expected norms is unclear, since many oncologic patients are subjected to aggressive follow-up testing that may reveal clinically unimportant sarcoidosis.

A local sarcoid-like reaction has also been known to occur in patients with cancer (Fig. 9.10). Therefore, it is important to consider the clinical situation carefully when making the diagnosis of sarcoidosis. For example, in one series, sarcoidosis-like reactions were estimated to occur in 0.5–1.1 % of cancers when FDG-PET scanning was used as the primary tool for ascertainment [147].

A frequent clinical question, especially when considering use of some types of immunosuppressive medications, is whether sarcoidosis increases the likelihood of subsequent malignancy. A population-based survey in Britain identified a relative risk ratio of 1.65 for development of cancer in sarcoidosis patients compared to controls over a 4-year time frame, but the risk was driven almost entirely by excess non-melanoma skin cancer [148]. An older Danish cohort from the 1960s suggested that lung cancer and lymphoma occurred 3 and 11 times more commonly than expected, but the estimates may be skewed by small numbers [149]. A separate cohort from Sweden suggested a doubling of overall risk, especially within the first decade after the diagnosis of sarcoidosis [150].

Management

Natural History and Prognosis

Although sarcoidosis is usually regarded as a benign disease, it can lead to death; historical estimates, largely from referral centers, estimated a 1–5 % attributable mortality risk [2]. The mortality rate for sarcoidosis patients in a British population survey from 1991 to 2003 was 5 and 7 % at 3 years and 5 years, respectively, compared to age- and gender-matched controls for whom mortality was 2 and 4 % [151]. An analysis of age-adjusted sarcoidosis mortality based on death certificates suggested that it has increased 51 % in women and 30 % in men in the United States in the last two decades from 1988 to 2007 [152]. In the United States and Europe, progressive pulmonary fibrosis leading to respiratory failure is the most common cause of death, followed by advanced myocardial or neurologic involvement [2]. In Japan, cardiac sarcoidosis is the leading cause of death [153].

The morbidity of sarcoidosis is frequently overlooked, perhaps due to the widespread perception that it is a spontaneously resolving disease and does not progress inexorably like idiopathic pulmonary fibrosis. However, at least 1/3 of those with sarcoidosis will develop persistent symptoms and organ damage [6, 154]. Since sarcoidosis tends to affect individuals in the prime years of life, the impact on employability, family structures, and comorbid diseases that develop from sarcoidosis or its therapies can be considerable. Preventing and ameliorating these outcomes are obvious goals of treatment, but these goals are complicated by the variable phenotypes and natural history of sarcoidosis.

Advanced pulmonary sarcoidosis develops in no more than 5–10 % of all sarcoidosis patients, generally over 1–2 decades [132, 155]. Nonetheless, most of the known prognostic factors for bothersome disease are apparent within 2 years of diagnosis [156–158]. While no specific risk factors for the development of advanced pulmonary disease have been identified, numerous factors for progressive and/or chronic disease have been defined. In the US ACCESS study, which was skewed to include a high proportion of patients with pulmonary sarcoidosis, the only independent variables predicting a requirement for ongoing therapy at 2 years after diagnosis were higher dyspnea scores and a requirement for therapy within the first 6 months [159]. Although sarcoidosis that is progressive or chronic does not always eventuate in end-stage disease, it is clear that those phenotypes are markers for those who will develop end-stage disease. For example, in a survey of 500 patients from ten tertiary centers specialized in treating the most severe patients, only 57 % of patients with persistent disease required any therapy at 5 years after the diagnosis [160]. Therefore, currently, decisions about prognosis and management must necessarily rely on the surrogate phenotypes of chronic or progressive sarcoidosis.

The Scadding chest radiographic (CXR) pattern is a widely used tool for predicting the overall likelihood for resolution at the 5-year time point after diagnosis [84]. A Spanish study of 209 patients demonstrated that the presence of parenchymal involvement and lack of lymphadenopathy at the time of diagnosis were independently associated with persistent disease at 2 years, even after adjustment for other possible prognostic variables [158]. Long-term studies utilizing CT (computed tomography) of the chest to determine potentially reversible lesions have been conducted. They showed that cystic spaces and architectural changes of the lung parenchyma are irreversible with or without treatment [161]. However, it is important to note that some patients with substantial pulmonary fibrosis have normal lung function or require no therapy [162, 163]. Therefore, the radiographic features of sarcoidosis must be interpreted in the context of longitudinal follow-up and symptoms.

Effect of Therapy on Natural History

Most authors do not believe that early treatment of sarcoidosis, regardless of Scadding stage or other putative prognostic features, necessarily results in a higher likelihood of spontaneous remission or substantially improved medium-term outcomes [164]. For most organs, including the lung, there does not seem to be a worse outcome when initiation of therapy is deferred [165]. As previously stated, a requirement for early institution of systemic therapy correlates with a worse prognosis, but it is unclear whether that observation is due to the severity of the disease or an adverse effect of treatment. In a cohort of Swedish patients with Löfgren's syndrome, 80 % of HLA-DRB1*03 negative patients treated with steroids had disease persistence at 2 years versus only 37 % of untreated patients [166]. Similarly, in a series of primarily African-American patients, those individuals who received steroids to control their disease had a 74 % likelihood of relapse when therapy was tapered [167].

Indications for Treatment

There are two broad indications for treatment: significant organ dysfunction, especially when a poor outcome is likely, and substantial impairment of quality of life due to symptoms caused by granulomatous inflammation. For the lungs, outcome is likely to be worse when sarcoidosis is chronic, when there is fibrosis, when the patient is dyspneic, and when there is progressive deterioration of the PFTs [102, 158, 159, 162]. Management of extrapulmonary sarcoidosis is beyond the scope of this chapter, but as a general rule, the prognosis is worse when more organs are involved, so that the treatment approach is typically more aggressive when pulmonary disease is combined with extrapulmonary disease.

Therapy

Inhaled corticosteroids (ICS) have a limited role in the management of symptomatic pulmonary sarcoidosis. Both budesonide and fluticasone have been studied for symptomatic pulmonary sarcoidosis, with most trials indicating little benefit on either PFTs or need for escalation of therapy [168–173]. Based on the currently available data, the main role of ICS appears to be for treatment of cough or bronchospasm.

Figure 9.11 presents a suggested algorithm for the management of pulmonary sarcoidosis. Due to the expectation of spontaneous resolution and the fact that many patients can be managed chronically with low daily doses [132, 174], corticosteroids are still generally accepted as the first-line approach for systemic treatment of sarcoidosis. However, the steroid-centric approach has been challenged for failing to sufficiently recognize the burden of steroid toxicities that occur in clinical practice [175].

There have been no prospective, randomized studies to determine the optimal dose, duration of therapy, or rate of tapering for glucocorticoids [176]. Most experts initiate therapy with prednisone 20–40 mg daily [176–178]. The benefits of corticosteroids (CS) on pulmonary disease are best established for chest radiographic improvement [179]. In contrast, there are data suggesting that the use of steroids may actually cause deterioration rather than improvement of quality of life [180].

For pulmonary sarcoidosis, the maximum improvement usually occurs within 3–4 weeks, and tapering to a maintenance dose can be accomplished in 1–3 months [165, 176, 181–184]. The dose of steroids should be tapered to the minimum level that will reasonably control symptoms and disease progression. The goal dose for maintenance therapy must be individualized for each patient but also must consider the likelihood of spontaneous remission. In one institution, 65 % of patients with chronic sarcoidosis were successfully maintained on 10 mg or less of prednisone daily [174]. As mentioned previously, serological markers such as ESR or ACE are not generally useful for adjustment of therapy. Some authors have suggested treatment can be discontinued after 6 months, whereas others have noted that relapse is less common when treatment is continued for at least 1 year

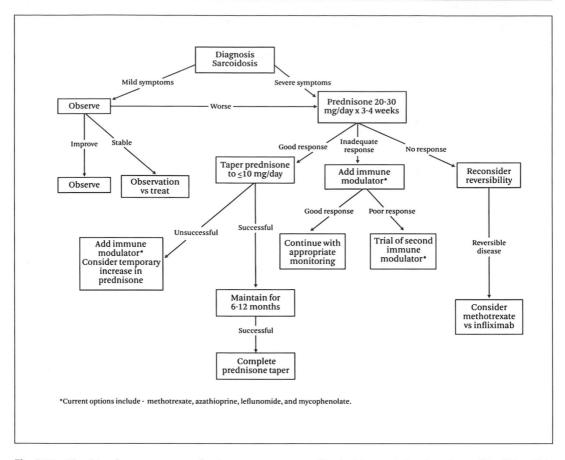

Fig. 9.11 Algorithm for management of pulmonary sarcoidosis. Other organs may require differing intensities or durations of therapy. The modern corticosteroid doses and time to initiate tapering are less aggressive than in the past. (Used with permission from Lazar CA, Culver DA. Treatment of sarcoidosis. Semin Respir Crit Care Med. 2010; 31:501–18.)

[165, 182]. Attempts to taper corticosteroids off should account for the chronicity of the disease, its severity, and the risk-benefit ratio of the extant treatment.

The side effect profile of steroids may limit their use in individual patients. The most common toxicities include weight gain, worsening of diabetes, and osteoporosis. In a randomized US trial, the median weight gain after 6 months of steroid therapy was 24 lb (11 kg) [185]. In contrast, the median weight gain after 12 months in the steroid-treated arm of a British steroid trial was only 3.6 kg [186]. For chronic treatment, Johns et al. reported that 24 % of patients gained 9 kg or more and 8 % of patients developed new diabetes [132]. Obviously, the risks of these toxicities must be considered individually for each patient.

Steroid-Sparing Agents

A range of alternative therapies are available for patients with inadequate responses to or excessive toxicities from corticosteroids. There are no prospective head-to-head comparisons of any of these agents, but methotrexate (MTX) is probably the most commonly advocated steroid-sparing medication [178]. A recent two-center study retrospectively compared the effectiveness of MTX versus azathioprine (AZA) for second-line treatment of pulmonary sarcoidosis [187]. Both agents were similarly effective for reduction of prednisone dose, which decreased by an average of 6.3 mg/day/year of MTX/AZA use, and for improvement of forced vital capacity (+95 mL/year) [187]. Infectious complications were more common in the AZA group, but otherwise the medications were tolerated similarly well [187].

In a double-blind, placebo-controlled trial comparing MTX to placebo in patients with acute pulmonary sarcoidosis on corticosteroids, MTX was well tolerated and exerted a significant steroid-sparing effect [185]. Up to 6 months may be needed prior to evidence of a benefit after starting MTX [188]. For sarcoidosis the typical dose is 10–20 mg orally once a week [189, 190]. Serious toxicities of MTX include hepatotoxicity, pneumonitis, and cytopenias. Common side effects include nausea, diarrhea, fatigue, rash, and headache, which are often temporally related to the weekly dose and may resolve by administration of the next dose. Risk for most of these side effects can be mitigated by supplementation with folic acid of 1–2 mg/day. The World Association of Sarcoidosis and Other Granulomatous Disorders guideline provides suggestions for monitoring and dosing MTX in sarcoidosis [191]. Some highlights of that guideline are that routine liver biopsies are not recommended and that MTX is deemed to be very safe for long-term use, even in patients with hepatic sarcoidosis [191].

AZA, a lymphocyte inhibitor, is theoretically attractive for sarcoidosis given the necessity of CD4+ lymphocyte-mediated immune activation to maintain the sarcoidosis granuloma. Despite its widespread use, there are no prospective controlled trials of AZA in sarcoidosis. The typical dose for sarcoidosis is 2–2.5 g/day in divided doses. Another antilymphocyte agent, leflunomide, has been evaluated in two retrospective series involving a total of 108 patients [192, 193]. Those reports suggested that leflunomide is effective for stabilizing lung function and may improve extrapulmonary disease in chronic sarcoidosis refractory to corticosteroids and MTX. It was also able to allow reduction in prednisone from a median dose of 10 to 0 mg/day [192]. Leflunomide appears to be more effective when used in combination with MTX [192].

A number of other agents have been used in pulmonary sarcoidosis. The antimalarial agent, chloroquine, was studied in a single randomized placebo-controlled trial of eighteen patients with refractory pulmonary sarcoidosis [194]. Chronic chloroquine use slowed deterioration of forced expiratory volume in 1 s (51 mL/year versus 196 mL/year) and reduced the frequency of relapses [194]. Some other medications that are frequently considered but for which there is little evidence of benefit for pulmonary sarcoidosis include mycophenolate, cyclophosphamide, thalidomide, rituximab, hydroxychloroquine, and pentoxifylline. In some cases, these options have not been well studied yet.

Biologic Anti-TNF Agents

Tumor necrosis factor (TNF) is critical for maintenance of granulomas in experimental models [195, 196]. Biologic TNF antagonists have been increasingly used for third-line therapy of pulmonary sarcoidosis, generally when patients have failed at least one steroid-sparing medication. A randomized, double-blind, placebo-controlled trial of 138 subjects demonstrated effectiveness of infliximab in chronic treatment-requiring pulmonary disease [197]. In that trial, the mean FVC increased by 2.5 % compared to placebo. Patients with FVC <70 %, higher dyspnea scores, and reticulonodular changes on CXR were more likely to respond [82, 197]. Although the magnitude of the FVC change has been criticized as small, the effects in the more severe group were similar to those reported in controlled trials of corticosteroids in untreated patients.

Benefits from adalimumab have also been reported, mainly in uncontrolled series [198–200]. However, its effect is less rapid and less robust than infliximab. When given for sarcoidosis, many experts administer a loading dose, similar to that for Crohn's disease, starting with 160 mg, followed by 80 mg 2 weeks later, and then 40 mg either weekly or every other week. Potential toxicities from use of TNF antagonists include infection, especially atypical reactivation syndromes from granulomatous organisms, risks of malignancy, and worsening of cardiomyopathy. Given the toxicity concerns and expense of TNF antagonists, their use is generally reserved for patients with moderate to severe disease who are failing conventional therapy.

Lung Transplantation

Patients with sarcoidosis make up 3.5 % of the total population of patients listed for transplantation [201]. According to the 2012 official report from the registry of the International Society for Heart & Lung Transplantation, 2.5 % of the patients who receive lung transplants and 1.6 % of the patients who receive heart-lung transplants have sarcoidosis, making it the seventh leading cause for lung transplantation [202]. Compared to the overall lung transplant population in the United States, patients with sarcoidosis are more likely to be younger (45.8 ± 8.8 years versus 48.9 ± 12.3 years; $p < 0.001$), female, and African-American [203]. These characteristics mirror the population that is affected by sarcoidosis in the United States.

Intermediate and long-term survival is similar to the reported overall worldwide lung transplant survival data [115, 203–205]. However, mortality in the first year after transplantation is higher in those with sarcoidosis. It is unclear whether the increased early mortality is due to complications such as SAPH and aspergilloma, preexisting immunosuppression, the presence of extrapulmonary sarcoidosis, or other factors.

Sarcoidosis can recur in the allograft, although the clinical implications are usually very modest [206, 207]. Sarcoidosis is estimated to recur in approximately one-half to two-thirds of lung allografts, as early as 14 days after transplantation [208]. The estimated average time to recurrence is 15 months [207]. Interestingly transmission of sarcoidosis from donor to recipient is also described [209].

Calcium Metabolism and Bone Health in Sarcoidosis

Patients with sarcoidosis are at risk for osteoporosis due to chronic inflammation, granuloma-derived osteoclast-stimulating factor, direct stimulation of osteoclasts by excessive levels of 1,25-dihydroxyvitamin D, and the pervasive use of glucocorticoid therapy [210]. Bone loss can be further exacerbated by limited mobility in patients with poor exercise tolerance due to compromised pulmonary function and in those with darker skin color.

Hypercalciuria and hypercalcemia are present in 3–11 % and 7–20 % of patients, respectively [211]. Renal lithiasis occurs in up to 5 % of patients [212]. Deranged calcium metabolism is the only "organ" manifestation that occurs more frequently in white than black patients [10]. Although most patients with sarcoidosis have low to very low levels of the inactive form of vitamin D (25-hydroxy vitamin D, vit D-25), most have normal or elevated levels of the active form of vitamin D (vit D-1,25), likely a result of the conversion of vit D-25 to vit D-1,25 by the enzyme 1α-hydroxylase contained in the sarcoid granuloma [210, 213]. Macrophages that make up sarcoid granulomas also have been reported to produce vit D-1,25, and the cytokines TNF-α and INF-γ seen in inflammation further amplify its production [214]. Therefore, serum levels of both vitamin D-25 and vitamin D-1,25 should be measured before starting vitamin D supplementation. Patients with low vitamin D-25, but normal vitamin D-1,25, do not need supplementation and may be at risk of developing symptomatic hypercalcemia with supplementation [215]. In patients with a 24-h urine calcium higher than 250 mg, avoidance of exogenous vitamin D and calcium supplementation has been recommended [215]. It is also widely promulgated among patient advocacy groups that high-dose vitamin D supplementation may provoke flares of sarcoidosis although there are little data to confirm this association.

Using the smallest dose of glucocorticoid for the shortest duration possible is an important strategy to minimize osteoporosis risk. Bisphosphonate therapy has been shown to successfully prevent osteoporosis in corticosteroid-treated sarcoidosis patients [216]. Therefore, all patients with sarcoidosis beginning glucocorticoids with an expected duration of at least 3 months should be evaluated and counseled for other risk factors for osteoporosis, and bone density should be measured. In postmenopausal women and men over the age of 50 years, the risk of fracture should be determined using the FRAX tool [217], and low-risk patients on glucocorticoids $\geq$7.5 mg/daily or those in a medium- or high-risk FRAX category should be considered for bisphosphonate therapy. Patients in a high-risk category alternatively could be considered for teriparatide. Premenopausal women or men less than 50 should be evaluated for a preexisting fragility fracture as the FRAX is not valid in this patient population. Premenopausal women that are not of childbearing potential or men <50 years with a prevalent fragility fracture should be started on a bisphosphonate if they are treated with any dose of glucocorticoids for at least 1 month. Women of childbearing potential should be started on a bisphosphonate if there is a planned prednisone dose of at least 7.5 mg daily for at least 3 months. There is no consensus for women of childbearing potential with less than 3 months of glucocorticoid duration, and there are no data to inform treatment recommendations for premenopausal women or men <50 years without a fragility fracture [218].

Conclusion

Sarcoidosis is a multisystem disease, implying that diagnosis and management often entail a team approach. Attempts to compartmentalize patients with sarcoidosis into separate organ systems are likely to lead to mistakes in pattern recognition and fragmentation of therapeutic priorities. Collaboration between rheumatologists and pulmonologists can facilitate comprehensive care of patients with sarcoidosis.

When managing patients with sarcoidosis, it is important to confirm the diagnosis and assess which aspects of the patient's symptoms relate to active sarcoidosis. A number of consequences of sarcoidosis, such as sleep apnea and pulmonary hypertension, may be more important contributors to morbidity than is active granulomatous inflammation. Therapy should be tailored to each patient, considering the expected disease course, the patient's comorbidities, and the impact of the sarcoidosis on either organ function or quality of life. In general, steroid-sparing therapies should be instituted with increasing alacrity as the burden of poor prognostic features, steroid toxicities, and chronicity of disease mounts.

Case Vignette

A 49-year-old female was evaluated for a 3-month history of fatigue, cough, arthralgias involving the hands and ankles and mild exertional dyspnea. Her past medical history was remarkable only for a history of diet-controlled diabetes, depression, and obesity. She had a single episode of renal lithiasis 5 years previously. She was a never smoker, and she drank alcohol only on social occasions several times a year. She worked as a claims processor for an insurance company. There were no relevant exposures except for an indoor hot tub that she used regularly during the cooler months. She did not notice worsening respiratory symptoms after using the hot tub.

Her physical exam was unremarkable, with no evidence of peripheral lymph node enlargement, normal cardiopulmonary exam, normal abdominal exam, and no joint abnormalities. Her complete metabolic panel, complete blood count, thyroid-stimulating hormone, rheumatoid factor, ESR, and CRP level were all within normal limits. Here ANA was weakly positive (1:80 titer) in a speckled pattern, but her extractable nuclear antigen panel was negative. Her 25-OH-vitamin D level was 17 ng/mL. A chest radiograph showed bilateral hilar prominence and mid-lung zone predominant infiltrates (Fig. 9.12). Ultrasound-guided bronchoscopic transbronchial needle aspiration of the enlarged lymph nodes revealed granulomatous inflammation; a transbronchial biopsy also demonstrated well-formed non-necrotizing granulomas in the bronchiolar mucosa. Special stains and cultures were negative. A diagnosis of sarcoidosis was conferred.

Discussion

As mentioned previously, the management of sarcoidosis requires careful consideration of the accuracy of the diagnosis, assessment of the extent of organ involvement, and

(continued)

Case Vignette (continued)

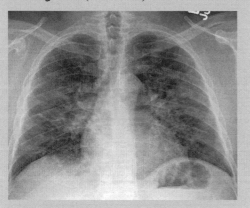

Fig. 9.12 Posteroanterior chest radiograph demonstrating bilateral reticulonodular infiltrates predominantly in the mid-lung zones. There is also bilateral hilar lymph node enlargement

determination of the goals of therapeutic intervention. In this case, there were some features that should lead to reconsideration of the diagnosis. The history of hot tub exposure suggests an alternate potential cause for granulomatous pulmonary inflammation—i.e., "hot tub lung," caused by a hypersensitivity reaction to inhaled nontuberculous mycobacteria. Finding granulomatous inflammation without obvious infectious triggers on needle aspirate specimens from intrathoracic lymph nodes does not conclusively establish a diagnosis of sarcoidosis, since lymph node granulomas can be reactive from several diseases that affect the lung parenchyma, including hypersensitivity pneumonitis. However, the diagnosis of sarcoidosis was secured in this case by the addition of transbronchial biopsies, which were typical of sarcoidosis. In the case of hot tub lung, granulomas would be expected to be less well formed, with more interstitial infiltrates and also with more substantial neutrophilic inflammation. Establishing the diagnosis required careful discussion between the bronchoscopist, the pulmonologist, and the pathologist.

The assessment of sarcoidosis in this case included a complete ophthalmologic exam, PFTs, and a 24-h urine calcium measurement, given the history of renal lithiasis. The 24-urine calcium excretion was 393 mg/day (normal 100–250 mg/day). The PFTs showed mild obstruction without a bronchodilator response (FEV1 74 % predicted). Consultation with a rheumatology colleague was requested to evaluate the cause of the arthralgias, the significance of the elevated ANA, and to assist with management of the calcium derangements. The rheumatologist found no evidence of an alternate explanation for the arthralgias and no features to establish a diagnosis of a connective tissue disorder related to the elevated ANA. Further laboratory testing ordered by the rheumatologist demonstrated an elevated 1,25 dihydroxyvitamin D level (86 pg/mL) and evidence of osteoporosis at the hip (T-score −2.7).

The management of sarcoidosis in this case required collaboration between the considerations of how aggressively to treat the lungs and the arthralgias, the management of the calcium metabolism issues, and the comorbidities of the patient. Importantly, the patient was adamant about avoiding potential toxicities of oral corticosteroids but was also so severely affected by the arthralgias that her daily activities were hampered. After discussion, she was treated with a combination of high-dose inhaled budesonide (1,600 mcg/day) and oral hydroxychloroquine (400 mg/day). An oral bisphosphonate agent was started without supplemental calcium or exogenous vitamin D. After 4 weeks, her cough was substantially improved, but her pulmonary function testing remained unchanged. Her repeat 24-h urine calcium level was 218 mg/day. Her 1,25 dihydroxyvitamin D level was now 62 pg/mL, with a 25-OH-vitamin D level of 15 ng/mL. Her arthralgias were moderately improved, to the degree that they no longer interfered with her quality of life. Her rheumatologist started low-dose vitamin D and calcium supplementation,

(continued)

Case Vignette (continued)

with careful follow-up to ensure that the hydroxychloroquine was maintaining control of her deranged vitamin D metabolism. A discussion with the patient led to a decision not to escalate therapy just for the purpose of trying to normalize her lung function and chest radiograph. Rather, it was determined that serial observation of pulmonary symptoms and PFTs would be sufficient to manage her pulmonary sarcoidosis. Of note, she was successfully managed without any measurements of serum ACE or other putative serological markers of disease activity.

In this case, it is clear that multiple competing priorities, including the patient's own preferences, needed to be considered for management of sarcoidosis. Ongoing longitudinal collaboration between the pulmonologist and rheumatologist will be necessary to provide comprehensive care for this individual.

References

1. James DG. Descriptive definition and historic aspects of sarcoidosis. Clin Chest Med. 1997;18: 663–79.
2. Hunninghake GW, Costabel U, Ando M, et al. ATS/ERS/WASOG statement on sarcoidosis. American Thoracic Society/European Respiratory Society/World Association of Sarcoidosis and other granulomatous disorders. Sarcoidosis Vasc Diffuse Lung Dis. 1999;16:149–73.
3. Bresnitz EA, Strom BL. Epidemiology of sarcoidosis. Epidemiol Rev. 1983;5:124–56.
4. Mayock RL, Bertrand P, Morrison CE, et al. Manifestations of sarcoidosis. Analysis of 145 patients, with a review of nine series selected from the literature. Am J Med. 1963;35:67–89.
5. Edmondstone WM, Wilson AG. Sarcoidosis in Caucasians, Blacks and Asians in London. Br J Dis Chest. 1985;79:27–36.
6. Siltzbach LE, James DG, Neville E, et al. Course and prognosis of sarcoidosis around the world. Am J Med. 1974;57:847–52.
7. Rybicki BA, Major M, Popovich Jr J, et al. Racial differences in sarcoidosis incidence: a 5-year study in a health maintenance organization. Am J Epidemiol. 1997;145:234–41.

8. Keller AZ. Hospital, age, racial, occupational, geographical, clinical and survivorship characteristics in the epidemiology of sarcoidosis. Am J Epidemiol. 1971;94:222–30.
9. McNicol MW, Luce PJ. Sarcoidosis in a racially mixed community. J R Coll Physicians Lond. 1985;19:179–83.
10. Baughman RP, Teirstein AS, Judson MA, et al. Clinical characteristics of patients in a case control study of sarcoidosis. Am J Respir Crit Care Med. 2001;164:1885–9.
11. Gideon NM, Mannino DM. Sarcoidosis mortality in the United States 1979–1991: an analysis of multiple-cause mortality data. Am J Med. 1996;100: 423–7.
12. Hosoda Y, Yamaguchi M, Hiraga Y. Global epidemiology of sarcoidosis. What story do prevalence and incidence tell us? Clin Chest Med. 1997;18:681–94.
13. Reid JD. Sarcoidosis in coroner's autopsies: a critical evaluation of diagnosis and prevalence from Cuyahoga County, Ohio. Sarcoidosis Vasc Diffuse Lung Dis. 1998;15:44–51.
14. Henke CE, Henke G, Elveback LR, et al. The epidemiology of sarcoidosis in Rochester, Minnesota: a population-based study of incidence and survival. Am J Epidemiol. 1986;123:840–5.
15. Milman N, Selroos O. Pulmonary sarcoidosis in the Nordic countries 1950–1982. II. Course and prognosis. Sarcoidosis. 1990;7:113–8.
16. Hillerdal G, Nou E, Osterman K, et al. Sarcoidosis: epidemiology and prognosis. A 15-year European study. Am Rev Respir Dis. 1984;130:29–32.
17. Cozier YC, Berman JS, Palmer JR, et al. Sarcoidosis in black women in the United States: data from the Black Women's Health Study. Chest. 2011;139: 144–50.
18. James DG. Epidemiology of sarcoidosis. Sarcoidosis. 1992;9:79–87.
19. Culver DA, Thomassen MJ, Kavuru MS. Pulmonary sarcoidosis: new genetic clues and ongoing treatment controversies. Cleve Clin J Med. 2004;71:88. 90, 92 passim.
20. Culver DA, Newman LS, Kavuru MS. Gene-environment interactions in sarcoidosis: challenge and opportunity. Clin Dermatol. 2007;25:267–75.
21. Newman KL, Newman LS. Occupational causes of sarcoidosis. Curr Opin Allergy Clin Immunol. 2012;12:145–50.
22. Gentry JT, Nitowsky HM, Michael Jr M. Studies on the epidemiology of sarcoidosis in the United States: the relationship to soil areas and to urban–rural residence. J Clin Invest. 1955;34:1839–56.
23. Newman LS, Rose CS, Bresnitz EA, et al. A case control etiologic study of sarcoidosis: environmental and occupational risk factors. Am J Respir Crit Care Med. 2004;170:1324–30.
24. Rybicki BA, Amend KL, Maliarik MJ, et al. Photocopier exposure and risk of sarcoidosis in African-American sibs. Sarcoidosis Vasc Diffuse Lung Dis. 2004;21:49–55.

25. Kajdasz DK, Lackland DT, Mohr LC, et al. A current assessment of rurally linked exposures as potential risk factors for sarcoidosis. Ann Epidemiol. 2001;11: 111–7.

26. Song Z, Marzilli L, Greenlee BM, et al. Mycobacterial catalase-peroxidase is a tissue antigen and target of the adaptive immune response in systemic sarcoidosis. J Exp Med. 2005;201:755–67.

27. Oswald-Richter KA, Culver DA, Hawkins C, et al. Cellular responses to mycobacterial antigens are present in bronchoalveolar lavage fluid used in the diagnosis of sarcoidosis. Infect Immun. 2009;77: 3740–8.

28. Chen ES, Wahlstrom J, Song Z, et al. T cell responses to mycobacterial catalase-peroxidase profile a pathogenic antigen in systemic sarcoidosis. J Immunol. 2008;181:8784–96.

29. Drake W, Richmond BW, Oswald-Richter K, et al. Effects of broad-spectrum antimycobacterial therapy on chronic pulmonary sarcoidosis. Sarcoidosis Vasc Diffuse Lung Dis. 2013;30:201–11.

30. Drake WP, Oswald-Richter K, Richmond BW, et al. Oral antimycobacterial therapy in chronic cutaneous sarcoidosis: a randomized, single-masked, placebo-controlled study. JAMA Dermatol. 2013;149:1040–9.

31. Chen ES, Song Z, Willett MH, et al. Serum amyloid A regulates granulomatous inflammation in sarcoidosis through Toll-like receptor-2. Am J Respir Crit Care Med. 2010;181:360–73.

32. Eishi Y. Etiologic link between sarcoidosis and Propionibacterium acnes. Respir Investig. 2013;51:56–68.

33. Oswald-Richter KA, Beachboard DC, Seeley EH, et al. Dual analysis for mycobacteria and propionibacteria in sarcoidosis BAL. J Clin Immunol. 2012;32:1129–40.

34. Culver DA. What is sarcoidosis? Respir Med. 2013;107:1285–6.

35. Grunewald J. Review: role of genetics in susceptibility and outcome of sarcoidosis. Semin Respir Crit Care Med. 2010;31:380–9.

36. Sverrild A, Backer V, Kyvik KO, et al. Heredity in sarcoidosis: a registry-based twin study. Thorax. 2008;63:894–6.

37. Rybicki BA, Iannuzzi MC, Frederick MM, et al. Familial aggregation of sarcoidosis. A case–control etiologic study of sarcoidosis (ACCESS). Am J Respir Crit Care Med. 2001;164:2085–91.

38. McGrath DS, Daniil Z, Foley P, et al. Epidemiology of familial sarcoidosis in the UK. Thorax. 2000;55:751–4.

39. Rossman MD, Thompson B, Frederick M, et al. HLA-DRB1*1101: a significant risk factor for sarcoidosis in blacks and whites. Am J Hum Genet. 2003;73:720–35.

40. Spagnolo P, Grunewald J. Recent advances in the genetics of sarcoidosis. J Med Genet. 2013;50:290–7.

41. Culver DA, Costabel U. EBUS-TBNA for the diagnosis of sarcoidosis: is it the only game in town? J Bronchology Interv Pulmonol. 2013;20:195–7.

42. Baughman RP, Culver DA, Judson MA. A concise review of pulmonary sarcoidosis. Am J Respir Crit Care Med. 2011;183:573–81.

43. Grunewald J, Eklund A. Sex-specific manifestations of Lofgren's syndrome. Am J Respir Crit Care Med. 2007;175:40–4.

44. Highland KB, Retalis P, Coppage L, et al. Is there an anatomic explanation for chest pain in patients with pulmonary sarcoidosis? South Med J. 1997;90:911–4.

45. Judson MA, Thompson BW, Rabin DL, et al. The diagnostic pathway to sarcoidosis. Chest. 2003;123:406–12.

46. Sweiss NJ, Patterson K, Sawaqed R, et al. Rheumatologic manifestations of sarcoidosis. Semin Respir Crit Care Med. 2010;31:463–73.

47. Yanardag H, Caner M, Papila I, et al. Diagnostic value of peripheral lymph node biopsy in sarcoidosis: a report of 67 cases. Can Respir J. 2007;14:209–11.

48. Culver DA. Sarcoidosis. Immunol Allergy Clin North Am. 2012;32:487–511.

49. Fireman E, Haimsky E, Noiderfer M, et al. Misdiagnosis of sarcoidosis in patients with chronic beryllium disease. Sarcoidosis Vasc Diffuse Lung Dis. 2003;20:144–8.

50. Studdy PR, Lapworth R, Bird R. Angiotensin-converting enzyme and its clinical significance—a review. J Clin Pathol. 1983;36:938–47.

51. Lieberman J, Nosal A, Schlessner A, et al. Serum angiotensin-converting enzyme for diagnosis and therapeutic evaluation of sarcoidosis. Am Rev Respir Dis. 1979;120:329–35.

52. Borowsky SA, Lieberman J, Strome S, et al. Elevation of serum angiotensin—converting enzyme level. Occurrence in alcoholic liver disease. Arch Intern Med. 1982;142:893–5.

53. Ainslie GM, Benatar SR. Serum angiotensin converting enzyme in sarcoidosis: sensitivity and specificity in diagnosis: correlations with disease activity, duration, extra-thoracic involvement, radiographic type and therapy. Q J Med. 1985;55:253–70.

54. Biller H, Zissel G, Ruprecht B, et al. Genotype-corrected reference values for serum angiotensin-converting enzyme. Eur Respir J. 2006;28:1085–90.

55. Bargagli E, Bennett D, Maggiorelli C, et al. Human chitotriosidase: a sensitive biomarker of sarcoidosis. J Clin Immunol. 2013;33:264–70.

56. Bargagli E, Bianchi N, Margollicci M, et al. Chitotriosidase and soluble IL-2 receptor: comparison of two markers of sarcoidosis severity. Scand J Clin Lab Invest. 2008;68:479–83.

57. Rothkrantz-Kos S, van Dieijen-Visser MP, Mulder PG, et al. Potential usefulness of inflammatory markers to monitor respiratory functional impairment in sarcoidosis. Clin Chem. 2003;49:1510–7.

58. Studdy PR, Bird R, Neville E, et al. Biochemical findings in sarcoidosis. J Clin Pathol. 1980;33: 528–33.

59. Hedfors E, Holm G, Pettersson D. Lymphocyte subpopulations in sarcoidosis. Clin Exp Immunol. 1974;17:219–26.

60. Winterbauer RH, Belic N, Moores KD. Clinical interpretation of bilateral hilar adenopathy. Ann Intern Med. 1973;78:65–71.

61. Reich JM, Brouns MC, O'Connor EA, et al. Mediastinoscopy in patients with presumptive stage I sarcoidosis: a risk/benefit, cost/benefit analysis. Chest. 1998;113:147–53.

62. Teirstein AS, Machac J, Almeida O, et al. Results of 188 whole-body fluorodeoxyglucose positron emission tomography scans in 137 patients with sarcoidosis. Chest. 2007;132:1949–53.

63. Keijsers RG, Grutters JC, Thomeer M, et al. Imaging the inflammatory activity of sarcoidosis: sensitivity and inter observer agreement of (67)Ga imaging and (18)F-FDG PET. Q J Nucl Med Mol Imaging. 2011;55:66–71.

64. Teirstein AS, Judson MA, Baughman RP, et al. The spectrum of biopsy sites for the diagnosis of sarcoidosis. Sarcoidosis Vasc Diffuse Lung Dis. 2005;22:139–46.

65. Agarwal R, Aggarwal AN, Gupta D. Efficacy and safety of conventional TBNA in sarcoidosis: a systematic review and meta-analysis. Respir Care. 2013;58(4):683–93.

66. von Bartheld MB, Dekkers OM, Szlubowski A, et al. Endosonography vs conventional bronchoscopy for the diagnosis of sarcoidosis: the GRANULOMA randomized clinical trial. JAMA. 2013;309:2457–64.

67. Costabel U, Bonella F, Ohshimo S, et al. Diagnostic modalities in sarcoidosis: BAL, EBUS, and PET. Semin Respir Crit Care Med. 2010;31:404–8.

68. Trisolini R, Lazzari Agli L, Cancellieri A, et al. The value of flexible transbronchial needle aspiration in the diagnosis of stage I sarcoidosis. Chest. 2003;124:2126–30.

69. Shorr AF, Torrington KG, Hnatiuk OW. Endobronchial biopsy for sarcoidosis: a prospective study. Chest. 2001;120:109–14.

70. Bilaceroglu S, Perim K, Gunel O, et al. Combining transbronchial aspiration with endobronchial and transbronchial biopsy in sarcoidosis. Monaldi Arch Chest Dis. 1999;54:217–23.

71. Plit M, Pearson R, Havryk A, et al. Diagnostic utility of endobronchial ultrasound-guided transbronchial needle aspiration compared with transbronchial and endobronchial biopsy for suspected sarcoidosis. Intern Med J. 2012;42:434–8.

72. Nagai S, Izumi T. Bronchoalveolar lavage. Still useful in diagnosing sarcoidosis? Clin Chest Med. 1997;18:787–97.

73. Meyer KC, Raghu G, Baughman RP, et al. An official American Thoracic Society clinical practice guideline: the clinical utility of bronchoalveolar lavage cellular analysis in interstitial lung disease. Am J Respir Crit Care Med. 2012;185:1004–14.

74. Rosen Y, Vuletin JC, Pertschuk LP, et al. Sarcoidosis: from the pathologist's vantage point. Pathol Annu. 1979;14(Pt 1):405–39.

75. Ohara K, Okubo A, Kamata K, et al. Transbronchial lung biopsy in the diagnosis of suspected ocular sarcoidosis. Arch Ophthalmol. 1993;111:642–4.

76. Sartin JS, Walker RC. Granulomatous hepatitis: a retrospective review of 88 cases at the Mayo Clinic. Mayo Clin Proc. 1991;66:914–8.

77. Morimoto Y, Routes JM. Granulomatous disease in common variable immunodeficiency. Curr Allergy Asthma Rep. 2005;5:370–5.

78. Brincker H. Granulomatous lesions of unknown significance: the GLUS syndrome. In: James D, editor. Sarcoidosis and other granulomatous disorders. New York: Marcel Dekker; 1994. p. 69–76.

79. Judson MA. The diagnosis of sarcoidosis. Clin Chest Med. 2008;29:415–27. viii.

80. Rose CD, Martin TM, Wouters CH. Blau syndrome revisited. Curr Opin Rheumatol. 2011;23:411–8.

81. Wallaert B, Ramon P, Fournier EC, et al. Activated alveolar macrophage and lymphocyte alveolitis in extrathoracic sarcoidosis without radiological mediastinopulmonary involvement. Ann N Y Acad Sci. 1986;465:201–10.

82. Baughman RP, Shipley R, Desai S, et al. Changes in chest roentgenogram of sarcoidosis patients during a clinical trial of infliximab therapy: comparison of different methods of evaluation. Chest. 2009;136(2):526–35.

83. Bergin CJ, Bell DY, Coblentz CL, et al. Sarcoidosis: correlation of pulmonary parenchymal pattern at CT with results of pulmonary function tests. Radiology. 1989;171:619–24.

84. Scadding JG. Prognosis of intrathoracic sarcoidosis in England. A review of 136 cases after five years' observation. Br Med J. 1961;5261:1165–72.

85. Baughman RP, Drent M, Culver DA, et al. Endpoints for clinical trials of sarcoidosis. Sarcoidosis Vasc Diffuse Lung Dis. 2012;29:90–8.

86. Lynch III JP, Ma YL, Koss MN, et al. Pulmonary sarcoidosis. Semin Respir Crit Care Med. 2007;28:53–74.

87. Sharma OP, Johnson R. Airway obstruction in sarcoidosis. A study of 123 nonsmoking black American patients with sarcoidosis. Chest. 1988;94:343–6.

88. Harrison BD, Shaylor JM, Stokes TC, et al. Airflow limitation in sarcoidosis—a study of pulmonary function in 107 patients with newly diagnosed disease. Respir Med. 1991;85:59–64.

89. Shorr AF, Torrington KG, Hnatiuk OW. Endobronchial involvement and airway hyperreactivity in patients with sarcoidosis. Chest. 2001;120:881–6.

90. Mihailovic-Vucinic V, Zugic V, Videnovic-Ivanov J. New observations on pulmonary function changes in sarcoidosis. Curr Opin Pulm Med. 2003;9:436–41.

91. Lynch III JP, Kazerooni EA, Gay SE. Pulmonary sarcoidosis. Clin Chest Med. 1997;18:755–85.

92. Marcellis RG, Lenssen AF, Elfferich MD, et al. Exercise capacity, muscle strength and fatigue in sarcoidosis. Eur Respir J. 2011;38:628–34.

93. Spruit MA, Thomeer MJ, Gosselink R, et al. Skeletal muscle weakness in patients with sarcoidosis and its relationship with exercise intolerance and reduced health status. Thorax. 2005;60:32–8.

94. Panselinas E, Halstead L, Schlosser RJ, et al. Clinical manifestations, radiographic findings, treatment options, and outcome in sarcoidosis patients with upper respiratory tract involvement. South Med J. 2010;103:870–5.

95. Aubart FC, Ouayoun M, Brauner M, et al. Sinonasal involvement in sarcoidosis: a case–control study of 20 patients. Medicine (Baltimore). 2006;85:365–71.

96. McCaffrey TV, McDonald TJ. Sarcoidosis of the nose and paranasal sinuses. Laryngoscope. 1983;93: 1281–4.

97. Yanardag H, Enoz M, Papila I, et al. Upper respiratory tract involvement of sarcoidosis in the Turkish population. Otolaryngol Head Neck Surg. 2006;134:848–51.

98. Carasso B. Sarcoidosis of the larynx causing airway obstruction. Chest. 1974;65:693–5.

99. Krespi YP, Mitrani M, Husain S, et al. Treatment of laryngeal sarcoidosis with intralesional steroid injection. Ann Otol Rhinol Laryngol. 1987;96:713–5.

100. Marks SC, Goodman RS. Surgical management of nasal and sinus sarcoidosis. Otolaryngol Head Neck Surg. 1998;118:856–8.

101. Neville E, Mills RG, Jash DK, et al. Sarcoidosis of the upper respiratory tract and its association with lupus pernio. Thorax. 1976;31:660–4.

102. Neville E, Walker AN, James DG. Prognostic factors predicting the outcome of sarcoidosis: an analysis of 818 patients. Q J Med. 1983;52:525–33.

103. Viskum K, Vestbo J. Vital prognosis in intrathoracic sarcoidosis with special reference to pulmonary function and radiological stage. Eur Respir J. 1993; 6:349–53.

104. Chambellan A, Turbie P, Nunes H, et al. Endoluminal stenosis of proximal bronchi in sarcoidosis: bronchoscopy, function, and evolution. Chest. 2005;127: 472–81.

105. Udwadia ZF, Pilling JR, Jenkins PF, et al. Bronchoscopic and bronchographic findings in 12 patients with sarcoidosis and severe or progressive airways obstruction. Thorax. 1990;45:272–5.

106. Davies CW, Tasker AD, Padley SP, et al. Air trapping in sarcoidosis on computed tomography: correlation with lung function. Clin Radiol. 2000;55: 217–21.

107. Lavergne F, Clerici C, Sadoun D, et al. Airway obstruction in bronchial sarcoidosis: outcome with treatment. Chest. 1999;116:1194–9.

108. Polychronopoulos VS, Prakash UB. Airway involvement in sarcoidosis. Chest. 2009;136:1371–80.

109. Battesti JP, Georges R, Basset F, et al. Chronic cor pulmonale in pulmonary sarcoidosis. Thorax. 1978;33:76–84.

110. Gluskowski J, Hawrylkiewicz I, Zych D, et al. Pulmonary haemodynamics at rest and during exercise in patients with sarcoidosis. Respiration. 1984;46:26–32.

111. Preston IR, Klinger JR, Landzberg MJ, et al. Vasoresponsiveness of sarcoidosis-associated pulmonary hypertension. Chest. 2001;120:866–72.

112. Shorr AF, Helman DL, Davies DB, et al. Pulmonary hypertension in advanced sarcoidosis: epidemiology and clinical characteristics. Eur Respir J. 2005;25: 783–8.

113. Emirgil C, Sobol BJ, Herbert WH, et al. The lesser circulation in pulmonary fibrosis secondary to sarcoidosis and its relationship to respiratory function. Chest. 1971;60:371–8.

114. Baughman RP, Engel PJ, Taylor L, et al. Survival in sarcoidosis-associated pulmonary hypertension: the importance of hemodynamic evaluation. Chest. 2010;138:1078–85.

115. Arcasoy SM, Christie JD, Pochettino A, et al. Characteristics and outcomes of patients with sarcoidosis listed for lung transplantation. Chest. 2001;120:873–80.

116. Diaz-Guzman E, Farver C, Parambil J, et al. Pulmonary hypertension caused by sarcoidosis. Clin Chest Med. 2008;29:549–63.

117. Sulica R, Teirstein AS, Kakarla S, et al. Distinctive clinical, radiographic, and functional characteristics of patients with sarcoidosis-related pulmonary hypertension. Chest. 2005;128:1483–9.

118. Swigris JJ, Olson AL, Huie TJ, et al. Increased risk of pulmonary embolism among US decedents with sarcoidosis from 1988 to 2007. Chest. 2011;140:1261–6.

119. Bourbonnais JM, Samavati L. Clinical predictors of pulmonary hypertension in sarcoidosis. Eur Respir J. 2008;32:296–302.

120. Gluskowski J, Hawrylkiewicz I, Zych D, et al. Effects of corticosteroid treatment on pulmonary haemodynamics in patients with sarcoidosis. Eur Respir J. 1990;3:403–7.

121. Baughman RP, Culver DA, Cordova FC, et al. Bosentan for sarcoidosis associated pulmonary hypertension: a double-blind placebo controlled randomized trial. Chest. 2013 Oct 31. doi: 10.1378/chest.13-1766.

122. Baughman RP, Judson MA, Lower EE, et al. Inhaled iloprost for sarcoidosis associated pulmonary hypertension. Sarcoidosis Vasc Diffuse Lung Dis. 2009;26:110–20.

123. Barnett CF, Bonura EJ, Nathan SD, et al. Treatment of sarcoidosis-associated pulmonary hypertension. A two-center experience. Chest. 2009;135:1455–61.

124. Soskel NT, Sharma OP. Pleural involvement in sarcoidosis. Curr Opin Pulm Med. 2000;6:455–68.

125. De Vuyst P, De Troyer A, Yernault JC. Bloody pleural effusion in a patient with sarcoidosis. Chest. 1979;76:607–9.

126. Aberg H, Bah M, Waters AW. Sarcoidosis: complicated by chylothorax. Minn Med. 1966;49:1065–70.

127. Poe RH. Middle-lobe atelectasis due to sarcoidosis with pleural effusion. N Y State J Med. 1978;78:2095–7.

128. Chusid EL, Siltzbach LE. Sarcoidosis of the pleura. Ann Intern Med. 1974;81:190–4.

129. Beekman JF, Zimmet SM, Chun BK, et al. Spectrum of pleural involvement in sarcoidosis. Arch Intern Med. 1976;136:323–30.

130. Huggins JT, Doelken P, Sahn SA, et al. Pleural effusions in a series of 181 outpatients with sarcoidosis. Chest. 2006;129:1599–604.

131. Judson MA, Boan AD, Lackland DT. The clinical course of sarcoidosis: presentation, diagnosis, and treatment in a large white and black cohort in the United States. Sarcoidosis Vasc Diffuse Lung Dis. 2012;29:119–27.

132. Johns CJ, Michele TM. The clinical management of sarcoidosis. A 50-year experience at the Johns Hopkins Hospital. Medicine (Baltimore). 1999;78: 65–111.

133. Hours S, Nunes H, Kambouchner M, et al. Pulmonary cavitary sarcoidosis: clinico-radiologic characteristics and natural history of a rare form of sarcoidosis. Medicine (Baltimore). 2008;87:142–51.

134. Jewkes J, Kay PH, Paneth M, et al. Pulmonary aspergilloma: analysis of prognosis in relation to haemoptysis and survey of treatment. Thorax. 1983;38:572–8.

135. Rockoff SD, Rohatgi PK. Unusual manifestations of thoracic sarcoidosis. AJR Am J Roentgenol. 1985;144:513–28.

136. Rubinstein I, Baum GL, Rosenthal T. Fungal infections complicating pulmonary sarcoidosis. J Infect Dis. 1985;152:1360.

137. Waldhorn RE, Tsou E, Kerwin DM. Invasive pulmonary aspergillosis associated with aspergilloma in sarcoidosis. South Med J. 1983;76:251–3.

138. Stevens DA, Kan VL, Judson MA, et al. Practice guidelines for diseases caused by Aspergillus. Infectious Diseases Society of America. Clin Infect Dis. 2000;30:696–709.

139. Jackson M, Flower CD, Shneerson JM. Treatment of symptomatic pulmonary aspergillomas with intracavitary instillation of amphotericin B through an indwelling catheter. Thorax. 1993;48:928–30.

140. Kravitz JN, Steed LL, Judson MA. Intracavitary voriconazole for the treatment of hemoptysis complicating Pseudallescheria angusta pulmonary mycetomas in fibrocystic sarcoidosis. Med Mycol. 2011;49:198–201.

141. Dar MA, Ahmad M, Weinstein AJ, et al. Thoracic aspergillosis (Part I). Overview and aspergilloma. Cleve Clin Q. 1984;51:615–30.

142. Crawshaw AP, Wotton CJ, Yeates DG, et al. Evidence for association between sarcoidosis and pulmonary embolism from 35-year record linkage study. Thorax. 2011;66:447–8.

143. Perez RL, Duncan A, Hunter RL, et al. Elevated D dimer in the lungs and blood of patients with sarcoidosis. Chest. 1993;103:1100–6.

144. Turner GA, Lower EE, Corser BC, et al. Sleep apnea in sarcoidosis. Sarcoidosis Vasc Diffuse Lung Dis. 1997;14:61–4.

145. Patterson KC, Huang F, Oldham JM, et al. Excessive daytime sleepiness and obstructive sleep apnea in patients with sarcoidosis. Chest. 2013;143:1562–8.

146. de Kleijn WP, De Vries J, Lower EE, et al. Fatigue in sarcoidosis: a systematic review. Curr Opin Pulm Med. 2009;15(5):499–506.

147. Chowdhury FU, Sheerin F, Bradley KM, et al. Sarcoid-like reaction to malignancy on whole-body integrated (18)F-FDG PET/CT: prevalence and disease pattern. Clin Radiol. 2009;64:675–81.

148. Le Jeune I, Gribbin J, West J, et al. The incidence of cancer in patients with idiopathic pulmonary fibrosis and sarcoidosis in the UK. Respir Med. 2007;101:2534–40.

149. Brincker H, Wilbek E. The incidence of malignant tumours in patients with respiratory sarcoidosis. Br J Cancer. 1974;29:247–51.

150. Askling J, Grunewald J, Eklund A, et al. Increased risk for cancer following sarcoidosis. Am J Respir Crit Care Med. 1999;160:1668–72.

151. Gribbin J, Hubbard RB, Le Jeune I, et al. Incidence and mortality of idiopathic pulmonary fibrosis and sarcoidosis in the UK. Thorax. 2006;61:980–5.

152. Swigris JJ, Olson AL, Huie TJ, et al. Sarcoidosis-related mortality in the United States from 1988 to 2007. Am J Respir Crit Care Med. 2011;183:1524–30.

153. Sekiguchi M, Yazaki Y, Isobe M, et al. Cardiac sarcoidosis: diagnostic, prognostic, and therapeutic considerations. Cardiovasc Drugs Ther. 1996;10:495–510.

154. Iannuzzi MC, Rybicki BA, Teirstein AS. Sarcoidosis. N Engl J Med. 2007;357:2153–65.

155. Nagai S, Shigematsu M, Hamada K, et al. Clinical courses and prognoses of pulmonary sarcoidosis. Curr Opin Pulm Med. 1999;5:293–8.

156. Judson MA, Baughman RP, Thompson BW, et al. Two year prognosis of sarcoidosis: the ACCESS experience. Sarcoidosis Vasc Diffuse Lung Dis. 2003;20:204–11.

157. Chappell AG, Cheung WY, Hutchings HA. Sarcoidosis: a long-term follow up study. Sarcoidosis Vasc Diffuse Lung Dis. 2000;17:167–73.

158. Mana J, Salazar A, Manresa F. Clinical factors predicting persistence of activity in sarcoidosis: a multivariate analysis of 193 cases. Respiration. 1994;61:219–25.

159. Baughman RP, Judson MA, Teirstein A, et al. Presenting characteristics as predictors of duration of treatment in sarcoidosis. QJM. 2006;99:307–15.

160. Baughman RP, Nagai S, Balter M, et al. Defining the clinical outcome status (COS) in sarcoidosis: results of the WASOG task force. Sarcoidosis Vasc Diffuse Lung Dis. 2011;28:56–64.

161. Akira M, Kozuka T, Inoue Y, et al. Long-term follow-up CT scan evaluation in patients with pulmonary sarcoidosis. Chest. 2005;127:185–91.

162. Baughman RP, Winget DB, Bowen EH, et al. Predicting respiratory failure in sarcoidosis patients. Sarcoidosis Vasc Diffuse Lung Dis. 1997;14:154–8.

163. Brauner MW, Lenoir S, Grenier P, et al. Pulmonary sarcoidosis: CT assessment of lesion reversibility. Radiology. 1992;182:349–54.

164. Lazar CA, Culver DA. Treatment of sarcoidosis. Semin Respir Crit Care Med. 2010;31:501–18.

165. Hunninghake GW, Gilbert S, Pueringer R, et al. Outcome of the treatment for sarcoidosis. Am J Respir Crit Care Med. 1994;149:893–8.

166. Grunewald J, Eklund A. Lofgren's syndrome: human leukocyte antigen strongly influence the disease course. Am J Respir Crit Care Med. 2009;179(4):307–12.

167. Gottlieb JE, Israel HL, Steiner RM, et al. Outcome in sarcoidosis. The relationship of relapse to corticosteroid therapy. Chest. 1997;111:623–31.

168. Alberts C, van der Mark TW, Jansen HM. Inhaled budesonide in pulmonary sarcoidosis: a double-blind, placebo-controlled study. Dutch Study Group on Pulmonary Sarcoidosis. Eur Respir J. 1995;8: 682–8.

169. Erkkila S, Froseth B, Hellstrom PE, et al. Inhaled budesonide influences cellular and biochemical abnormalities in pulmonary sarcoidosis. Sarcoidosis. 1988;5:106–10.

170. Milman N, Graudal N, Grode G, et al. No effect of high-dose inhaled steroids in pulmonary sarcoidosis: a double-blind, placebo-controlled study. J Intern Med. 1994;236:285–90.

171. Zych D, Pawlicka L, Zielinski J. Inhaled budesonide vs prednisone in the maintenance treatment of pulmonary sarcoidosis. Sarcoidosis. 1993;10:56–61.

172. du Bois RM, Greenhalgh PM, Southcott AM, et al. Randomized trial of inhaled fluticasone propionate in chronic stable pulmonary sarcoidosis: a pilot study. Eur Respir J. 1999;13:1345–50.

173. Baughman RP, Iannuzzi MC, Lower EE, et al. Use of fluticasone in acute symptomatic pulmonary sarcoidosis. Sarcoidosis Vasc Diffuse Lung Dis. 2002;19:198–204.

174. Johns CJ, Schonfeld SA, Scott PP, et al. Longitudinal study of chronic sarcoidosis with low-dose maintenance corticosteroid therapy. Outcome and complications. Ann N Y Acad Sci. 1986;465:702–12.

175. Sweiss N, Yeager H. Sarcoidosis requiring systemic treatment: why not a steroid-sparing regimen upfront? Sarcoidosis Vasc Diffuse Lung Dis. 2010;27: 3–4.

176. Judson MA. An approach to the treatment of pulmonary sarcoidosis with corticosteroids: the six phases of treatment. Chest. 1999;115:1158–65.

177. Paramothayan NS, Lasserson TJ, Jones PW. Corticosteroids for pulmonary sarcoidosis. Cochrane Database Syst Rev. 2005:CD001114.

178. Schutt AC, Bullington WM, Judson MA. Pharmacotherapy for pulmonary sarcoidosis: a delphi consensus study. Respir Med. 2010;104(5): 717–23.

179. Paramothayan S, Jones PW. Corticosteroid therapy in pulmonary sarcoidosis: a systematic review. JAMA. 2002;287:1301–7.

180. Cox CE, Donohue JF, Brown CD, et al. Health-related quality of life of persons with sarcoidosis. Chest. 2004;125:997–1004.

181. Sharma OP. Pulmonary sarcoidosis and corticosteroids. Am Rev Respir Dis. 1993;147:1598–600.

182. Winterbauer RH, Kirtland SH, Corley DE. Treatment with corticosteroids. Clin Chest Med. 1997;18:843–51.

183. Goldstein DS, Williams MH. Rate of improvement of pulmonary function in sarcoidosis during treatment with corticosteroids. Thorax. 1986;41:473–4.

184. Siltzbach LE. Effects of cortisone in sarcoidosis; a study of thirteen patients. Am J Med. 1952;12: 139–60.

185. Baughman RP, Winget DB, Lower EE. Methotrexate is steroid sparing in acute sarcoidosis: results of a double blind, randomized trial. Sarcoidosis Vasc Diffuse Lung Dis. 2000;17:60–6.

186. Gibson GJ, Prescott RJ, Muers MF, et al. British Thoracic Society Sarcoidosis study: effects of long term corticosteroid treatment. Thorax. 1996;51: 238–47.

187. Vorselaars AD, Wuyts WA, Vorselaars VM, et al. Methotrexate versus azathioprine in second line therapy of sarcoidosis. Chest. 2013;144(3):805–12.

188. Baughman RP, Lower EE. A clinical approach to the use of methotrexate for sarcoidosis. Thorax. 1999; 54:742–6.

189. Lower EE, Baughman RP. Prolonged use of methotrexate for sarcoidosis. Arch Intern Med. 1995;155:846–51.

190. Webster GF, Razsi LK, Sanchez M, et al. Weekly low-dose methotrexate therapy for cutaneous sarcoidosis. J Am Acad Dermatol. 1991;24:451–4.

191. Cremers JP, Drent M, Bast A, et al. Multinational evidence-based World Association of Sarcoidosis and other granulomatous disorders recommendations for the use of methotrexate in sarcoidosis: integrating systematic literature research and expert opinion of sarcoidologists worldwide. Curr Opin Pulm Med. 2013;19:545–61.

192. Sahoo DH, Bandyopadhyay D, Xu M, et al. Effectiveness and safety of leflunomide for pulmonary and extrapulmonary sarcoidosis. Eur Respir J. 2011;38:1145–50.

193. Baughman RP, Lower EE. Leflunomide for chronic sarcoidosis. Sarcoidosis Vasc Diffuse Lung Dis. 2004;21:43–8.

194. Baltzan M, Mehta S, Kirkham TH, et al. Randomized trial of prolonged chloroquine therapy in advanced pulmonary sarcoidosis. Am J Respir Crit Care Med. 1999;160:192–7.

195. Kindler V, Sappino AP, Grau GE, et al. The inducing role of tumor necrosis factor in the development of bactericidal granulomas during BCG infection. Cell. 1989;56:731–40.

196. Marino MW, Dunn A, Grail D, et al. Characterization of tumor necrosis factor-deficient mice. Proc Natl Acad Sci U S A. 1997;94:8093–8.

197. Baughman RP, Drent M, Kavuru M, et al. Infliximab therapy in patients with chronic sarcoidosis and pulmonary involvement. Am J Respir Crit Care Med. 2006;174:795–802.

198. Erckens RJ, Mostard RL, Wijnen PA, et al. Adalimumab successful in sarcoidosis patients with refractory chronic non-infectious uveitis. Graefes Arch Clin Exp Ophthalmol. 2012;250:713–20.

199. Kamphuis LS, Lam-Tse WK, Dik WA, et al. Efficacy of adalimumab in chronically active and symptomatic patients with sarcoidosis. Am J Respir Crit Care Med. 2011;184:1214–6.

200. Milman N, Graudal N, Loft A, et al. Effect of the TNF-alpha inhibitor adalimumab in patients with recalcitrant sarcoidosis: a prospective observational study using FDG-PET. Clin Respir J. 2012;6(4): 238–47.

201. Nathan SD. Lung transplantation: disease-specific considerations for referral. Chest. 2005;127: 1006–16.

202. Christie JD, Edwards LB, Kucheryavaya AY, et al. The Registry of the International Society for Heart and Lung Transplantation: 29th adult lung and heart-lung transplant report-2012. J Heart Lung Transplant. 2012;31:1073–86.

203. Shorr AF, Helman DL, Davies DB, et al. Sarcoidosis, race, and short-term outcomes following lung transplantation. Chest. 2004;125:990–6.

204. Nunley DR, Hattler B, Keenan RJ, et al. Lung transplantation for end-stage pulmonary sarcoidosis. Sarcoidosis Vasc Diffuse Lung Dis. 1999;16: 93–100.

205. Milman N, Burton C, Andersen CB, et al. Lung transplantation for end-stage pulmonary sarcoidosis: outcome in a series of seven consecutive patients. Sarcoidosis Vasc Diffuse Lung Dis. 2005;22:222–8.

206. Ionescu DN, Hunt JL, Lomago D, et al. Recurrent sarcoidosis in lung transplant allografts: granulomas are of recipient origin. Diagn Mol Pathol. 2005;14: 140–5.

207. Padilla ML, Schilero GJ, Teirstein AS. Sarcoidosis and transplantation. Sarcoidosis Vasc Diffuse Lung Dis. 1997;14:16–22.

208. Johnson BA, Duncan SR, Ohori NP, et al. Recurrence of sarcoidosis in pulmonary allograft recipients. Am Rev Respir Dis. 1993;148:1373–7.

209. Heatly T, Sekela M, Berger R. Single lung transplantation involving a donor with documented pulmonary sarcoidosis. J Heart Lung Transplant. 1994;13:720–3.

210. Burke RR, Rybicki BA, Rao DS. Calcium and vitamin D in sarcoidosis: how to assess and manage. Semin Respir Crit Care Med. 2010;31:474–84.

211. James DG, Neville E, Siltzbach LE. A worldwide review of sarcoidosis. Ann N Y Acad Sci. 1976;278:321–34.

212. Muther RS, McCarron DA, Bennett WM. Renal manifestations of sarcoidosis. Arch Intern Med. 1981;141:643–5.

213. Rizzato G, Fraioli P. Natural and corticosteroid-induced osteoporosis in sarcoidosis: prevention, treatment, follow up and reversibility. Sarcoidosis. 1990;7:89–92.

214. Stoffels K, Overbergh L, Giulietti A, et al. Immune regulation of 25-hydroxyvitamin-D3-1alpha-hydroxylase in human monocytes. J Bone Miner Res. 2006;21:37–47.

215. Sweiss NJ, Lower EE, Korsten P, et al. Bone health issues in sarcoidosis. Curr Rheumatol Rep. 2011;13: 265–72.

216. Gonnelli S, Rottoli P, Cepollaro C, et al. Prevention of corticosteroid-induced osteoporosis with alendronate in sarcoid patients. Calcif Tissue Int. 1997;61:382–5.

217. FRAX. WHO Fracture Risk Assessment Tool, 2013.

218. Grossman JM, Gordon R, Ranganath VK, et al. American College of Rheumatology 2010 recommendations for the prevention and treatment of glucocorticoid-induced osteoporosis. Arthritis Care Res (Hoboken). 2010;62:1515–26.

Pulmonary Manifestations of Vasculitis

10

Ulrich Specks

Introduction

The term "pulmonary vasculitis" has been used in different ways. Primarily, it refers simply to inflammation of the walls of vessels of any size in the lower respiratory tract. The term is, however, also used for the systemic vasculitis syndromes that commonly or predominantly present with involvement of the respiratory tract, such as the vasculitis syndromes associated with antineutrophil cytoplasmic antibodies (ANCA). Pulmonary vasculitis is usually associated with a systemic disorder caused by a variety of immunologic mechanisms. In the context of a vasculitis syndrome, the lungs and lower airways can be affected by three major pathologic processes: (1) inflammatory cell infiltration and necrosis of the pulmonary parenchyma; (2) inflammation of the tracheobronchial tree often leading to stenoses; and (3) pulmonary capillaritis causing diffuse alveolar hemorrhage (DAH). Beyond capillaritis, inflammation of vessels of different sizes in the lung, including pulmonary arteries, veins, and bronchial arteries, are comparably rare manifestations of some unique vasculitis syndromes. Clinicians should also remember that not all respiratory symptoms occurring in patients

with vasculitis are caused by inflammation of pulmonary vessels or the underlying vasculitis syndrome, infection being the most important alternative diagnosis. This chapter reviews the pulmonary manifestations of the various vasculitis syndromes using the recently revised Chapel Hill Consensus definitions and nomenclature [1].

Pulmonary Manifestations of Small Vessel Vasculitis

ANCA-Associated Vasculitis

Microscopic polyangiitis (MPA), granulomatosis with polyangiitis (Wegener's; GPA), and eosinophilic granulomatosis with polyangiitis (Churg–Strauss; EGPA) are the three primary systemic small vessel vasculitis syndromes with prominent respiratory tract involvement [1]. In contrast to the other forms of vasculitis with predilections for larger vessels, most patients with active MPA and GPA as well as the majority of patients with active EGPA have ANCA. MPA and GPA will be discussed together as the same diagnostic and therapeutic principles apply. EGPA will be covered separately.

Microscopic Polyangiitis and Granulomatosis with Polyangiitis

MPA is defined as necrotizing vasculitis with few or no immune deposits, affecting small vessels

U. Specks, M.D. (✉)
Division of Pulmonary and Critical Care Medicine,
Mayo Clinic Rochester, 200 First Street SW,
Rochester, MN 55905, USA
e-mail: specks.ulrich@mayo.edu

P.F. Dellaripa et al. (eds.), *Pulmonary Manifestations of Rheumatic Disease: A Comprehensive Guide*,
DOI 10.1007/978-1-4939-0770-0_10, © Springer Science+Business Media New York 2014

including capillaries, venules, or arterioles (polyangiitis). Necrotizing arteritis involving small- and medium-sized arteries may be present. Necrotizing glomerulonephritis is very common; pulmonary capillaritis resulting in alveolar hemorrhage occurs frequently [1]. GPA is characterized by necrotizing granulomatous inflammation involving the respiratory tract and necrotizing vasculitis affecting small- to medium-sized vessels. The most commonly affected vessels are capillaries, venules, arterioles, and arteries, but the wall of the aorta can also be affected by necrotizing granulomatous inflammation [1]. For these reasons the term "polyangiitis" is used for these syndromes [1]. It is the necrotizing granulomatous inflammation that sets GPA apart from MPA. The diagnosis of GPA depends on the presence of clinical, pathologic, or radiographic evidence or surrogates of granulomatous inflammation. The vasculitis of MPA is indistinguishable from that of GPA, and there may be substantial overlap between the syndromes. For these reasons, the therapeutic approach to patients with GPA and MPA is governed by the same principles, and most clinical studies and therapeutic trials have combined both diseases.

The following paragraphs will focus on respiratory manifestations of MPA and GPA other than pulmonary capillaritis. Other organ manifestations will be covered briefly as they pertain to general treatment decisions. The pulmonary capillaritis of MPA and GPA will be discussed in more detail in the section on DAH.

The pathognomonic histopathologic features of GPA include neutrophilic microabscesses, fibrinoid necrosis, palisading histiocytes, and giant cells forming a granulomatous inflammation pattern that is often referred to as "geographic necrosis" [2]. Focal vasculitis, thrombosis, and fibrous obliteration of vascular lumina may be seen in areas affected by this type of inflammation which affects predominantly the upper respiratory tract and lungs, but may involve any organ. Atypical and rare histopathologic features of GPA include organizing pneumonia, bronchocentric inflammation, and occasionally a marked number of eosinophils in the inflammatory infiltrates [3]. Tracheobronchial inflammation, often representing unique treatment challenges, is another feature of GPA not shared with MPA [4, 5].

The etiology of MPA and GPA remains unknown. A multifactorial genetic predisposition for the development of ANCA-associated vasculitis seems to be required [6, 7]. Environmental triggers such as exposure to silica and more commonly infections appear to be linked to the onset of the disease as well as to relapses by initiating and perpetuating an inflammatory environment that leads to the production of ANCA, which in turn appear instrumental for the development of capillaritis [8].

Greater than 90 % of patients with GPA are Caucasian. The clinical presentation of GPA varies from subacute nonspecific respiratory illness to rapidly progressive alveolar hemorrhage syndrome. The majority of disease manifestations of GPA affecting the upper and lower respiratory tract are caused by the necrotizing granulomatous inflammation. Ear, nose, and throat symptoms affect more than 85 % of patients [9]. These may include rhinorrhea, purulent or bloody nasal discharge, nasal mucosal drying and crust formation, epistaxis, and serous otitis media. Deep facial pain from paranasal sinus involvement, nasal septal perforation, and ulceration of the vomer are important signs. *Staphylococcus aureus* is frequently detected in the nose and sinuses and has been linked to relapses of the disease [10]. Aphthous lesions of the nasal and oral mucosa and inflammation and destruction of the nasal cartilage lead to a "saddle-nose deformity." Ulcerated lesions of the larynx and trachea are present in 30 % of untreated cases [4]. These may cause hemoptysis.

The diagnostic evaluation of patients suspected of having GPA or MPA should include screening for all possible organ manifestations and treatment toxicities and then be adjusted based on patient-specific symptoms. Measurement of nonspecific markers of inflammation including erythrocyte sedimentation rate and C-reactive protein, complete blood count, serum chemistry panel, urine analysis, and microscopy and testing for ANCA and chest imaging constitutes the core of diagnostic screening. Pulmonary function testing should be performed if the patient has any respiratory symptoms or chest roentgenographic abnormalities.

Respiratory symptoms such as cough, hemoptysis, dyspnea, stridor, or chest wall pain are usually associated with roentgenographic abnormalities, but roentgenographic abnormalities may be asymptomatic [11]. Lung nodules or mass lesions which may or may not cavitate, can be singular, but are usually multiple and bilateral. They can range in size from a few millimeters to several centimeters. Alveolar infiltrates should prompt consideration of DAH even in the absence of hemoptysis (see discussion later in this chapter). Unusual manifestations include lymphadenopathy, lobar consolidation, and large pleural effusions. Tracheobronchial lesions are common, may be asymptomatic, and only detectable by bronchoscopy. When airway stenoses occur, symptoms that can be mistaken for asthma include stridor or localized wheezes. Pulmonary function testing including inspiratory and expiratory flow-volume loops may provide important clues to the presence of airway narrowing. Bronchoscopic inspection of the tracheobronchial tree is recommended for patients with unexplained respiratory symptoms, abnormalities on pulmonary function test results, or radiographic abnormalities [5, 12].

MPA with MPO-ANCA can occasionally be associated with lung fibrosis, predominantly of the usual interstitial pneumonia (UIP) and sometimes of the nonspecific interstitial pneumonitis (NSIP) variety [13]. The causal relationship between the interstitial lung disease and MPA remains unclear. In most instances the lung fibrosis precedes the development of vasculitis or is detected at the time of first vasculitis disease manifestations. In such patients the MPA disease manifestations respond to immunosuppressive therapy as expected, whereas the lung fibrosis generally does not.

Treatment of MPA and GPA follows several general principles. First is the distinction of disease categories based on disease severity. Second is the separation of treatment phases into a remission induction phase, followed by a remission maintenance phase. Third is the distinction between symptoms caused by damage from the disease itself or treatment and those attributable to active inflammation. Lastly, all therapeutic interventions need to be paired with adjunctive measures aimed at minimizing treatment toxicities, or designed to repair damage.

To stratify remission induction therapy, patients' disease activity is categorized as "limited or non-severe disease" or "severe disease." "Severe disease" is either life-threatening or threatening an affected organ with irreversible loss of function. This includes alveolar hemorrhage, glomerulonephritis, eye involvement (except mere episcleritis), and nervous system involvement including sensorineural hearing loss. "Limited or non-severe disease" includes essentially all patients with disease activity that does not qualify as "severe" by our definitions. The term "limited disease" used in the United States comprises what European investigators have referred to as "early-systemic disease" as well as "localized disease." Even though this separation is not based on well-defined biological distinctions, most disease manifestations leading to the categorization as "severe disease" are caused by capillaritis. In contrast, most symptoms leading to the classification as "limited or non-severe" disease are the result of necrotizing granulomatous inflammation. Patients with limited GPA have a more protracted disease course, a greater likelihood of experiencing a disease relapse following a period of remission, and a higher prevalence of destructive upper respiratory tract disorders (e.g., saddle-nose deformity).

Therapy for MPA and GPA follows similar principles and is based on randomized controlled trial results. Methotrexate (MTX) given once a week at a dose of up to 25 mg in combination with daily oral prednisone is considered the standard of care for patients with non-severe GPA [14]. For remission induction in severe GPA and MPA, CYC at a dose of 2 mg/kg/day in combination with prednisone has been the standard of care until recently [9, 15]. Rituximab (RTX) has now been proven to be an effective and safe alternative for CYC, and for patients presenting with a severe disease relapse RTX was shown to be superior to CYC [16, 17].

Once remission has been induced and the prednisone taper is well under way, CYC should be switched to either azathioprine (AZA, preferred in patients with renal involvement and any degree of renal insufficiency) or MTX [18]. MTX and AZA are equivalent for remission maintenance, whereas another randomized controlled trial showed that mycophenolate mofetil (MMF) is not as effective as AZA for remission maintenance [19]. Thus, the use of MMF for remission maintenance can only be supported for patients who have failed MTX and AZA, or who have contraindications for both agents. The Wegener's Granulomatosis Etanercept trial (WGET), in which MTX was used for remission maintenance, confirmed that long-term remission remains an elusive goal for many patients, as remission was maintained in less than half of the patients [20]. The RTX in ANCA-associated Vasculitis (RAVE) trial showed that a single 4-week infusion series of RTX was as effective as 18 months of conventional cytotoxic therapy with CYC followed by AZA, even though patients in the RTX treatment arm of that trial received no further therapy following the original infusion therapy [17]. Several recent studies including the RAVE trial have shown that PR3-ANCA (versus MPO-ANCA), the diagnosis of GPA (versus MPA), and relapsing disease (versus new diagnosis) represent risk factors for subsequent relapses even when patients are maintained on AZA for maintenance therapy [17, 21, 22].

Large airway involvement in GPA may call for specialized management beyond standard immunosuppression [5]. Subglottic stenosis is often addressed with dilation procedures paired with local injection of long-acting glucocorticoids with or without mitomycin C [23]. Stenosis of the large airways may require bronchoscopic interventions, including dilation by rigid bronchoscope, YAG-laser treatment, and the placement of silicone airway stents, or balloon dilations which can be performed with the flexible bronchoscope [5]. Tracheobronchial infections, like nose or sinus infections, are thought to play a role in the pathogenesis of the disease by promoting relapses. For this reason, it is advisable to provide antimicrobial therapy based on culture and susceptibility results from bronchial washings. The application of topical glucocorticoids may spare patients with tracheobronchial involvement from ongoing oral glucocorticoid therapy. Lastly, pneumocystis *jerovecii* pneumonia is a well recognized and potentially fatal complication of immunosuppressive therapy for

GPA that can easily be prevented [24]. Pneumocystis pneumonia prophylaxis is recommended for all patients with GPA receiving any kind of immunosuppression including being B-cell depleted after RTX therapy [25].

Eosinophilic Granulomatosis with Polyangiitis (Churg–Strauss)

The Chapel Hill Consensus defines EGPA as "eosinophil-rich and granulomatous inflammation involving the respiratory, and necrotizing vasculitis affecting small to medium-sized vessels, and associated with asthma and eosinophilia" [1]. EGPA is included among the ANCA-associated vasculitides, but only 40–70 % of patients with active EGPA have detectable ANCA prior to treatment. If ANCA is detectable it is usually of the P-ANCA/MPO-ANCA type [26, 27]. EGPA is primarily distinguished from GPA and MPA by a high prevalence of asthma and peripheral blood and tissue eosinophilia. Three distinct disease phases which may not always follow in sequence have been described for the disease [28]. A *prodromal allergic phase* with asthma may last for a number of years. The *eosinophilic phase* with prominent peripheral and tissue eosinophilia may also last a number of years, and the manifestations may remit and recur over this time period. The differential diagnosis for patients in this phase of the disease includes parasitic infection and chronic eosinophilic pneumonia. The *vasculitic phase* consisting of systemic vasculitis may be life-threatening. This is usually the last phase and may be masked or prevented by glucocorticoid therapy used for the management of earlier phases. Asthma usually predates the vasculitic phase by a mean of 7 years (range 0–61). "Formes frustes" of EGPA have also been described with eosinophilic vasculitis and/or eosinophilic granulomas in isolated organs without evidence of systemic disease [29].

Pulmonary parenchymal involvement in the form of transient alveolar-type infiltrates occurs in 38 % of patients. These have a predominantly peripheral distribution and are indistinguishable from infiltrates seen in chronic eosinophilic pneumonia [26]. Nodular lesions are rare in EGPA. In contrast to GPA and MPA, alveolar hemorrhage is exceedingly rare (<5 % of cases). Renal involvement in EGPA is less prominent than in GPA or MPA and does not generally lead to renal failure [30]. In contrast, peripheral nerve involvement, typically in the form of mononeuritis multiplex, is more frequent [26, 27, 31]. Skin, heart, central nervous system, and abdominal viscera may also be involved.

The classic histopathologic picture consists of necrotizing vasculitis, eosinophilic tissue infiltration, and extravascular granulomas. However, not all features are found in every case, and they are not pathognomonic of the condition. Particularly the finding of a "Churg–Strauss granuloma" on skin biopsy should not be confused with the diagnosis of EGPA. This type of necrotizing extravascular granuloma may be seen in EGPA as well as in other systemic autoimmune diseases including GPA and rheumatoid arthritis. Recent studies suggest that a more vasculitic disease phenotype is associated with the presence of ANCA, but this was not confirmed by all studies. There remains substantial overlap of organ manifestations between patients with EGPA who are ANCA positive and those who are ANCA negative [26, 27, 31].

Several case studies and limited population-based incidence estimates have indicated that leukotriene receptor blocking agents may lead to unmasking of vasculitic symptoms in asthmatics, by allowing dose reductions or discontinuation of oral glucocorticoid therapy. There is currently no evidence suggesting that these agents directly cause the disease or need to be avoided in EGPA.

The overall mortality of EGPA is lower than that of GPA or MPA and not significantly different from the normal population [26]. Most reported deaths are secondary to cardiac involvement [31].

Systemic glucocorticoids remain the mainstay of therapy. There are no randomized controlled trials that provide clear guidance. Treatment approaches following the principles applied to the management of ANCA-associated vasculitis have been adopted for EGPA. Accordingly, CYC should be added to glucocorticoids for remission induction in all patients with disease manifestations that threaten the patient's life or the function of a vital organ, i.e., particularly those with central- or peripheral nerve involvement, glomerulonephritis, heart involvement, or alveolar hemorrhage [32]. MTX, AZA, and MMF have all been used as glucocorticoid-sparing agents in less severe disease and for remission maintenance. Refractory disease, and disease dominated by difficult-to-control eosinophilic inflammation, has been reported to respond to interferon-alpha therapy, and more recently anti-interleukin-5 therapy [33, 34]. RTX has also been used successfully in EGPA, particularly ANCA-positive patients with renal disease, but the data are still scarce, and it cannot be recommended to use RTX instead of CYC for patients with severe EGPA [35].

IgA Vasculitis (Henoch–Schönlein)

IgA vasculitis is an immune-complex-mediated disease characterized by IgA1-dominant immune deposits affecting predominantly capillaries, venules, and arterioles leading to acute purpura, arthritis, colicky abdominal pain, and nephritis. Proliferative and necrotizing glomerulonephritis is usually mild. Immunofluorescence microscopy shows large deposits of IgA in the skin and kidney. IgA vasculitis is more common in children (mean age of patients, 17 years), but adults can also be affected. The triad of purpura, arthritis, and abdominal pain is present in approximately 80 % of patients. Joint involvement affecting the large joints is typically monoarticular and transient causing pain that is out of proportion to the objective evidence of synovitis. Peritonitis and melena are common.

Pulmonary manifestations of IgA vasculitis are rare. Only 36 cases have been reported to date, and capillaritis has been documented histopathologically only in a minority of them. As in the skin and glomeruli, IgA deposits along the pulmonary capillary walls are pathognomonic for the disease. Half of the patients with IgA vasculitis associated DAH required mechanical ventilation and almost a third of the reported patients died [36].

Cryoglobulinemic Vasculitis

Cryoglobulinemic vasculitis is characterized by circulating cryoglobulins and their deposits in small vessels including capillaries, venules, and arterioles. Half of all cases are linked to *Hepatitis C Virus* infection [37]. Compared to skin, peripheral nerve, and renal involvement, capillaritis of the lung leading to DAH is rare (3 %), but associated with a high mortality (80 %) [37]. RTX is now the preferred immunosuppressive agent for cryoglobulinemic vasculitis [38].

Hypocomplementemic Urticarial Vasculitis (Anti-C1q Vasculitis)

Another rare small vessel vasculitis is hypocomplementemic urticarial vasculitis (HUV). HUV is characterized by urticaria, hypocomplementemia, anti-C1q antibodies, and vasculitis of small vessels [1]. Signs and symptoms consist of fever, arthralgias, arthritis, angioedema, uveitis, episcleritis, abdominal pain, glomerulonephritis, and seizures occurring at variable frequencies and combinations. The reported pulmonary complications of HUV are not directly caused by vasculitis. Obstructive pulmonary disease, often severe, occurs in up to 66 % patients [39]. Its immunologic etiology remains unclear, and cannot always be related to smoking.

Pulmonary Manifestations of Medium-Sized Vessel Vasculitis

Classic Polyarteritis Nodosa

Polyarteritis nodosa (PAN) is not associated with ANCA and does not affect capillaries. Therefore, it does not cause glomerulonephritis or alveolar hemorrhage. However, case reports of classic PAN affecting the bronchial or bronchiolar arteries have been reported as the cause of occasional lung hemorrhage. Most cases of classic PAN diagnosed today are associated with viral infections, specifically hepatitis B and C. Consequently, antiviral therapy plays a prominent role in the management of such cases in addition to immunosuppression [40]. In contrast to MPA, classic PAN rarely relapses.

Pulmonary Manifestations of Large Vessel Vasculitis

Giant Cell Arteritis

Giant cell arteritis (GCA) represents a generalized inflammatory disorder involving large- and medium-sized arteries. GCA is the most common form of vasculitis in elderly patients of the Northern hemisphere. Granulomatous inflammation of vessel walls can be found in 60 % of temporal artery biopsy specimens, and the aorta may also be affected possibly leading to thoracic aortic aneurysms in the elderly.

Respiratory symptoms have been reported in up to 25 % of patients, but are usually mild and of little consequence. However, respiratory symptoms can sometimes be the initial presentation of GCA. Therefore, GCA should be considered in elderly patients presenting with new onset of cough, hoarseness, or throat pain without other identifiable cause [41]. An elevated sedimentation rate may lead to the correct diagnosis, and cough, hoarseness, and throat pain usually resolve promptly with glucocorticoid therapy. Pleural effusion or multinodular pulmonary lesions associated with GCA have also been reported on rare occasions raising questions about a possible overlap with GPA since the latter may also involve the temporal arteries. Therapy of GCA continues to be based on the use of glucocorticoids without proven alternative. The glucocorticoid-sparing role of MTX for GCA remains controversial.

Takayasu's Arteritis

Takayasu's arteritis (TA) is a large vessel vasculitis affecting predominantly the aorta and its major branches in young patients most commonly affecting women [1]. It is not limited to patients of Asian descent. Constitutional symptoms, low grade fever, and arthralgias are often early disease manifestations. More characteristic features of this chronically relapsing disease include variable pulses of the extremities and claudication of affected vascular territories. Renovascular hypertension, pulmonary hypertension, and ischemia of affected organs can be disabling.

The pulmonary manifestations are caused by a unique arteriopathy affecting the large- and medium-sized pulmonary vessels. Pulmonary artery stenoses and occlusion as well as pulmonary hypertension can occur in up to half of all patients as a result of progressive defects in the outer media of the arteries and ingrowth of granulation tissue-like capillaries associated with thickened intima and subendothelial smooth muscle proliferation. The inflammatory infiltrate of the vessel wall consists of lymphocytes, plasma cells, and giant cells. The involvement of pulmonary arteries which is often asymptomatic can be detectable by conventional angiography, perfusion scan, magnetic resonance angiography, or PET scanning [42]. Chest roentgenograms are usually normal, but computed tomography may show areas of low attenuation as a result of regional hypoperfusion, subpleural reticulolinear changes, and pleural thickening. Fistulas can form between pulmonary artery branches and bronchial arteries. Nonspecific inflammatory interstitial lung disease has also been reported.

Therapy for TA relies on immunosuppression with glucocorticoids and MTX [43]. Unfortunately, many patients relapse when the glucocorticoid dose is reduced below 15 mg daily. Antitumor necrosis factor-alpha agents may also be useful. Vascular bypass procedures may restore perfusion to areas affected by severe arterial stenoses, but the results are only temporary [44].

Behçet's Disease

Behçet's disease (BD) is a rare chronically relapsing systemic inflammatory disorder characterized by aphthous oral ulcers and at least two or more of the following: aphthous genital ulcers, uveitis, cutaneous nodules or pustules, or meningoencephalitis [1]. The reported prevalence varies widely between different ethnic groups, for instance 1:16,000 in Japan but 1:200,000 in the United States. The disease is associated with the major histocompatibility complex antigen HLA-B51. The mean age of patients at the onset of BD is 35 years, and men are predominantly affected. Respiratory manifestations of BD consist of cough, hemoptysis, chest pain, and dyspnea [45]. The vasculitis of BD is immune-complex mediated, and may affect vessels of all sizes. Secondary thrombosis with major venous occlusion can occur. Anticoagulation may not be effective for prevention of thrombosis, but aspirin 80 mg/day has been advocated. Destruction of the elastic lamina of pulmonary arteries causing aneurysm formation, secondary erosion of bronchi, and arterial-bronchial fistulae may result in massive hemoptysis, which can be fatal. Computed tomography or magnetic resonance angiography is recommended for detection of pulmonary artery aneurysms. Recurrent pneumonia, organizing pneumonia, and bronchial obstruction resulting from mucosal inflammation have also been described.

Therapy of the underlying disease consists of immunosuppression. Prednisone alone may not be sufficient to control the vasculitis. The addition of other drugs, such as colchicine, chlorambucil, MTX, cyclosporin, or AZA, is recommended. The use of biologic agents, in particular anti-TNF agents and RTX, has also been reported recently. The addition of AZA or CYC to glucocorticoids may result in resolution of pulmonary aneurysms. Anticoagulation should be avoided once pulmonary artery aneurysms have been identified, but coil embolization of identified aneurysms may prevent fatal hemorrhage. The prognosis of pulmonary involvement overall remains poor. About one third of patients die within 2 years of developing pulmonary involvement, most from fatal pulmonary hemorrhage.

Secondary Vasculitis

Infectious processes, particularly infections with *Aspergillus* and *Mucor* species, invade vascular structures and produce secondary vasculitis. Certain drugs and chemicals can induce a systemic vasculitis picture that mimics MPA. Other uncommon secondary vasculitic entities include benign lymphocytic angiitis and granulomatosis, bronchocentric granulomatosis, and necrotizing sarcoid angiitis.

Clinical Approach to DAH

Diffuse hemorrhage into the alveolar spaces is often referred to as *DAH syndrome*. The clinical course of DAH is unpredictable and, therefore, should always be considered potentially life-threatening. Patients usually seek care because of nonspecific symptoms, including dyspnea, cough, and possibly fever. Diffuse alveolar filling defects on chest roentgenogram are usually found, and anemia and hypoxemia may be prominent at the time of presentation. Hemoptysis is common, but DAH should be considered in the differential diagnostic evaluation of any patient with alveolar infiltrates on chest roentgenogram even in the absence of hemoptysis. DAH can result from a variety of underlying or associated conditions that cause a disruption of the alveolar-capillary basement membrane integrity including immunological inflammatory conditions causing immune-complex deposition or capillaritis (e.g., anti-GBM disease (Goodpasture's), systemic lupus erythematosus (SLE), ANCA-associated vasculitis), direct chemical/toxic injury (e.g., from toxic or chemical inhalation, abciximab use, all-trans-retinoic acid, trimellitic anhydride, or smoked crack cocaine), physical trauma (e.g., pulmonary contusion), and increased vascular pressure within the capillaries (e.g., mitral stenosis or severe left ventricular failure) (Table 10.1). Pulmonary alveolar hemorrhage can also be associated with thrombocytopenia (<50,000 cells/µL), other abnormal coagulation variables, renal failure (creatinine concentration, ≥2.5 mg/dL), and occasionally with a history of heavy smoking. Only the vasculitis syndromes giving rise to DAH will be discussed here.

Bronchoalveolar lavage (BAL) is the best diagnostic modality to confirm the presence of DAH. Progressively more bloody return indicates alveolar origin of active bleeding. A positive iron stain in more than 20 % of all alveolar macrophages

Table 10.1 Causes of diffuse alveolar hemorrhage

Immune-mediated capillaritis and vasculitis
Pauci-immune small vessel vasculitides
Microscopic polyangiitis
Granulomatosis with polyangiitis (Wegener's)
Eosinophilic granulomatosis with polyangiitis (Churg–Strauss)
Idiopathic pauci-immune pulmonary capillaritis
Drug-induced ANCA-associated vasculitis
Immune-complex-mediated disease
Systemic lupus erythematosus (rarely other collagen vascular diseases)
Antiphospholipid syndrome
IgA vasculitis (Henoch–Schönlein)
Cryoglobulinemic vasculitis
Anti-glomerular basement membrane disease
Drug-induced immune-complex-mediated vasculitis
Immune mediated without capillaritis
Anti-glomerular basement membrane disease
Celiac disease (Lane-Hamilton syndrome)
Idiopathic pulmonary hemosiderosis
Nonimmune mediated
Mitral valve disease
Coagulopathy (anticoagulation, thrombocytopenia, renal failure)[a]
Diffuse alveolar damage
Chest trauma (pulmonary contusion)
Other rare causes

[a]Usually requires "second hit" such as pulmonary inflammation or inhalational injury

recovered by BAL is indicative of DAH, even in the absence of ongoing active bleeding. In patients with an established diagnosis of vasculitis, BAL should be performed in any patient with new alveolar infiltrates to differentiate infection, DAH, and other inflammatory infiltrates such as eosinophilic pneumonia. Once DAH is established the additional diagnostic approach is aimed at the rapid identification of the underlying cause and at prompt implementation of appropriate therapy.

History and physical examination can provide important first clues about the specific etiology of DAH. Exposure to inhalational toxins including trimellitic anhydride or pyromellitic dianhydrate, drug abuse such as crack cocaine abuse, and smoking should be identified. The past medical history may reveal comorbidities that can cause DAH, including mitral stenosis, coagulation disorders, recent bone marrow or hematopoietic stem cell transplantation, preexisting autoimmune disorders, and therapeutic drugs. The initial physical exam findings may also point towards a specific systemic autoimmune disease as cause of the DAH.

Laboratory testing performed during an evaluation of DAH should assess the acuity, progression, or stability of the disease process, uncover potential other organ involvement, and help to identify a specific underlying cause. Thus, initial laboratory testing should consist of a complete blood count, metabolic panel, urine analysis, and microscopy, and determine the current coagulation status (APTT, INR). Baseline markers of inflammation (erythrocyte sedimentation rate and C-reactive protein) are helpful to monitor subsequent responses to therapy. Specific autoantibody testing for a potential underlying systemic disease process should also be initiated promptly, including testing for ANCA, anti-GBM antibodies, antinuclear antibodies, anti-double-stranded DNA antibodies, and antiphospholipid antibodies, as well as determination of cryoglobulins, complement, and creatinine kinase levels.

A lung biopsy is not always necessary to obtain a specific diagnosis for a DAH syndrome. Factors deserving careful consideration before performing a biopsy include the risks of the biopsy procedure, the likelihood of obtaining a diagnostic piece of tissue, the likelihood of the biopsy findings to alter the therapeutic approach, and the risks associated with the chosen therapy. Most lung biopsies obtained from patients with DAH will show either pulmonary capillaritis or a "bland histology" in which the pulmonary architecture is well preserved and inflammatory changes are minimal. The histopathologic diagnosis of pulmonary capillaritis requires the findings of alveolar wall infiltration with inflammatory cells centered on capillary walls and small veins and fibrinoid necrosis of alveolar and vessel walls. The inflammatory cells are usually neutrophils, but can be eosinophils or monocytes. Leukocytoclasis, a phenomenon describing pyknotic cells and nuclear fragments from neutrophils associated with cell apoptosis, is also an important feature of capillaritis. Capillaritis usually causes and may culminate in the destruction of the underlying lung architecture. Capillaritis needs to be distinguished from the predominant intra-alveolar neutrophilic infiltration associated with active infections and from mere neutrophil margination related to surgical trauma.

Most of the syndromes associated with pulmonary capillaritis leading to DAH have been discussed in the previous sections of this chapter. The subsequent paragraphs will describe a few unique syndromes or conditions that may also be associated with DAH and variable degrees of capillaritis.

ANCA-Associated Vasculitis and DAH

MPA and GPA combined represent the most common causes of pulmonary capillaritis. Alveolar hemorrhage caused by capillaritis in the setting of MPA or GPA may be subtle or rapidly progressive. Its course is unpredictable and this condition should always be considered life-threatening or severe disease regardless of how well maintained oxygenation may be at the time of presentation. The presence of renal disease, the requirement of mechanical ventilation, and advanced age have all been identified as factors portending a worse prognosis [46–48]. Early implementation of definitive therapy is crucial, and the application of 1–3 daily doses of 1 g of methyl-prednisolone intravenously is considered standard prior to implementation of additional standard therapy for severe disease. The RAVE trial had shown that patients with severe GPA or MPA with DAH achieve the same outcomes as all other patients with severe GPA or MPA [16]. However, patients requiring mechanical ventilation because of their DAH were excluded from participation in the trial.

For some patients with GPA and MPA the combination of glucocorticoids and CYC or RTX may not be sufficient to induce a remission quickly. Plasma exchange (PLEX) has been advocated for early consideration in patients who present with DAH as well as for those presenting with rapidly progressive glomerulonephritis and renal failure. The MEPEX (Methyl-prednisolone versus Plasma Exchange) trial compared three pulses of intravenous methyl-prednisolone to 2 weeks of PLEX (7×60 mL/kg) in addition to standard therapy for severe disease (oral prednisone and CYC) in 156 patients who presented with a serum creatinine level of 5.5 mg/dL or greater [49]. Even though this trial showed significantly better patient and renal survival at 6 months, there was no long-term advantage of PLEX and there were too few patients with DAH to allow a subset analysis. Only one single-center cohort study focusing on MPA with DAH in 20 patients admitted to an intensive care unit described 100 % survival of these patients when PLEX was added to standard immunosuppressive therapy [50]. The role of PLEX in severe AAV is currently undergoing further investigation. If DAH is uncontrolled despite aggressive immunosuppressive therapy and PLEX, the endobronchial application of recombinant-activated factor VII may be considered as salvage therapy. In patients who survive DAH caused by MPA or GPA, lung function usually recovers well.

Idiopathic Pauci-Immune Pulmonary Capillaritis

This rare condition is by definition not a systemic form of vasculitis [51]. This isolated pulmonary capillaritis of unknown etiology is histopathologically indistinguishable from the pauci-immune capillaritis seen in ANCA-associated vasculitis. No specific autoantibodies have been identified in these patients. This disorder represents a diagnosis of exclusion, and these patients are best treated with an immunosuppressive regimen that follows the guidelines for severe MPA.

Anti-glomerular Basement Membrane Antibody Disease (Goodpasture Syndrome)

Anti-glomerular basement membrane antibody disease (anti-GBM disease) or Goodpasture syndrome is a rare autoimmune disease caused by autoantibodies directed against the NC1-domain of the alpha-3 chain of basement membrane collagen type IV. This epitope is only accessible for autoantibodies in the basement membranes of kidneys and lungs. DAH occurs in about half of patients with anti-GBM disease and requires an additional inhalational injury, particularly smoking, to render the antigen accessible for the autoantibodies and for the development of the pulmonary

disease manifestation. Anti-GBM disease rarely causes isolated alveolar hemorrhage in the absence of renal disease. Even though patients usually have serum anti-GBM autoantibodies, the diagnosis of anti-GBM disease cannot be established without histopathologic documentation of linear immunoglobulin G deposits along the basement membranes in lung or kidney. Whether anti-GBM disease represents a true vasculitis is a matter of definition. As the glomerulus is a capillary structure, its inflammation by definition represents a form of capillaritis. This is the main reason for the inclusion of anti-GBM disease in the nomenclature and definitions of the Chapel Hill classification. Yet, the prominent histopathologic finding in the lung of patients with anti-GBM disease is the "bland histopathology," whereas capillaritis represents a secondary histopathologic feature that has also been described in some patients [52]. Early implementation of immunosuppressive therapy in conjunction with PLEX is the key to a favorable outcome in patients with anti-GBM disease [53]. Lung function usually recovers fully from anti-GBM disease, but chronic renal failure is common and defines the overall outcome of the disease.

SLE and Other Collagen Vascular Disorders

DAH as a result of immune-complex-mediated pulmonary capillaritis is a rare but usually severe complication of SLE. The onset of DAH in patients with SLE is usually abrupt, but hardly ever the first sign of the disease. The disease presentation is usually rapidly progressive with pulmonary infiltrates and fever, mimicking infection, and hemoptysis may be absent. Consequently, the differentiation of DAH from infection in SLE usually requires a diagnostic BAL. Mechanical ventilation, infection, and CYC therapy were reported as negative prognostic factors in one report. The reported mortality of DAH in SLE varies between 0 and 90 % [54–56]. Treatment consists of glucocorticoids and CYC. The use of PLEX has been suggested, but its benefit remains unproven.

Respiratory complications are very common in most other types of collagen vascular or connective tissue disorders. Yet, pulmonary capillaritis presenting as DAH is rare. Isolated cases have been reported with polymyositis, rheumatoid arthritis, and mixed connective tissue disease. Consequently, serologic testing performed as part of an evaluation of DAH should include studies aimed at the identification of these potential underlying disease entities.

Antiphospholipid Syndrome

DAH resulting from capillaritis can also be a rare complication of primary antiphospholipid syndrome (APS). Other respiratory complications include pulmonary embolism and infarction, pulmonary microthrombosis, and pulmonary arterial thrombosis with secondary pulmonary hypertension, all resulting from the hypercoagulability characterizing this disorder. However, primary pulmonary hypertension as well as adult respiratory distress syndrome can also occur.

The clinical presentation of DAH in primary APS is nonspecific and consists of cough, dyspnea, fever, and bilateral pulmonary infiltrates. As DAH can also occur in the context of adult respiratory distress syndrome, and hemoptysis is absent in over half of the reported patients with APS and DAH, BAL should be performed early to establish the diagnosis. Tissue necrosis from microthrombosis as well as pulmonary capillaritis has been implicated as causes of DAH in APS. The capillaritis of APS is immune-complex mediated. The coexistence of thrombosis and capillaritis with DAH represents a therapeutic dilemma, as anticoagulation may need to be interrupted to control the hemorrhage, and patients often require placement of an inferior vena cava filter. The largest single-center report comprising 17 patients and review of 24 cases published in the literature indicates a high mortality of about 40 % despite aggressive immunosuppressive therapy [57]. Glucocorticoid therapy alone is usually ineffective, as is monotherapy with agents like AZA or MMF. PLEX in addition to immunosuppressive therapy is often considered, but its efficacy remains questionable in patients with APS and DAH. Best results were obtained with cyclophosphamide or RTX, sometimes in combination.

> **Case Vignette: 20-Year-Old Young Man with Granulomatosis with Polyangiitis (GPA, Wegener's)**
>
> Five months prior to presentation at the emergency room of a tertiary care center, this young man had developed maxillary sinusitis, unresponsive to broad spectrum antibiotics. This lingered until he experienced significant worsening of sinusitis symptoms 3 months later. At that time he also developed epistaxis prompting an evaluation by an allergist. A couple of weeks later he developed acute left-sided hearing loss, night sweats, and migratory large joint arthralgias. By this time he had already lost 10 lb of weight due to malaise and lack of appetite. Four months after the onset of first symptoms he was hospitalized at a local rural hospital, where he was found to have dry cough, bilateral episcleritis, lower extremity palpable purpura, and nodular lesions on chest roentgenogram. A rheumatology evaluation at the local hospital led to testing for ANCA, and a nasal biopsy was obtained. Renal function and urinary sediment were normal. The ANCA test was positive for C-ANCA and PR3-ANCA, and the nasal biopsy reportedly showed "granulomas." The patient was treated for 3 days with intravenous methylprednisolone and dismissed on oral prednisone 40 mg twice daily to be tapered to 30 mg daily over the course of the next 3 weeks. He was scheduled for initiation of RTX infusions 375 mg/m^2 as an outpatient. Scheduling difficulties led to a delay in initiation of the infusions. Three weeks later, while on prednisone 30 mg daily he had noted significant worsening of symptoms consisting of cough and malaise.
>
> At this time he presented to the emergency room of a tertiary referral center with cough, malaise, and bilateral alveolar infiltrates on chest roentgenogram (Fig. 10.1a). He denied hemoptysis. The patient's room air oxygenation was 93 %, respiratory rate 20 per minute, temperature

(continued)

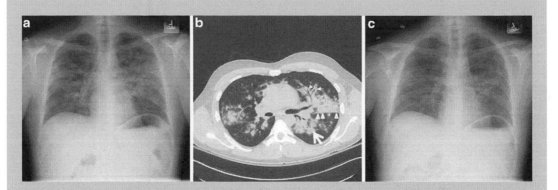

Fig. 10.1 (**a**) Chest roentgenogram of 20-year-old man with recently diagnosed granulomatosis with polyangiitis (GPA) presenting with diffuse alveolar hemorrhage. (**b**) Computed tomography of the chest obtained 1 day later shows diffuse alveolar infiltrates respecting the lobar plains (*white triangles*), nodular lesions distinguishing GPA from MPA (*thick white arrow*), and prominent peribronchial inflammation (*thin white arrows*) frequently seen in GPA. (**c**) Follow-up chest roentgenogram obtained 14 days later shows resolution of diffuse alveolar infiltrates caused by hemorrhage, but nodular lesions and peribronchial inflammation are still detectable on this imaging study

36.6 °C, pulse 78 beats per minute, blood pressure 114/64. Physical examination of eyes, ears, nose, heart, and lungs was unremarkable. Hemoglobin was 11.0 g/dL, white blood count 23.3×10^9/L, platelet count 405×10^9/L, and lymphocyte and CD4 count are normal. An electrolyte panel and urinalysis and microscopy were normal. The patient's only medications consisted of prednisone and trimethoprim-sulfamethoxazole for pneumocystis pneumonia prophylaxis. The patient was dismissed from the emergency room for further outpatient evaluation by rheumatology the next day. A CT scan of the chest is obtained (Fig. 10.1b) and after consultation with a pulmonologist a bronchoscopy with BAL is performed. This shows progressively bloody return indicative of alveolar hemorrhage. Over the next several hours the patient's respiratory status worsens, hemoglobin drops to 8.8 g/dL, and patient is admitted to the medical intensive care unit and requires mechanical ventilation. His course is complicated by the development of bilateral pneumothoraces requiring bilateral chest tube placement. Methyl-prednisolone is given at a dose of 1 g/day for 3 days, and one dose of RTX, 375 mg/m², is given, followed 48 h later by eight daily sessions of PLEX. Ten days after admission to the intensive care unit he is transferred to the general ward where the second chest tube is removed (Fig. 10.1c). Following completion of PLEX, he receives completion of the RTX course (the remaining three once weekly doses). Following recovery he completes the taper of the prednisone dose to complete discontinuation before month 6. He has not relapsed over the course of the last 3 years. However, he has been retreated once with RTX without glucocorticoids following reconstitution of B-cells and recurrence of PR3-ANCA positivity.

This case offers the following teaching and discussion points:

- The development of symptoms and disease manifestations is quite typical in this patient. Despite this, the diagnosis of GPA is often delayed.
- Glucocorticoids alone can only temporize and do not control this systemic disease process very well at doses below 60 mg daily without prompt implementation of definitive therapy.
- Even though the combination of ENT disease with pulmonary nodules could be

(continued)

interpreted as "non-severe" disease allowing the choice of MTX in combination with glucocorticoids as first remission induction regimen, the severe constitutional symptoms (night sweats and weight loss) and the presence of palpable purpura suggest a rapidly progressive disease process with developing features of capillaritis. The provided information does not allow the distinction between conductive or sensorineural hearing loss, and we don't know whether the eye inflammation was merely episcleritis or early scleritis. Sensorineural hearing loss and scleritis are clearly severe disease manifestations. The classification as severe disease for treatment purposes made at the outside hospital is certainly appropriate. For a newly diagnosed patient with severe GPA, cyclophosphamide or RTX is equally effective. However, in this young man who wanted to preserve his fertility, RTX is the preferred choice for that reason.

- Without prompt implementation of definitive therapy, the disease progresses, and in this case DAH developed.
- DAH presents without hemoptysis in a large proportion of patients, and the absence of hemoptysis should not dissuade from suspecting it, particularly in a patient with preexisting diagnosis of GPA. Infection is the alternative explanation for the chest roentgenographic changes at the time of presentation to the emergency room.
- DAH of any degree of severity should be considered as potentially life-threatening, and patients should be closely monitored until a definitive diagnosis is established, definitive therapy has been initiated, and control of disease activity has been ascertained.
- Bronchoscopy with BAL for the evaluation of suspected DAH should be conducted in a safe setting, where worsening of the respiratory status that can be associated with the procedure can be treated with the necessary supportive measures.
- Once disease activity is controlled and the pulmonary bleeding stops, alveolar hemorrhagic infiltrates clear fast, unless diffuse alveolar damage with ARDS develops.
- Survivors of DAH usually experience complete recovery of lung function.
- The role of PLEX in this patient's course remains unclear. There is currently no data from a randomized controlled trial that applies to patients with DAH caused by ANCA-associated vasculitis.

References

1. Jennette JC, Falk RJ, Bacon PA, et al. 2012 revised International Chapel Hill Consensus Conference nomenclature of vasculitides. Arthritis Rheum. 2013;65(1):1–11.
2. Colby TV, Specks U. Wegener's granulomatosis in the 1990s—a pulmonary pathologist's perspective. Monogr Pathol. 1993;36:195–218.
3. Travis WD. Common and uncommon manifestations of Wegener's granulomatosis. Cardiovasc Pathol. 1994;3(3):217–25.
4. Daum DE, Specks U, Colby TV, et al. Tracheobronchial involvement in Wegener's granulomatosis. Am J Respir Crit Care Med. 1995;151:522–6.
5. Polychronopoulos VS, Prakash UB, Golbin JM, Edell ES, Specks U. Airway involvement in Wegener's granulomatosis. Rheum Dis Clin North Am. 2007; 33(4):755–75.
6. Willcocks LC, Lyons PA, Rees AJ, Smith KG. The contribution of genetic variation and infection to the pathogenesis of ANCA-associated systemic vasculitis. Arthritis Res Ther. 2010;12(1):202.
7. Lyons PA, Rayner TF, Trivedi S, et al. Genetically distinct subsets within ANCA-associated vasculitis. N Engl J Med. 2012;367(3):214–23.
8. Cartin-Ceba R, Peikert T, Specks U. Pathogenesis of ANCA-associated vasculitis. Curr Rheumatol Rep. 2012;14(6):481–93.
9. Hoffman GS, Kerr GS, Leavitt RY, et al. Wegener granulomatosis: an analysis of 158 patients. Ann Intern Med. 1992;116:488–98.

10. Stegeman CA, Cohen Tervaert JW, Sluiter WJ, Manson WL, de Jong PE, Kallenberg CGM. Association of chronic nasal carriage of Staphylococcus aureus and higher relapse rates in Wegener granulomatosis. Ann Intern Med. 1994;120:12–7.

11. Ananthakrishnan L, Sharma N, Kanne JP. Wegener's granulomatosis in the chest: high-resolution CT findings. AJR Am J Roentgenol. 2009;192(3):676–82.

12. Koldingsnes W, Jacobsen EA, Sildnes T, Hjalmarsen A, Nossent HC. Pulmonary function and high-resolution CT findings five years after disease onset in patients with Wegener's granulomatosis. Scand J Rheumatol. 2005;34(3):220–8.

13. Tzelepis GE, Kokosi M, Tzioufas A, et al. Prevalence and outcome of pulmonary fibrosis in microscopic polyangiitis. Eur Respir J. 2010;36(1):116–21.

14. Specks U. Methotrexate for Wegener's granulomatosis: what is the evidence? Arthritis Rheum. 2005;52(8):2237–42.

15. Jayne D, Rasmussen N, Andrassy K, et al. A randomized trial of maintenance therapy for vasculitis associated with antineutrophil cytoplasmic autoantibodies. N Engl J Med. 2003;349(1):36–44.

16. Stone JH, Merkel PA, Spiera R, et al. Rituximab versus cyclophosphamide for ANCA-associated vasculitis. N Engl J Med. 2010;363(3):221–32.

17. Specks U, Merkel PA, Seo P, et al. Efficacy of remission-induction regimens for ANCA-associated vasculitis. N Engl J Med. 2013;369(5):417–27.

18. Pagnoux C, Mahr A, Hamidou MA, et al. Azathioprine or methotrexate maintenance for ANCA-associated vasculitis. N Engl J Med. 2008;359(26):2790–803.

19. Hiemstra TF, Walsh M, Mahr A, et al. Mycophenolate mofetil vs azathioprine for remission maintenance in antineutrophil cytoplasmic antibody-associated vasculitis: a randomized controlled trial. JAMA. 2010;304(21):2381–8.

20. TheWGETResearchGroup. Etanercept plus standard therapy for Wegener's granulomatosis. N Engl J Med. 2005;352(4):351–61.

21. Lionaki S, Blyth ER, Hogan SL, et al. Classification of antineutrophil cytoplasmic autoantibody vasculitides: the role of antineutrophil cytoplasmic autoantibody specificity for myeloperoxidase or proteinase 3 in disease recognition and prognosis. Arthritis Rheum. 2012;64(10):3452–62.

22. Mahr A, Katsahian S, Varet H, et al. Revisiting the classification of clinical phenotypes of anti-neutrophil cytoplasmic antibody-associated vasculitis: a cluster analysis. Ann Rheum Dis. 2013;72(6):1003–10.

23. Langford CA, Sneller MC, Hallahan CW, et al. Clinical features and therapeutic management of subglottic stenosis in patients with Wegener's granulomatosis. Arthritis Rheum. 1996;39(10):1754–60.

24. Ognibene FP, Shelhamer JH, Hoffman GS, et al. Pneumocystis carinii pneumonia: a major complication of immunosuppressive therapy in patients with Wegener's granulomatosis. Am J Respir Crit Care Med. 1995;151(3 Pt 1):795–9.

25. Martin-Garrido I, Carmona EM, Specks U, Limper AH. Pneumocystis pneumonia in patients treated with rituximab. Chest. 2013;144(1):258–65.

26. Keogh KA, Specks U. Churg-Strauss syndrome: clinical presentation, antineutrophil cytoplasmic antibodies, and leukotriene receptor antagonists. Am J Med. 2003;115(4):284–90.

27. Sinico RA, Di Toma L, Maggiore U, et al. Prevalence and clinical significance of antineutrophil cytoplasmic antibodies in Churg-Strauss syndrome. Arthritis Rheum. 2005;52(9):2926–35.

28. Lanham JG, Elkon KB, Pusey CD, Hughes GR. Systemic vasculitis with asthma and eosinophilia: a clinical approach to the Churg-Strauss syndrome. Medicine. 1984;63:65–81.

29. Churg A, Brallas M, Cronin SR, Churg J. Formes frustes of Churg-Strauss syndrome. Chest. 1995;108(2):320–3.

30. Sinico RA, Di Toma L, Maggiore U, et al. Renal involvement in Churg-Strauss syndrome. Am J Kidney Dis. 2006;47(5):770–9.

31. Comarmond C, Pagnoux C, Khellaf M, et al. Eosinophilic granulomatosis with polyangiitis (Churg-Strauss): clinical characteristics and long-term followup of the 383 patients enrolled in the French Vasculitis Study Group cohort. Arthritis Rheum. 2013;65(1):270–81.

32. Guillevin L, Pagnoux C, Seror R, Mahr A, Mouthon L, Le Toumelin P. The five-factor score revisited: assessment of prognoses of systemic necrotizing vasculitides based on the French Vasculitis Study Group (FVSG) cohort. Medicine. 2011;90(1):19–27.

33. Tatsis E, Schnabel A, Gross WL. Interferon-a treatment of four patients with the Churg-Strauss syndrome. Ann Intern Med. 1998;129:370–4.

34. Kim S, Marigowda G, Oren E, Israel E, Wechsler ME. Mepolizumab as a steroid-sparing treatment option in patients with Churg-Strauss syndrome. J Allergy Clin Immunol. 2010;125(6):1336–43.

35. Cartin-Ceba R, Fervenza FC, Specks U. Treatment of antineutrophil cytoplasmic antibody-associated vasculitis with rituximab. Curr Opin Rheumatol. 2012;24(1):15–23.

36. Rajagopala S, Shobha V, Devaraj U, D'Souza G, Garg I. Pulmonary hemorrhage in Henoch-Schonlein purpura: case report and systematic review of the english literature. Semin Arthritis Rheum. 2013;42(4):391–400.

37. Amital H, Rubinow A, Naparstek Y. Alveolar hemorrhage in cryoglobulinemia—an indicator of poor prognosis. Clin Exp Rheumatol. 2005;23(5):616–20.

38. Ferri C, Cacoub P, Mazzaro C, et al. Treatment with rituximab in patients with mixed cryoglobulinemia syndrome: results of multicenter cohort study and review of the literature. Autoimmun Rev. 2011;11(1):48–55.

39. Wisnieski JJ, Baer AN, Christensen J, et al. Hypocomplementemic urticarial vasculitis syndrome. Clinical and serologic findings in 18 patients. Medicine. 1995;74(1):24–41.

40. de Menthon M, Mahr A. Treating polyarteritis nodosa: current state of the art. Clin Exp Rheumatol. 2011;29(1 Suppl 64):S110–6.

41. Larson TS, Hall S, Hepper NGG, Hunder GG. Respiratory tract symptoms as a clue to giant cell arteritis. Ann Intern Med. 1984;101:594–7.

42. Addimanda O, Spaggiari L, Pipitone N, Versari A, Pattacini P, Salvarani C. Pulmonary artery involvement in Takayasu arteritis. PET/CT versus CT angiography. Clin Exp Rheumatol. 2013;31(1 Suppl 75): S3–4.

43. Liang P, Hoffman GS. Advances in the medical and surgical treatment of Takayasu arteritis. Curr Opin Rheumatol. 2005;17(1):16–24.

44. Maksimowicz-McKinnon K, Clark TM, Hoffman GS. Limitations of therapy and a guarded prognosis in an American cohort of Takayasu arteritis patients. Arthritis Rheum. 2007;56(3):1000–9.

45. Uzun O, Akpolat T, Erkan L. Pulmonary vasculitis in behcet disease: a cumulative analysis. Chest. 2005; 127(6):2243–53.

46. Lauque D, Cadranel J, Lazor R, et al. Microscopic polyangiitis with alveolar hemorrhage. A study of 29 cases and review of the literature. Medicine. 2000; 79(4):222–33.

47. Kostianovsky A, Hauser T, Pagnoux C, et al. Alveolar haemorrhage in ANCA-associated vasculitides: 80 patients' features and prognostic factors. Clin Exp Rheumatol. 2012;30(1 Suppl 70):S77–82.

48. Hruskova Z, Casian AL, Konopasek P, et al. Long-term outcome of severe alveolar haemorrhage in ANCA-associated vasculitis: a retrospective cohort study. Scand J Rheumatol. 2013;42(3):211–4.

49. Jayne DR, Gaskin G, Rasmussen N, et al. Randomized trial of plasma exchange or high-dosage methylprednisolone as adjunctive therapy for severe renal vasculitis. J Am Soc Nephrol. 2007;18(7):2180–8.

50. Klemmer PJ, Chalermskulrat W, Reif MS, Hogan SL, Henke DC, Falk RJ. Plasmapheresis therapy for diffuse alveolar hemorrhage in patients with small-vessel vasculitis. Am J Kidney Dis. 2003;42(6):1149–53.

51. Jennings CA, King Jr TE, Tuder R, Cherniack RM, Schwarz MI. Diffuse alveolar hemorrhage with underlying isolated, pauciimmune pulmonary capillaritis. Am J Respir Crit Care Med. 1997;155(3):1101–9.

52. Lombard CM, Colby TV, Elliott CG. Surgical pathology of the lung in anti-basement membrane antibody-associated Goodpasture's syndrome. Hum Pathol. 1989;20(5):445–51.

53. Levy JB, Turner AN, Rees AJ, Pusey CD. Long-term outcome of anti-glomerular basement membrane antibody disease treated with plasma exchange and immunosuppression. Ann Intern Med. 2001;134(11): 1033–42.

54. Zamora MR, Warner ML, Tuder R, Schwarz MI. Diffuse alveolar hemorrhage and systemic lupus erythematosus. Clinical presentation, histology, survival, and outcome. Medicine. 1997;76(3):192–202.

55. Santos-Ocampo AS, Mandell BF, Fessler BJ. Alveolar hemorrhage in systemic lupus erythematosus: presentation and management. Chest. 2000;118(4): 1083–90.

56. Chang MY, Fang JT, Chen YC, Huang CC. Diffuse alveolar hemorrhage in systemic lupus erythematosus: a single center retrospective study in Taiwan. Ren Fail. 2002;24(6):791–802.

57. Cartin-Ceba R, Peikert T, Ashrani A, et al. Primary antiphospholipid syndrome-associated diffuse alveolar hemorrhage. Arthritis Care Res (Hoboken). 2014; 66(2):301–10.

Pulmonary Hypertension Associated with Connective Tissue Disease

11

Stephen C. Mathai and Laura K. Hummers

Introduction

Pulmonary hypertension (PH) is a chronic disease of the pulmonary vasculature characterized by pulmonary vascular remodeling; leading to increased pulmonary vascular resistance (PVR) that ultimately causes right ventricular dysfunction, failure, and death [1]. PH can develop in association with many different diseases and can result from processes that primarily affect systems distinct from the pulmonary vasculature, such as the heart, lung parenchyma, liver, and kidneys, in addition to processes that affect the pulmonary vasculature directly, such as thromboembolism [2]. Patients with connective tissue disease are at particularly high risk for the development of PH not only related to the involvement of the aforementioned organ systems, but also to the possibility of direct pulmonary vascular involvement in the absence of thromboembolism, known as pulmonary arterial hypertension (PAH) [3]. The presence of PH in any form is nearly

S.C. Mathai, M.D., M.H.S. (✉)
Division of Pulmonary and Critical Care Medicine, Johns Hopkins University School of Medicine, 1830 East Monument Street, 5th Floor, Baltimore, MD 21205, USA
e-mail: smathai4@jhmi.edu

L.K. Hummers, M.D., Sc.M.
Department of Medicine/Rheumatology, Johns Hopkins University School of Medicine, 5200 Eastern Avenue, Suite 4000, Mason F. Ford Building, Center Tower, Baltimore, MD 21224, USA

uniformly associated with increased morbidity and mortality. Unfortunately, patients with CTD-associated PH have variable response to therapy and tend to have poorer survival compared to PH patients without CTD. The reasons for the increased risk of development of PH, attenuated response to therapy, and poorer outcomes are poorly understood.

Definition and Classification of Pulmonary Hypertension

According to the most recent consensus guidelines, pulmonary hypertension is defined hemodynamically as a mean pulmonary artery pressure (mPAP) greater than or equal to 25 mmHg [2]. Thus, right heart catheterization (RHC) is required to diagnose PH as mPAPs cannot be directly measured by echocardiography. In hemodynamic terms, PH is often divided into pre-capillary and post-capillary disease based upon measurements; namely, if the PVR is greater than 3 Wood units and the pulmonary capillary wedge pressure (PCWP) is less than or equal to 15 mmHg, pre-capillary PH is present. If the PCWP is greater than 15 mmHg, post-capillary PH is present. This results from elevated left atrial pressures passively transmitted backwards into the pulmonary veins and arteries, leading to an elevated PAP with normal PVR and transpulmonary gradient (TPG, TPG = mPAP-PCWP, normal ≤12) [4]. So-called "mixed-PH" or "reactive PH" refers to mixed pre- and post-capillary PH in which chronic elevation

Table 11.1 Clinical classification of pulmonary hypertension

1. Pulmonary arterial hypertension (PAH)
(a) Idiopathic PAH (IPAH)
(b) Heritable
(c) Drug-and toxin-induced
(d) Associated with (APAH)
– Connective tissue disease
– HIV infection
– Portal hypertension
– Congenital heart disease
– Schistosomiasis
1. Pulmonary veno-occlusive disease, pulmonary capillary hemangiomatosis
Persistent pulmonary hypertension of the newborn
2. Pulmonary hypertension owing to left heart disease
(a) Systolic dysfunction
(b) Diastolic dysfunction
(c) Valvular disease
3. Pulmonary hypertension owing to lung diseases and/or hypoxia
(a) Chronic obstructive lung disease
(b) Interstitial lung disease
(c) Other pulmonary diseases with mixed restrictive and obstructive patterns
(d) Sleep disordered breathing
(e) Alveolar hypoventilation
(f) Chronic exposure to high altitude
(g) Developmental abnormalities
4. Chronic thromboembolic pulmonary hypertension (CTEPH)
5. Pulmonary hypertension with unclear multifactorial mechanisms
(a) Hematologic disorders, chronic hemolytic anemias
(b) Systemic disorders
(c) Metabolic disorders
(d) Others

of the pulmonary venous pressure leads to pulmonary arterial vasoconstriction with pulmonary vascular remodeling [5]. Current guidelines further refine this classification and incorporate hemodynamic criteria with clinical and associated characteristics (Table 11.1).

Distinguishing between the various forms of PH is imperative to properly diagnose and treat the disease and to appropriately risk-stratify patients. The initial classification schema included only two groups: primary pulmonary hypertension and secondary pulmonary hyper-

tension [6]. However, this schema and terminology has been abandoned in favor of the current classification system. As shown in Table 11.1, PH is divided into five groups, referred to as World Health Organization groups (WHO). PAH (WHO Group 1 disease) is defined hemodynamically by a mPAP greater than or equal to 25 mmHg with a PCWP less than or equal to 15 mmHg in the absence of chronic thromboembolic disease or other chronic respiratory disease. Included within this group is idiopathic PAH (IPAH), which was formerly known as primary pulmonary hypertension, and associated pulmonary arterial hypertension (APAH), which includes PAH related to CTD. Identifying Group I disease is particularly important as most of the current therapies for PH are approved only for use in this patient population [2, 7]. Group IV disease, PH related to chronic thrombotic or embolic disease, is also imperative to diagnose given the possibility of a surgical cure [8, 9]. Similarly, proper classification into the other WHO groups informs treatment strategies and management [10].

Because CTD in general can affect multiple organ systems, PH related to CTD can be associated with any of the five WHO groups (Fig. 11.1) [3, 11–18]. The most common CTDs associated with PH are listed in the figure and include mixed connective tissue disease (MCTD), polymyositis/dermatomyositis (PM/DM), rheumatoid arthritis (RA), Sjogren syndrome (SS), systemic lupus erythematosus (SLE), and systemic sclerosis (SSc). The risk of development of PH of any form varies by underlying CTD; the risk of PAH in particular seems to be higher in certain CTDs such as SSc. Thus, recommendations for screening for PH in CTD vary by CTD. Further, the evaluation of patients with suspected CTD-PAH can slightly differ from evaluation for other forms of PAH. For instance, since patients with CTD-PAH rarely demonstrate a significant response to acute vasodilator testing during RHC and are even less likely to demonstrate a sustained response to calcium channel blocker therapy, routine acute vasodilator challenges during RHC are not recommended [2]. Similarly, treatment recommendations and treatment response also depend in part upon the underlying CTD.

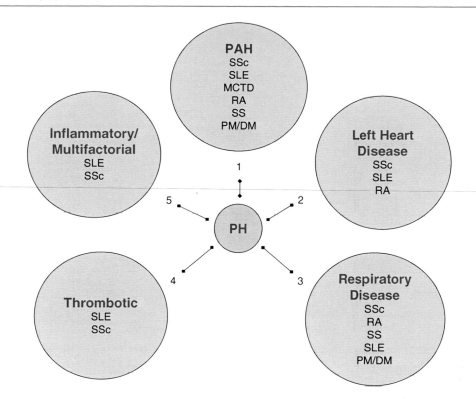

Fig. 11.1 Types of pulmonary hypertension in various connective tissue diseases

In general, the presence of PH complicating any of these CTDs is associated with a poorer prognosis [12, 19–23].

Pathophysiology and Pathobiology

The pathophysiology and pathobiology of pulmonary hypertension remain poorly understood. Further, there appears to be significant differences in the pathobiology of PAH compared to most other forms of PH, with notable distinctions between PAH and PH related to lung disease, for example [24–26]. However, given the substantial overlap between proposed mechanisms for CTD, ILD, and PAH, there may be commonality in the pathobiology that could be informative for therapeutic strategies [27].

PAH develops as a consequence of progressive remodeling of the small-to-medium sized pulmonary vasculature. Plexiform lesions, medial hypertrophy with muscularization of the arterioles, concentric intimal proliferation, and in situ

thrombosis are the pathologic hallmarks of the disease (Fig. 11.2) [28]. While the exact mechanisms of this remodeling remain unclear, multiple factors are thought to be involved [2, 25]. Functionally, there is an imbalance between vasoactive mediators such as thromboxane A2 and endothelin-1 and vasodilatory factors such as prostaglandins and nitric oxide in the vascular endothelium. Pulmonary artery vasoconstriction ensues in tandem with cellular proliferation; increased shear stress on the vasculature propagates endothelial injury. With this, sympathetic activity and hypoxemia follow, leading to further pulmonary vasoconstriction and eventually in situ thrombosis. These changes in the pulmonary vasculature cause a progressive increase in PVR and right ventricular afterload. Compensatory mechanisms in the right ventricle (RV) initially maintain cardiac function, however, in the face of prolonged increased afterload, the RV decompensates and cardiac failure ensues.

Genetic factors contribute to not only the predisposition to the development of PAH but also

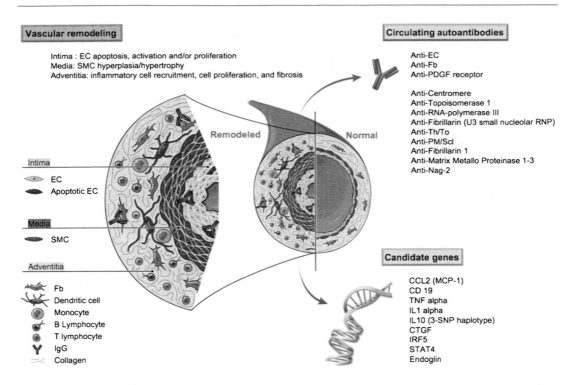

Fig. 11.2 Pulmonary vascular remodeling in CTD-PAH. This schematic features inflammatory mediators, cells, and mechanisms involved in the pulmonary vascular remodeling of SSc-PAH. Vascular changes affect all three layers (intima, media, and adventitia) of the pulmonary vessel and involve endothelial cell (EC) apoptosis, EC activation with increased expression of cell adhesion molecules, and inflammatory cell recruitment leading to vessel obliteration. A number of circulating auto-antibodies including classic autoantibodies, such as anti-centromere, anti-topoisomerase 1, anti-RNA-polymerase III, anti-fibrillarin (U3 small nucleolar ribonucleoprotein [RNP]), anti-Th/To, and antipolymyositis/scleroderma (PM/Scl), and more recently anti-fibrillarin 1, anti-matrix metalloproteinases (MMP) 1-3, anti-novel antigen(nag)-2 (non-steroidal anti-inflammatory drug-activated gene), and evidence that anti-fibroblast (Fb) antibodies, anti-EC antibodies (AECA), and anti-platelet derived growth factor (PDGF) receptor antibodies might exert a pathogenic role.

An increasing number of candidate genes have been reported to be associated with SSc in different cohorts, including, among others, a variant in the promoter of chemokine (C-C motif) ligand 2 (monocytes chemotactic protein-1) (CCL2 [MCP-1]), two variants in cluster of differentiation 19 (CD 19), a promoter and coding polymorphism in tumor necrosis factor (TNF)-α, a variant in the promoter of IL-1α gene, a three-single-nucleotide polymorphism (SNP) haplotype in IL-10, a polymorphism in the connective tissue growth factor (CTGF) promoter region, the interferon regulatory factor 5 (IRF5) rs2004640 GT substitution, and the signal transducer and activator of transcription 4 (STAT4) rs 7574865 single nucleotide polymorphism. *SMC* smooth muscle cell. (Used with permission from Le Pavec J, Humbert M, Mouthon L, Hassoun PM. Systemic sclerosis-associated pulmonary arterial hypertension. Am J Respir Crit Care Med 2010; 181[12]: 1285-93)

may contribute to the progression of disease and disease severity. Specific mutations in the transforming growth factor-β (TGF-β) superfamily, involved in regulation of fibrosis and angiogenesis, have been described in PAH patients. Mutations of the bone morphogenic protein type II receptor (BMPR2) gene are highly prevalent in patients with the familial/hereditary form of PAH; a smaller proportion of patients without the

familial/hereditary form of PAH also demonstrate mutations in this gene [29]. Other TGF-β pathways are associated with PAH; mutations in the type I TGF-β receptor, activin A receptor type-II like-1 (ALK-1), are found in patients with hereditary hemorrhagic telangiectasias who develop PAH [30]. Other more rare mutations in the downstream mediators of BMPR2 signaling have also been described [31]. In general, these mutations in the BMPR2 pathway lead to loss of function or reduced expression [32]. While mechanistic studies of BMPR2 mutations show that these mutations are permissive but not necessary for the development of PAH, the genetic data to date suggest a role for BMPR2 in the maintenance of the pulmonary vasculature. Interestingly, there are limited data demonstrating mutations in the TGF-β pathway in PAH related to CTD. Two small studies failed to show BMPR2 mutations in cohorts of patients with SSc-PAH and CTD-PAH [33, 34]. However, another study reported an association between a mutation in endoglin, a glycoprotein present on vascular endothelium that is part of the TGF-β superfamily, and risk of PAH in a cohort of SSc patients with and without PAH [35]. Still, this association remains to be recapitulated in other cohorts and highlights the potential differences in pathogenesis and pathobiology between various forms of PAH.

Inflammation and autoimmunity are thought to play a central role in the development of PAH, both in the IPAH and in CTD-PAH [36, 37]. In human PAH, plexiform lesions have been found to contain macrophages, T lymphocytes, B lymphocytes, and dendritic cells [38]. Tertiary lymphoid follicles containing these cells have recently been identified in patients with IPAH, located adjacent to remodeled pulmonary arteries [39]. Circulating factors, including inflammatory mediators, such as macrophage inflammatory protein-1 α, interleukin (IL)-1, IL-6, and P-selectin are increased in IPAH. Involvement of inflammatory cells is also a prominent feature of pulmonary vascular remodeling in CTD-PAH [40].

Autoimmunity and subsequent immune dysregulation may lead to activation of pathogenic autoreactive B cells and T cells and thus may be involved in the pathobiology of PAH and in particular, CTD-PAH. In SSc in particular, a number of specific autoantibodies are found, including anti-centromere, anti-topoisomerase 1, anti-RNA-polymerase III, anti-fibrillarin (U3 small nucleolar ribonucleoprotein), anti-Th/To, and anti-polymyositis/scleroderma; these autoantibodies typically correlate strongly with particular clinical phenotypes including the presence of various forms of PH [41]. More recently, anti-fibrillarin 1, anti-matrix metalloproteinases 1-3, anti-novel antigen 2, and anti-fibroblast antibodies have been identified [42]. Anti-fibroblast antibodies, thought to be important mediators of fibroblast activation and thus collagen synthesis that contributes to vascular remodeling, have been found in the serum of both SSc-PAH and IPAH patients [43]. Anti-endothelial cell antibodies (AECA) and antibodies to fibrin-bound tissue plasminogen activator are also present in patients with SSc-PAH. AECA have been shown to activate endothelial cells, induce the expression of adhesion molecules, and trigger apoptosis; thus these antibodies may be implicated in the pathogenesis of PAH [44]. In a recent study, antibodies to angiotensin II type 1(AT1R) receptor and endothelin-1 type A (ET1R) receptors were found to be significantly elevated in the serum of patients with SSc when compared to other CTDs such as RA and SS; these levels were highest in patients with SSc-PAH and were strongly associated with risk of death [45]. Further, the authors showed AT1R and ET1R antibodies initiated canonic signaling mediated by ERK1/2 in vitro using microvascular endothelial cells, suggesting a potential link between autoimmunity, endothelial injury, and fibrosis and thus, a role in PAH pathogenesis. Taken together, these data support a role for autoimmunity in the development of PAH and may explain the higher prevalence of PAH in CTDs in general.

The pathobiology of other forms of pulmonary hypertension (non-PAH pulmonary hypertension) is less well characterized than for PAH. Patients with Group 2 PH (PH due to left heart disease) can have either passive PH (due solely to increased pressure downstream of the pulmonary arteries) or reactive/mixed PH (due to a combination of increased downstream pressure and structural and/or functional abnormalities of the pulmonary vasculature) [4]. Pathologically, pulmonary veins are enlarged, dilated, and thickened with pulmonary capillary dilatation, interstitial edema, alveolar hemorrhage, and enlarged lymphatics. Distal pulmonary arteries can show evidence of medial hypertrophy, smooth muscle cell proliferation, and eccentric intimal lesions, without the classic plexiform lesions. Chronic elevation of pulmonary venous pressures leads to excessive production and accumulation of collagen IV in the extracellular matrix that leads to structural changes in the pulmonary vasculature from the capillaries to the arterioles and arteries [46]. Patients with CTD may be particularly prone to developing Group 2 PH due to high prevalence of diastolic or non-systolic dysfunction of the left ventricle; additionally, valvular disorders, particularly affecting the mitral valve, may also be present in certain CTDs and lead to increased pulmonary venous pressures [3].

Group 3 PH can result from several entities, including obstructive lung disease, restrictive lung disease, neuromuscular disease, or obstructive sleep apnea. Within this category, PH related to restrictive lung disease from interstitial lung disease is most commonly encountered clinically. While vascular obliteration related to parenchymal destruction can contribute to the development of PH in ILD, this mechanism is not thought to be sufficient to cause PH. While hypoxia clearly contributes to the development of PH related to ILD, there is a growing interest in commonalities in pathobiology between PH and ILD, and in particular, SSc related ILD (SSc-ILD), that may explain the frequent co-presentation of these two entities [27]. Endothelial apoptosis possibly due to circulating AECA and anti-fibrillarin antibodies represent the initial insult in the pathogenesis of SSc [47]. This process is followed by inflammation and dysregulated angiogenesis initially that ultimately progresses to obliterative vasculopathy with intimal proliferation. The same factors that lead to fibrosis in the vasculature may be influencing fibrosis in the interstitium, mediated by several pathways including the TGF-β superfamily, and factors such as the CXC chemokines, platelet-derived growth factor, and angiotensin II, among others [48–50]. Whether or not endothelial injury in SSc predisposes these patients to a higher risk of development of PH-ILD compared to other forms of ILD remains to be determined [51].

Characteristics of PH by CTD Type

Scleroderma

SSc is a heterogeneous disorder characterized by endothelial dysfunction, fibroblast dysregulation, and immune system abnormalities that lead to progressive fibrosis of the skin and internal organs [42]. Genetic and environmental factors in the setting of immune dysregulation are thought to contribute to host susceptibility [23]. More accurate estimates of the incidence and prevalence of SSc have resulted from the use of a standard classification system [52]. These estimates vary by geographic location, suggesting a role for environmental factors in the disease pathogenesis [53, 54]. For instance, the prevalence of SSc ranges from 30 to 70 cases per million in Europe and Japan to approximately 240 per million in the United States [55–58]. Incidence also varies by geographic location; the highest rates occur in the United States with approximately 19 cases per million per year.

Typically classified as limited or diffuse based upon extent of skin involvement, SSc of both subtypes can involve multiple organs, such as the heart, lungs, kidneys, and gastrointestinal tract [53]. Pulmonary hypertension in SSc may result from PAH, left heart disease, lung disease, chronic thromboembolic disease, and renal disease and thus fall into any of the five WHO classification groups of PH. In addition, various forms of PAH can develop in patients with SSc. In an autopsy series, Dorfmuller and colleagues described pulmonary veno-occlusive disease-like changes in the pulmonary venules and veins in 75 % of CTD patients with clinically diagnosed PAH [40]. While technically not PVOD, the authors surmised that these changes in the pulmonary veins of SSc patients may lead to similar responses to pulmonary vasodilator therapy as in PVOD. The classification (i.e., limited vs. diffuse) along with extended antibody profile have been associated with certain types of PH within the WHO group schema.

PAH occurs in about 8–14 % of patients with SSc when the diagnosis is based upon RHC

Table 11.2 Clinical risk factors for the development of PAH in SSc

Limited SSc
Late age of onset of SSc
Duration of SSc
Post-menopausal time period
Raynaud phenomenon
Number of telangiectasia
Severe digital ulcers
Decreased DL_{CO}
$FVC/DL_{CO} > 1.6$
Increased NT-proBNP
Antibody profile (anti-centromere, anti-U3 RNP)
Increasing RVSP >2 mmHg/year

[59, 60]. Higher estimates of PAH (up to 45 % in certain series) have overestimated the prevalence because the diagnosis has relied upon echocardiography and not RHC [61–64]. While echocardiography can be useful to suggest the presence of PH and to identify potential etiologies of PH (e.g., valvular disease, left ventricular dysfunction, congenital heart disease), echocardiography cannot establish the diagnosis of PH due to the inaccuracy of the Doppler signal in assessing true right ventricular systolic pressure and the frequent inability to obtain an adequate Doppler signal, particularly in CTD patients [65–67]. In a recent study of SSc patients who were at risk of developing PH based upon clinical characteristics including echocardiography findings, less than two-thirds of patients had RHC-confirmed PAH; around 15 % had Group II PH and 20 % had Group III PH [68]. However, despite the potential for over-diagnosis of PAH based upon the limitations of echocardiography; SSc-PAH is still likely to be under-recognized and under-diagnosed as suggested by the lower than expected prevalence of SSc-PAH in PH registries [69–71].

Risk factors for the development of PAH in SSc patients are varied and range from immutable patient characteristics to SSc-specific features to cardiopulmonary manifestations of developing pulmonary vascular disease (Table 11.2). Typically, PAH develops in women more frequently than men with SSc, however, men have poorer outcomes with a nearly fourfold

increased risk of death [72]. Race may influence disease severity as blacks with SSc-PAH have poorer functional capacity, RV function, and more severe hemodynamics at diagnosis than whites [73]. Age also influences the risk of PAH. As shown by Schachna and colleagues, the risk of PAH increased over 20 % with every 10 years of age at onset of SSc and when dichotomized at 60 years of age, there was twofold increased risk of development of PAH for late onset rather than younger onset of SSc [74]. There may be effect modification between gender and age with respect to the risk of development of PAH; post-menopausal changes in estrogen levels may abrogate its cardioprotective effects and thus be linked to increased risk of development of PAH amongst older women [75, 76]. Duration of SSc has also been associated with risk of PAH [77].

SSc type may also be associated with risk of PAH. While historically, PAH has been associated with limited cutaneous SSc (lcSSc), more recent epidemiologic studies from France have suggested that patients with diffuse cutaneous SSc (dcSSc) may have a higher likelihood of developing PAH [59, 78, 79]. Still, these associations may be biased by the low prevalence overall of incident cases (only 8 total PAH cases out of 374 SSc patients followed for 3 years) and perhaps by differences in the overall prevalence of SSc by disease type since lcSSc is three to five times more prevalent than dcSSc in Western Europe [80]. Other disease-specific features of SSc that can be associated with the development of PAH include severe digital ischemia and higher number of telangiectasias [81, 82].

Decline in pulmonary function as assessed by pulmonary function testing has also been associated with the risk of development of PAH. Isolated decreases in diffusing capacity of carbon monoxide (DLCO) in lcSSc patients portends an increased risk of PAH; a retrospective study identified patients with SSc-PAH had significantly reduced DLCO almost 5 years prior to establishing the diagnosis of PAH [81]. Other parameters, such as a forced vital capacity (FVC) to DLCO ratio of greater than 1.6 and a DLCO to alveolar volume (VA) ratio of less than 70 % have been demonstrated to predict the presence of PAH [81, 83].

Screening and Early Detection

Because SSc patients are at high risk of developing PAH, routine screening for this disease has been recommended by several medical societies [2, 84]. However, the frequency of screening, type of test selected, and patient characteristics vary by screening program. Since some of the recommendations include patient symptoms as an indicator for screening, these programs actually represent early detection algorithms rather than true screening programs [85]. However, employing early detection algorithms can effectively identify patients with PAH earlier in the disease course [59, 86]. When compared to a cohort of patients identified with PAH in routine practice, employment of an algorithm based upon echocardiographic findings (tricuspid regurgitant (TR) jet velocity ≥2.5 m/s) in combination with patient symptoms identified patients with less severe hemodynamic disease and less severe symptoms. Survival was also significantly better in this small cohort of patients compared to those who underwent routine clinical evaluation [86]. However, reliance solely upon echocardiography as a screening tool has significant limitations, with both high false positive and false negative rates [87]. Incorporation of other tools, such as symptoms, PFTs, and serum biomarkers such as N-terminal pro-brain natriuretic peptide (NT-proBNP) may potentially enhance the effectiveness of early detection strategies [59, 83]. A recent multinational study employed a two-step algorithm incorporating PFT parameters, serum biomarkers, clinical characteristics (presence of telangiectasias), and EKG findings to generate a risk score to determine the need for echocardiography [88]. Subsequent findings on echocardiography (right atrial enlargement, TR jet ≥2.5 m/s) in combination with Step 1 score determined the need for RHC. Using this algorithm, the false negative rate for PAH was 4 % compared to nearly 30 % false negative rate when employing the European Society of Cardiology/European Respiratory Society guidelines for screening in this population [87]. A recent consensus statement on the screening and early detection of PAH in CTD endorsed this algorithm for SSc patients with DLCO <60 % predicted and >3 years duration of SSc (from first non-Raynaud's symptom) while recommending yearly PFTs and echocardiography in all SSc patients [89].

Outcomes

Outcomes in SSc-PAH are poor. While a recent study from the multicenter observational PHAROS cohort reports improved overall survival in the SSc-PAH population with 3 year survival of 75 %, other modern era cohort studies have reported 3-year survival less than 60 % [17, 60, 70, 72, 90–93]. The improved survival in the PHAROS registry may reflect inclusion of patients with less severe disease as more than half of the subjects had NYHA functional class I or II disease at enrollment. Prior studies have also demonstrated that survival remains worse in SSc-PAH than in patients with the idiopathic form of PAH, despite seemingly less severe hemodynamic perturbations at diagnosis [91, 94]. However, as recent research has shown, traditional measures of hemodynamic derangements in PAH (e.g., RAP and CO) may not be the best metrics to assess disease severity or outcomes in SSc-PAH [93]. For example, in one cohort study of SSc-PAH and IPAH patients, NT-proBNP levels were significantly higher in the SSc-PAH population despite less severe hemodynamic impairment; this difference persisted when controlling for potential confounders such as age and renal function [95]. Since NT-proBNP is released from the ventricles in response to increased wall stress, the observation suggested that responses to increased afterload on the RV may differ between SSc-PAH and IPAH. In line with this, recent physiologic studies have shown depressed RV function for a similar afterload in SSc-PAH compared to IPAH [96, 97]. Using pressure-volume measurements in the RV, Tedford and colleagues demonstrated significantly lower contractility in SSc-PAH compared to IPAH patients, despite similar pulmonary vascular resistive and pulsatile loading characteristics as assessed by resistance-compliance relationships and arterial elastance measures [97]. These findings suggest intrinsic RV dysfunction may contribute to the clinical differences in presentation and outcomes

Table 11.3 Predictors of survival in PAH-SSc

Male gender[a]
Age[a]
NYHA functional class at diagnosis[a]
Increased NT-proBNP
Right atrial pressure[a]
Mean pulmonary artery pressure[a]
Cardiac index
Stroke volume index
Pulmonary vascular resistance
Renal function

[a]Variable association with survival in PAH-SSc

noted between SSc-PAH and IPAH. Table 11.3 shows predictors of outcomes in patients with SSc-PAH.

PH Related to ILD in SSc

SSc patients can also develop PH related to ILD. However, there are few data describing the prevalence of PH in SSc-ILD. While the presence of ILD in SSc in the absence of PH portends a poor prognosis, survival is even worse in SSc patients with combined ILD and PH [12, 23, 70, 98]. In a cohort of 59 SSc-PH patients, 20 of whom had significant ILD (defined as a TLC <60 % predicted or TLC between 60 and 70 % predicted combined with moderate to severe fibrosis on high resolution CT of the chest), survival was significantly worse in the SSc-ILD cohort with 1-, 2-, and 3-year survival rates of 82 %, 49 %, and 39 % compared to 87 %, 79 %, and 64 % in the PH alone group, respectively ($p<0.01$) [12]. Presence of ILD portended a fivefold increased risk of death compared to PAH. Similar 3-year survival rates (47 %) were noted in another cohort of 47 SSc-PH-ILD patients [98].

Mixed Connective Tissue Disease

Patients with MCTD have clinical features of several connective tissue diseases including SSc, SLE, rheumatoid arthritis, and polymyositis. Symptoms include polyarthritis, myositis, sclerodactyly, Raynaud's phenomenon, esophageal dysmotility; less commonly serositis, rash, telangiectasias, and pigmentation abnormalities can

be found. The characteristic laboratory feature is presence of antibodies to uridine-rich (U1) RNP polypeptides. While several diagnostic classification schemas for this disease have been proposed, all require the presence of U1-RNP antibodies [99]. These U1-RNP antibodies are also implicated in the pathogenesis of PAH by inducing endothelial cell activation and damage, perhaps in association with AECA [100, 101].

While renal involvement in MCTD is less common than with SLE or SSc, lung involvement may be more common than either entity [102–104]. Lung disease in MCTD can manifest as parenchymal disease, pulmonary vascular disease, or both [15, 21]. In one single center series of 201 subjects with MCTD, over 50 % of patients had ILD; whereas nearly 24 % were reported to have PAH. However, this is likely an over-estimate of the prevalence of PAH given that the diagnosis was established by echocardiography using a non-standard definition of PH (right ventricular systolic pressure estimate greater than 25 mmHg). Further, the proportion of patients with PH-ILD in this study was not reported. Other cohort studies have provided estimates of the prevalence of PAH in MCTD ranging from 19 % to as high as 50 %; however, some of these studies were either single-center studies or defined PAH based upon echocardiographic findings alone [103, 105, 106]. A recent study from a Norwegian prospective registry of patients with MCTD suggested a much lower prevalence of PAH, with only 5/147 patients with PH and just 2/147 with PAH [15]. However, since this was an observational study without a specific screening protocol for PH, this is likely an underestimate of the prevalence of PH and PAH. For example, while all patients underwent a screening echo at the time of enrollment, only 64 % of patients underwent a repeat echo during a mean follow-up period of nearly 6 years. Thus, it is likely that incident cases were missed during the study follow-up. Therefore, a reliable estimate of both PAH and PH-ILD in MCTD remains to be defined.

Another potential contributor to pulmonary vascular disease may be more common in MCTD than SSc. In the prior study by Gunnarsson and colleagues, the authors report a remarkably high proportion of patients who develop thrombosis, both arterial (6.4 %) and venous (19.9 %) [107]. Whether these patients with venous thrombosis developed chronic thromboembolic disease and PH is unknown. Interestingly, anti-endothelial cell and anti-cardiolipin antibodies were frequently found in patients who developed thrombotic events, suggesting a possible common pathway for pulmonary vascular disease. This finding alone reinforces the importance of a thorough evaluation for chronic PE in MCTD patients with possible PH.

The REVEAL registry included 52 patients with MCTD-PAH and thus has added to our understanding of the particular characteristics of this disease [17]. These patients tended to be younger at enrollment than SSc-PAH patients (49.4 ± 16.1 vs. 61.8 ± 11.1 years, respectively). While there was no difference in gender distribution between MCTD-PAH and SSc-PAH, a higher proportion of MCTD-PAH patients were black and Hispanic. Serum biomarkers such as brain natriuretic peptide and creatinine were both significantly lower in the MCTD-PAH group compared to the SSc-PAH group. Interestingly, while there were no differences in spirometry or lung volume measurements between these groups, diffusion capacity for carbon monoxide (DLCO) was significantly higher in the MCTD-PAH group. On echocardiography, MCTD-PAH patients had less evidence of left ventricular systolic dysfunction; invasive hemodynamics did not significantly differ between groups, except for right atrial pressure that tended to be lower in the MCTD-PAH cohort.

Screening and Early Detection

In the REVEAL registry, nearly 70 % of patients with MCTD-PAH had functional class III symptoms at the time of diagnosis, highlighting the delay in diagnosis in this patient population [17]. A recent consensus statement suggests that MCTD patients with features of SSc should undergo the same screening protocol as patients with SSc alone to potentially mitigate the delay in diagnosis of PAH [89]. Whether this strategy will be effective in the early detection of PH in this population remains to be determined.

Outcomes

PAH is likely the most common cause of death in patients with MCTD. In a cluster analysis that divided patients into three groups based upon clinical features and antibody profiles, patients with either "PAH" (defined by echocardiography) or predominantly vascular involvement (thrombosis) had significantly poorer survival than the group with predominantly ILD and the group with predominantly articular manifestations [107]. PAH was the most common cause of death in both the vascular cohort (72 %) and in the overall cohort (50 %). Two recent cohort studies have reported outcomes in RHC-proven MCTD-PAH. In a national registry from the United Kingdom, survival in MCTD-PAH ($n = 28$) was similar to the survival observed in the SSc-PAH cohort ($n = 259$), at 1 year (83 % vs. 77 %) but perhaps better at 3 years (66 % vs. 47 %) [70]. In the REVEAL registry, 1-year survival did not differ between MCTD-PAH and SSc-PAH (88 % vs. 82 %) [17]. However, when compared to other forms of CTD-PAH, such as SLE-PAH, survival was worse in the MCTD-PAH cohorts in both studies.

Systemic Lupus Erythematous

SLE is also a multisystem disease that can affect the lungs and lead to several forms of pulmonary vascular disease including PH-ILD, PAH, and CTEPH. In addition, PH can result from SLE-associated cardiomyopathy or from renal failure requiring hemodialysis and placement of arteriovenous fistulas [108]. Thus, PH in SLE can also be classified in any of the five PH categories (Fig. 11.1).

Prevalence estimates of PH in SLE vary widely, from 0.0005 to 14 % of patients [19, 109–118]. Much of this variance in estimates can be attributed to the definition of PH and the method of detection employed. For example, three of the studies that employed RHC to diagnose PH utilized non-standard definitions of PH (mPAP >30 mmHg (one study) and mPAP >40 mmHg (two studies)) [19, 109, 110]. Furthermore, since screening protocols for PH are not recommended based upon the relative rarity of PH in the SLE population, only symptomatic patients undergo evaluation for PH. Thus, while it appears that the prevalence of PH in SLE is lower than that in other CTDs such as SSc and MCTD, the true prevalence may be significantly higher.

Patients who develop the disease tend to be young (average age around 30 at diagnosis) and often have Raynaud's phenomenon. On average, patients have SLE for nearly 5 years prior to the development of PAH [119]. Risk factors for the development of PAH related to SLE are not well described, but one retrospective cohort study that used echo to define PH (defined as a RVSP ≥35 mmHg) found that blacks were more likely to have PH. Further, patients with longer disease duration, peripheral nervous system involvement, and with pericarditis were more likely to have PH [118]. The authors also found patients with anti-smooth muscle antibodies and anticardiolipin antibodies were more likely to develop PH.

Outcomes

As expected, outcomes in SLE patients with PH are worse than for those without PH. While prior studies reported median survival for SLE-PAH patients ranging from 2 to 3 years, a more recent cohort study from the United Kingdom reported a 3-year survival of 75 % [19, 70, 113, 120]. PAH also appears to be a common cause of death in several cohorts from Korea and China, however, it is a rare cause of death in North American and European cohorts [121, 122]. These differences between cohorts suggest possible ethnic differences in the impact of PH on outcomes in SLE but remain to be confirmed or explained. In a recent systematic review of factors associated with outcomes in SLE-PAH, Johnson and colleagues found both PH-specific and SLE-specific parameters predicted survival [117]. Higher mPAP at diagnosis was associated with poorer outcomes. Vascular manifestations of SLE in particular, such as Raynaud's phenomenon, pulmonary vasculitis, thrombosis, thrombocytopenia, and presence of anti-cardiolipin antibodies, portended a poorer prognosis. Interestingly, neither lupus disease activity nor nephritis was associated with poorer outcomes.

Sjogren Syndrome

Sjogren syndrome (SS) is a chronic inflammatory disease characterized by lymphocytic infiltration of exocrine glands and extra-glandular tissues. The disease can present as primary disease or in association with other CTDs like RA or SSc. Up to 0.4 % of the general population has SS; the vast majority are women in the fourth and fifth decades of life [123]. While the sicca syndrome (xerophthalmia and/or keratoconjunctivits sicca and xerostomia) is most commonly present in patients with SS, extra-glandular involvement of the lungs is common, typically manifesting as ILD. Various types of ILD have been described in SS, including lymphocytic interstitial pneumonia, non-specific interstitial pneumonitis, usual interstitial pneumonitis, and organizing pneumonia [124].

In contrast, PAH is rare in SS; in fact, only 43 known cases of RHC-confirmed SS-PAH are reported in the literature. Relatively large cohort studies have estimated the prevalence of PH around 20 %, however, neither study distinguished between PH related to ILD and PAH and RHC was not used to establish the diagnosis [22, 125]. Thus, the true prevalence remains unknown. However, in the largest case series of patients with SS associated PH Launay and colleagues describe characteristics of patients with this disease, noting that these patients were more likely to have Raynaud's phenomenon, vasculitis, and ILD [14]. Antibody profiles suggested associations with anti-Ro and RNP antibodies; hypergammaglobulinemia was also noted to be more frequent in SS patients with PAH. Survival in this cohort was poor with 1- and 3-year survival at 73 % and 66 % respectively, similar to survival seen in patients with PAH-SSc.

Rheumatoid Arthritis

Rheumatoid arthritis (RA) is an autoimmune disease characterized by a symmetric, inflammatory polyarthritis that leads to joint destruction. RA is more prevalent than most other CTDs occurring in 40 out of 100,000 persons in the US.

Women in the US have a nearly 4 % lifetime risk of developing RA [126]. Extra-articular disease affects multiple organs including the skin, eyes, hematologic system, and kidneys; importantly, cardiopulmonary involvement is common. There is a high risk of coronary artery disease, myocardial infarction, heart failure, and sudden death compared to age-matched persons without RA [127]. Pulmonary manifestations include interstitial lung disease, rheumatoid nodules, airways disease with bronchiolitis obliterans and organizing pneumonia. Additionally, pleural disease with effusion, empyema, bronchopleural fistula, or pyopneumothorax is fairly common, occurring in up to 20 % of patients [128]. Lung disease may also result from disease-modifying antirheumatic drugs, with complications such as pneumonitis, fibrosis, obliterative bronchiolitis, infection, and bronchospasm, amongst others [129].

Pulmonary hypertension in RA has been reported in association with left heart disease, interstitial lung disease, and chronic thromboembolic disease [130, 131]. Isolated pulmonary hypertension, that is, PH in the absence of overt left heart disease, ILD, and chronic thromboembolic disease, has been infrequently reported in the literature [132–142]. In these case reports, PH has been attributed to pulmonary vasculitis [132, 135, 136, 138], hyperviscosity syndromes [134], and PAH [133, 137]. In a few of these studies, RHC was performed, confirming the diagnosis of PAH. Further, lung tissue obtained either by biopsy or at autopsy in these patients demonstrated some classic features of PAH, including intimal proliferation, medial hypertrophy, and even plexiform lesions in the small pulmonary arterioles [132, 135, 137]. In the UK registry, only 12 RA-PAH patients were identified while in the REVEAL registry, 28 cases of RHC-proven RA-PAH were included [17, 70]. When compared to patients with SSc-PAH in the REVEAL cohort, RA-PAH patients tended to be younger (54 ± 15.8 vs. 61.8 ± 11.1 years). Raynaud's phenomenon was less likely to be present (3.6 % vs. 32.6 % of the cohort); renal insufficiency was less frequent, and BNP levels were significantly lower. Functional class at baseline, 6 min walk distance, and hemodynamics were similar between RA-PAH and SSc-PAH

patients. Similar to the findings seen in the MCTD-PAH cohort in the REVEAL registry, while spirometry and lung volumes were similar when compared to SSc-PAH, diffusing capacity was higher in the RA-PAH cohort. Survival in the RA-PAH cohort was significantly better than the SSc-PAH cohort with 1-year survival at 96 % vs. 82 % in the SSc-PAH cohort (p-value = 0.01).

Polymyositis/Dermatomyositis

Polymyositis (PM) and dermatomyositis (DM) are idiopathic inflammatory myopathies that are characterized by proximal muscle weakness. DM has characteristic skin manifestations though clinical features of both DM and PM vary among affected individuals. The estimated prevalence of these diseases varies from 5 to 22 per 100,000 persons with an annual incidence of 2 per 100,000 [143, 144]. PM/DM are both multisystem disorders with the potential to affect the heart, GI tract, and lungs; there is also an increased rate of malignancy, particularly with DM [145]. The most common pulmonary manifestation of PM/DM is interstitial lung disease, occurring in about 10 % of patients, though respiratory symptoms such as dyspnea and orthopnea can also arise from muscle weakness affecting the diaphragm [146].

Pulmonary hypertension appears to be a rare complication of PM/DM and if present, may be related to underlying ILD [18]. In the UK registry, only seven patients (2 % of the entire CTD-PAH cohort) with PM/DM-PAH were identified; there were no cases of PM/DM-PAH in the REVEAL registry [17, 70]. No clinical demographic or hemodynamic characteristics of these patients were reported in the UK registry; however, the 1- and 3-year survival was 100 % for these patients, suggesting better outcomes for PM/DM-PAH compared to other CTD-PAH.

Treatment

With improved understanding of PAH, novel therapies targeting select pathways in the putative pathogenesis have been developed. These therapies focus on the chronically impaired endothelial function that affects pulmonary vascular tone and remodeling. Further, recent studies identifying aberrant proliferation of endothelial and smooth muscle cells and increased secretion of growth factors have drawn investigators to compare PAH to a neoplastic process and have paved the way for trials of antineoplastic agents in PAH [147–151].

Randomized clinical trials of novel therapeutics for PAH have included patients with various forms of CTD-PAH, although the majority of patients enrolled likely have SSc (Table 11.4). Sub-group analyses in the CTD-PAH cohorts of these studies have only been intermittently reported [152–156]. Given the differences in demographic and hemodynamic characteristics between CTD-PAH types, the results from these clinical trials are unlikely to be generalizable to all forms of CTD-PAH and thus should be interpreted with caution in most cases. Still, the PAH therapies discussed next are commonly used in all forms of CTD-PAH although the evidence base for diseases other than SSc is minimal.

General Measures

Despite a lack of specific data for PAH of any form, consensus guidelines recommend the use of supplemental oxygen in patients who are hypoxic (peripheral oxygen saturation <90 %) at rest or with exercise, largely based upon extrapolation of data from chronic obstructive lung disease [2, 157, 158]. In addition, diuretics are recommended for the management of volume overload and for right heart failure. Digoxin may also be useful for the management of refractory right heart failure complicated by atrial arrhythmias. Exercise, and in particular, pulmonary rehabilitation, may also be beneficial as demonstrated in a clinical trial of prescribed exercise in a population of patients with IPAH [159]. In this study, both quality of life and exercise capacity as assessed by the 6MWT were significantly improved in patients who completed a specific exercise program, with rather large effect sizes. Similar results were demonstrated in a smaller observational study of CTD-PAH [160].

Table 11.4 Inclusion of CTD-PAH patients in pivotal trials of PAH therapy

	CTD-PAH (n, overall %)	Type of CTD (n, % CTD)
Epoprostenol	111 (100 %)	lcSSc: 77 (69 %)
		dcSSc: 14 (13 %)
		Others: 20 (18 %)
Oral treprostinil	110 (19 %)	NR
Oral treprostinil add-on	92 (26 %)	NR
SC treprostinil	90 (19 %)	lcSSc: 20 (22 %)
		dcSSc: 25 (28 %)
		SLE: 25 (28 %)
		MCTD: 17 (19 %)
		Overlap: 3 (3 %)
Inhaled treprostinil	77 (33 %)	NR
Inhaled iloprost (AIR)	35 (17 %)	NR
Inhaled iloprost + bosentan	NR	NR
Beraprost	13 (10 %)	NR
Vardenafil (EVOLUTION)	20 (30 %)	NR
Tadalafil (PHIRST)	95 (29 %)	NR
Sildenafil + epoprostenol (PACES)	55 (21 %)	SSc: 31 (56 %)
		SLE: 14 (25 %)
		Other: 10 (18 %)
Sildenafil (SUPER)	84 (30 %)	SSc: 50 (60 %)*
		SLE: 19 (23 %)
		MCTD: 8 (10 %)
		SjS: 4 (5 %)
		RA: 1 (1 %)
Bosentan (EARLY)	33 (18 %)	SSc: 15 (46 %)
		SLE: 11 (6 %)
		MCTD: 3 (9 %)
		SjS: 1 (3 %)
		Other: 1 (3 %)
Bosentan (Study 351 + BREATHE)	66 (27 %)	SSc: 52 (78 %)
		SLE: 8 (12 %)
		Overlap: 4 (6 %)
		UCTD: 2 (3 %)
Bosentan + epoprostenol (BREATHE-2)	6 (18 %)	SSc: 5 (83 %)
		SLE: 1 (17 %)
Ambrisentan (ARIES 1 + ARIES 2)	136 (35 %)	NR
Sitaxsentan (STRIDE-1)	42 (24 %)	SSc: 19 (45 %)
		SLE: 15 (36 %)
		MCTD: 7 (17 %)

Anticoagulation

Anticoagulation is recommended in the treatment of IPAH based primarily upon retrospective, observational data showing improved survival in patients on warfarin therapy [2]. However, no such data exists for CTD-PAH. Despite the potential for increased risk of gastrointestinal bleeding due to vascular ectasias that may be common in certain forms of CTD, the current guidelines recommend therapy with oral anticoagulation in those without contraindications, particularly in those patients with more advanced disease who are receiving continuous intravenous therapy.

Immunosuppression

As discussed previously, inflammatory and immunological mechanisms are likely involved in the pathogenesis of both CTD and PAH. Given this potential commonality in pathobiology, anti-inflammatory agents have been employed in various types of CTD-PAH. However, there are no randomized clinical trials in patients with CTD-PAH to support its use in this patient population. Still, several case series have suggested efficacy in certain populations within CTD-PAH. In the report by Jais and colleagues, 23 patients with either SLE- or MCTD-associated PAH were treated with combination therapy including cyclophosphamide and glucocorticoids; nearly half of the SLE-PAH and MCTD-PAH patients demonstrated clinical improvement in functional capacity and hemodynamics [161]. However, the 6 SSc-PAH patients included in the cohort did not demonstrate response to immunosuppression. Still, these patients did experience improvement in these parameters once PAH-specific therapy was initiated. Other investigators have reported improvements in functional capacity, hemodynamics, and in certain cases, in expected survival, with immunosuppressant therapy [162–164]. Randomized clinical trials are needed to better understand the role of immunosuppressant therapy in patients with CTD-PAH, and in particular, in SSc-PAH in whom disease is often refractory to such interventions.

Prostaglandins

Prostacyclin is an endogenous vasodilator that inhibits platelet aggregation via activation of cyclic adenosine monophosphate. Exogenous prostanoids increase production of prostacyclins which in turn restores the balance between vasoconstrictors such as thromboxane A2 and vasodilators. The synthetic prostacyclin epoprostenol was the first drug approved for therapy for PAH and to date, remains the only therapy that has been shown to improve survival in a randomized clinical trial of PAH patients [165]. Epoprostenol has also been studied in patients with SSc-PAH [166]. However, while there were statistically significant improvements in exercise capacity and hemodynamics, no survival benefit was found. Still, this medication is considered the most efficacious for the treatment of PAH and thus, is used in patients with severe disease.

There are several important factors related to drug delivery and side effects that must be carefully considered prior to initiation of intravenous epoprostenol. Since the half-life of this medication is only 2–3 min, it must be delivered via continuous infusion through a tunneled catheter. Further, IV epoprostenol is only stable at room temperature for 8 h and thus must be kept cold to maintain its integrity. Recently, a room temperature stable formulation was approved for commercial use. Side effects are common and include headache, jaw pain, nausea, diarrhea, leg pain, heel pain, and flushing. Systemic hypotension is also common. These side effects can be dose-limiting in certain patients. Several reports of pulmonary edema in patients with SSc-PAH who were treated both acutely and chronically with prostaglandin derivatives raise the suspicion of occult pulmonary veno-occlusive disease and highlight the risks of therapy in these patients [167, 168].

Use of IV epoprostenol in patients with CTD-PAH seems to vary from use in IPAH patients. A recent study reporting the 15-year experience at the University of Michigan found that significantly fewer SSc-PAH patients received IV prostacyclins compared to IPAH patients in the cohort (38.5 % vs. 55.3 %, $p = 0.02$) despite nearly 80 %

of the SSc cohort demonstrating severe PAH (WHO functional class III/IV) [94]. We have a similar experience at our center, with less than 45 % of class III/IV SSc-PAH patients on IV prostacyclin therapy. This is in part related to patient factors including limited manual dexterity in our SSc population due to sclerodactyly and digital ulcers (DU); historically, the need for the use of cold packs also precipitated Raynaud's exacerbations and contributed to lower utilization in this patient population. However, this rate of use in severe PAH patients parallels use across the United States as shown in the REVEAL registry, where only 43 % of patients (all PAH types) who died were receiving IV prostacyclin therapy at the time of death [169].

There are several other formulations of prostacyclin analogues that are currently available for use in the treatment of PAH and have been studied in CTD-PAH. Iloprost is formulated in both intravenous and inhaled versions, though only the inhaled form is approved for therapy of PAH in the USA. IV iloprost has been studied in CTD patients without PAH for treatment of peripheral vascular complications and shown to improve exercise capacity and hemodynamics compared to baseline values; however no specific data exist in patients with CTD-PAH [170, 171]. Studies of inhaled iloprost in various forms of PAH, including CTD-PAH, have demonstrated significant improvements in functional class, exercise capacity, and hemodynamics compared to placebo [172].

Treprostinil is another prostacyclin analogue that is chemically stable at room temperature and is available in IV, subcutaneous (SC) and inhaled forms; trials with an oral form of treprostinil are currently underway. Similar to IV epoprostenol, IV treprostinil must be delivered via a central catheter and continuous infusion pump. The SC formulation is also delivered via continuous infusion, but through a needle placed in the subcutaneous space. Ninety patients with various types of CTD-associated PAH were included in the large randomized clinical trial of SC treprostinil (Table 11.4). The response in this subset, as reported by Oudiz and colleagues, suggested clinical efficacy, with improvements in dyspnea scores, functional capacity, and hemodynamics, though the change in 6MWD between treatment and placebo groups was of marginal statistical significance (25 m, $p=0.055$) [153]. Although patients with CTD-PAH were included in the TRIUMPH study investigating the addition of inhaled treprostinil to bosentan or sildenafil and significant improvement in functional capacity was found, no subgroup analyses on CTD-PAH patients were reported [173].

Endothelin Receptor Antagonists

Endothelin-1 (ET-1) is a potent vasoconstrictor that regulates vascular tone and cell proliferation in the pulmonary vasculature; perturbations in ET-1 balance are thought to contribute to the pathogenesis of PAH [174]. Further, ET-1 also may have a role in the pathogenesis of SSc contributing to vascular damage and fibrosis as prior studies have identified relationships between ET-1 levels and disease severity [175]. Thus, ET-1 remains an attractive target for therapy in CTD-PAH and SSc-PAH in particular.

Endothelin receptor antagonists (ERA) block ET receptors on vascular smooth muscle thereby promoting vasorelaxation in the pulmonary vasculature. Bosentan, a dual competitive ET receptor antagonist, was the first agent developed in this class. In the BREATHE-1 study, significant improvements in functional class, 6MWD, time to clinical worsening (TTCW), and hemodynamics were found in PAH subjects receiving bosentan compared to placebo. Almost a third of these subjects in this trial had CTD-PAH. In a subgroup analysis of this study, CTD-PAH patients, most of whom had SSc-PAH, did not exhibit a significant improvement in 6MWD; however, subjects in the treatment arm were less likely to experience deterioration. These findings were similar to observations from our experience with initial therapy with bosentan; when compared to IPAH patients, SSc-PAH patients had less robust response to therapy with no change in FC, poorer survival, and a higher incidence of side effects [176]. However, in a multicenter observational study of initial therapy with bosentan in a cohort of 53 CTD-PAH patients (80 % with SSc-PAH), after 48 weeks of therapy, a larger proportion of patients experienced an improvement in FC than a decline (27 % vs. 16 %), but the majority experiencing no change in FC (57 %) [156]. Further, 1-year survival was 92 %; improved when compared to historical controls, however, no improvement in health-related quality of life was noted. In a sub-group analysis of randomized clinical trials of bosentan in which CTD-PAH subjects were included, trends towards improvement in 6MWD and improved survival compared to historical controls were found [154]. However, this cohort included patients with various forms of CTD-PAH and thus may not accurately reflect the experience of a particular group within the CTD population. Bosentan has also been studied in the management of Raynaud's and digital ulcers (DU), but a recent meta-analysis suggests that while the number of new DU are reduced in SSc patients on bosentan, there is no effect on healing of existing DU [177]. Thus, bosentan therapy seems to stabilize and in some cases, improve symptoms and functional capacity in patients with CTD-PAH, but may not improve quality of life or other vascular complications of CTD such as DU. There may also be improvement in 1-year outcomes compared to historical controls, but this has not been evaluated in a prospective, randomized study.

Ambrisentan is another ERA with a high selectivity for ETA vs. ETB receptors (>4,000-fold). This selectively may target the vasoconstrictive effects of endothelin while preserving the vasodilatory action that is mediated by ETB receptors, however, the clinical relevance of this degree of selectivity is unknown. In large, randomized, double-masked, placebo-controlled clinical trials of PAH, patients receiving ambrisentan demonstrated significant improvement in 6MWD and a significant reduction in TTCW [178]. In the CTD-PAH subgroup, initially there was improvement in 6MWD, but by the end of the study at 24 weeks, no differences compared to baseline were found. In the long-term extension study, 124 of the 383 subjects (32 %) included had CTD-PAH, however, the type of CTD was not reported [179]. In this observational study, 1- and 2-year survival for CTD-PAH patients was 91 % and 83 % respectively; however, since nearly 20 % of subjects were on combination therapy with other PAH-specific medications at 2 years, the long-term effects of ambrisentan alone cannot be determined accurately. In another observational study that included 40 CTD-PAH patients who were either treatment-naïve or on background therapy with other PAH-specific medications, no significant improvement in 6MWD was noted after 24 weeks of therapy with ambrisentan. Still, in each of these studies, ambrisentan was well tolerated; however, nearly 33 % of patients experienced worsening lower extremity edema with initiation of therapy.

Macitentan is a tissue-targeting ERA that has been shown in vivo to remain active in local tissue environments leading to longer functional half-life than other ERAs [180]. A recent randomized, double blind, placebo controlled trial of macitentan at 3 and 10 mg demonstrated a significantly reduced risk of morbidity/mortality compared to placebo with 45 % reduction in the 10 mg group with a 30 % reduction in the 3 mg group [181]. In this study, 30.5 % of PAH patients had CTD-related disease; however, no data on specific effects in this population have been published to date. Macitentan was well tolerated, with no difference in lower extremity edema between the placebo and treatment arms.

Side effects with ERA are common and include peripheral edema, headache, dyspnea, upper respiratory tract infection, nasal congestion, fatigue, and nausea. ERAs may also cause hepatotoxicity. However, due to differences in formulation between bosentan, ambrisentan, and macitentan, there is no increased risk of liver dysfunction over placebo with ambrisentan and macitentan and thus, monthly monitoring for hepatotoxicity is not required for these agents, but is for bosentan [182]. Further, decreases in hemoglobin can occur and require monitoring. ERAs are teratogenic and thus pregnancy is a formal contraindication; further, due to drug–drug interactions, estrogen/progesterone contraception is not a reliable form of contraception in the presence of bosentan.

Phosphodiesterase Inhibitors

Phosphodiesterase type 5 inhibitors (PDE5I) inhibit the degradation of cyclic guanosine monophosphate (cGMP), a second messenger released by soluble guanylate cyclase (sGC) in response to nitric oxide (NO) stimulation. NO is a potent vasodilator that also inhibits platelet aggregation and vascular smooth muscle cell proliferation; deficiency of NO is thought to be an integral part of the pathogenesis of PAH [183]. By slowing the breakdown of cGMP, PDE5I enhance vascular smooth muscle cell dilation.

The expression and activity of PDE5 is considerably elevated in the lung and pulmonary vascular smooth muscle cells and is thus an attractive therapeutic target for treatment of PAH. Several agents initially used to treat erective dysfunction have been studied as therapy for PAH. Sildenafil was the first agent studied in a large, randomized clinical trial of PAH. In the SUPER study, subjects were randomized to 20, 40, or 80 mg of sildenafil three times a day or placebo [184]. Compared to placebo, there was a significant improvement in the primary outcome (6MWD) at all doses at the end of the 12-week study. Secondary outcomes, such as hemodynamics, also demonstrated significant improvement between groups, but no significant differences in dyspnea or TTCW were noted between groups. A sub-group analysis of CTD-PAH subjects in the SUPER study showed statistically significant improvements in 6MWD with the 20 and 40 mg doses (42 m, 95 % CI 20–64 m, $p < 0.01$ and 36 m, 95 %CI 14–58, $p < 0.01$, respectively) [156]. In addition, functional class improved with each dose, but a higher proportion of patients in the 40 and 80 mg dose groups experienced improvement compared to the 20 mg group (40 % and 42 % vs. 29 %, respectively). Hemodynamic improvements with all treatment doses were also noted. Based upon the conglomeration of data, the FDA approved dose of sildenafil for the treatment of PAH is 20 mg TID, though some clinicians advocate higher doses in practice.

Tadalafil is another PDE5I that has been studied for the treatment of PAH. Tadalafil has a distinct chemical structure compared to sildenafil that leads to differences in selectivity for the PDE5 enzyme and in its pharmacokinetics [185]. Since tadalafil has a 17.5 h half-life, it can be administered once daily. In the PHIRST study, a double-blind, placebo-controlled trial of once daily tadalafil in either treatment naïve or patients on stable bosentan therapy, significant improvement in 6MWD was noted at the highest dose studied (40 mg daily) [186]. Further, improved TTCW and quality of life in the treatment arm was noted, though there was no significant improvement in functional class or in dyspnea. In CTD-PAH subjects, there was a dose-dependent improvement in 6MWD, with a placebo-adjusted improvement of 49 m (95 %CI 15–83) in the 40 mg group compared to placebo.

In general, PDE5I are well tolerated. Common side effects include flushing, headache, nasal congestion, myalgias, and gastrointestinal upset. Given some homology between PDE5 and PDE6 which is predominantly in the retina and integral in the phototransduction cascade, there is a potential for visual side effects, including light sensitivity, blue-greenish or blurred vision. Importantly, a recent study in patients on chronic therapy with PDE5I reported that sildenafil is well tolerated from an ocular perspective [187]. The authors' practice is to have patients undergo evaluation by an ophthalmologist prior to initiation of PDE5I therapy and then follow up on a yearly basis while on therapy to monitor for potential ocular problems.

Riociguat is a sGC stimulator that sensitizes sGC to low levels of bioavailable NO and leads to increased cGMP synthesis through NO-independent mechanisms [188]. This mechanism of action offers a potential benefit over PDE5I since PDE5I depends upon bioavailability of NO and NO is relatively deficient in PAH [189]. Thus, sGC stimulation by riociguat may be more effective in increasing NO bioavailability.

Two recent studies of riociguat in PH have been completed, one in PAH and one in CTEPH. PATENT-1 investigated the efficacy and safety of riociguat in PAH patients who were either treatment naïve or on background therapy with another

PAH-specific medication [190]. The primary outcome of change in 6MWD at 12 weeks was met, with a 36 m improvement in the treatment group compared to placebo (95 % CI 20–52 m, $p < 0.01$). Interestingly, significant improvements in 6MWD of nearly similar magnitude were noted in both treatment naïve patients and in those on background therapy. Statistically significant improvements in secondary outcomes, including functional class, TTCW, quality of life, dyspnea, NT-proBNP, and hemodynamics were also found. No data regarding efficacy in CTD-PAH subjects, who comprised 25 % of the study cohort, has been published to date. Side effects were generally mild and riociguat had a favorable safety profile.

Combination Therapy

Given the potential for synergistic effects between the available PAH therapies that target separate pathways involved in the pathogenesis of the disease, combination of therapies from different classes commonly occurs in clinical practice, though the evidence base for this practice is limited. As discussed previously, several therapies have been studied in clinical trials that enrolled a proportion of subjects on background PAH therapy with an agent from a different class than the drug of interest. Several on-going trials are examining the efficacy of combination therapy, including COMPASS (sildenafil and bosentan) and AMBITION (tadalafil and ambrisentan). In addition, there is an on-going investigator-initiated observational study of tadalafil and ambrisentan in treatment naïve SSc-PAH patients, which is nearing completion (clinicaltrials.gov identifier NCT01042158). Other completed studies examining the impact of combination therapy have demonstrated mixed results. In BREATHE-2, a study of adding bosentan or placebo to IV epoprostenol failed to achieve the primary endpoint of improvement in total pulmonary resistance on RHC and in secondary endpoints such as improvement in 6MWD [191]. Interestingly, the authors attribute the lack of clinical response in this study to a higher proportion of SSc-PAH patients in the treatment arm citing less robust response to therapy in general in the SSc-PAH population. In PACES, where subjects on IV epoprostenol therapy were randomized to sildenafil 80 mg TID or placebo, there were significant improvements in exercise capacity, TTCW, quality of life, and hemodynamics. However, only 17 % of the cohort had CTD-PAH and thus, no conclusions regarding the efficacy of this combination in this population can be drawn.

At our center, we have found poorer response to combination therapy in SSc-PAH compared to IPAH patients [192]. Although the addition of sildenafil to bosentan monotherapy improved functional class and 6MWD in IPAH subjects, no such effect was found in the SSc-PAH subjects. Furthermore, there were significantly more side effects in the SSc-PAH group, including hepatotoxicity. Drug–drug interactions have been described between bosentan and sildenafil and may be of clinical significance, particularly in the SSc-PAH population [193].

Novel Therapies

Recent insights into the pathobiology of PAH that emphasize the aberrant proliferation of endothelial and smooth muscle cells have led investigators to study anti-neoplastic agents that target these processes. In experimental models of PH, inhibition of proliferation and increased apoptosis of smooth muscle cells with the addition of various tyrosine kinase inhibitors (TKI) improved hemodynamics, reversed vascular remodeling, and improved survival [194, 195]. Several case reports of the TKI imatinib, a dual platelet-derived growth factor and vascular endothelial growth factor inhibitor, suggested utility in patients with PAH, including one patient with SS-PAH and one with PVOD [150, 196–199]. However, several large clinical trials of imatinib demonstrated mixed results and ultimately, the drug was not approved for use in PAH [148, 149]. In addition, the TKI dasatinib has recently been reported to induce PAH [200]. This is thought to be related to the wide-ranging targets of dasatinib, including Src kinase, that may be implicated in the development of PAH [201].

A multi-center study of the anti-neoplastic agent, rituximab, in PAH-SSc patients is ongoing. Rituximab is a chimeric monoclonal antibody against the B-cell surface protein CD20. Based upon pre-clinical data suggesting integral involvement of B-cells in SSc pathogenesis and in PAH pathogenesis, a Phase II clinical trial for the evaluation of rituximab in SSc-PAH was initiated and currently enrolling subjects [202]. The primary outcome of this trial is change in PVR at 24 weeks.

PH-Specific Therapy in PH-ILD-CTD

As discussed previously, patients with CTD often develop PH related to concomitant ILD and this may be more common in SSc compared to other CTDs. While treatment of PH-ILD with PAH-specific medications is appealing from a therapeutics standpoint, differences in the mechanism of development of PH in the presence vs. absence of ILD may influence the response to specific pulmonary vasodilator therapy. Hypoxic vasoconstriction, one of the predominant mechanisms of development of PH in ILD, is also an important regulator of ventilation perfusion (VQ) matching in the presence of parenchymal lung disease. Currently, all commercially available PAH medications work by causing pulmonary vascular dilation; thus, it is highly likely that addition of such medications would worsen VQ matching by releasing appropriate hypoxic vasoconstriction. Still, given the high prevalence of pulmonary vascular disease in SSc, there may be a population of patients with some degree of ILD who will respond to PAH-specific therapy (Fig. 11.3). Unfortunately, identification of these patients is challenging.

Several investigators have reported their experience with off-label use of PAH-specific therapies in SSc patients with PH-ILD. Le Pavec and colleagues recently reviewed the response to PAH-specific therapy in 70 SSc patients with PH-ILD who were treated with various PAH-specific therapies [203]. After a mean follow up of 7.7 years, there were no changes in functional class, 6MWD, or hemodynamics when compared

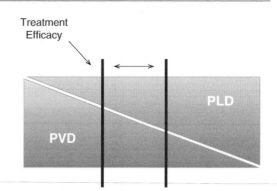

Fig. 11.3 Contributors to pulmonary hypertension in CTD and response to pulmonary vasodilator therapy. While clinically pulmonary hypertension in CTD is commonly attributed to either pulmonary vascular disease or parenchymal lung disease, typically, there are components of both contributing to elevated pulmonary pressures as demonstrated in this figure. Efficacy of pulmonary vasodilator therapy seems to be greatest in patients with predominantly pulmonary vascular disease, however, the "threshold" proportion of parenchymal lung involvement (represented here by the red lines) for which efficacy of these therapies can be demonstrated remains to be determined

to baseline values. One-, 2-, and 3-year survival rates were 71 %, 39 %, and 29 % respectively. In multivariable analyses, worsening of oxygenation with initiation of therapy and deterioration of renal function were associated with risk of death. There are few studies examining the response to PAH-specific therapies in PH-related to other forms of CTD.

Lung Transplantation in CTD-Related Pulmonary Hypertension

Many centers consider CTD to be relative contraindication to lung transplantation due to concerns about gastroesophageal reflux leading to bronchiolitis obliterans syndrome, renal impairment complicating management of immunosuppressive and antimicrobial agents commonly employed post-transplantation that are often nephrotoxic, and extrapulmonary organ involvement. Based upon these concerns, less than 2 % of all lung transplantation worldwide between 1995 and 2010 occurred in patients with underlying CTD [204]. However, as shown by several investigators, outcomes for CTD patients do not appear to be significantly different from patients with either IPAH or ILD in isolation [205–207]. Thus, lung transplantation should be considered for patients with severe PH who are failing therapy.

Response to Therapy in CTD-PAH

In general, clinical trials of PAH-specific therapies for the treatment of PAH have shown a blunted response in CTD-PAH, and in particular, SSc-PAH. For instance, a systematic review of treatment effect of PAH therapies in CTD-PAH using data from the pivotal clinical trials of these agents demonstrated a non-significant improvement in exercise capacity in the CTD population with smaller effect size estimates [208]. However, the presence of comorbidities and confounding factors in CTD-PAH may limit the interpretation of the currently employed outcome measures for clinical trials of therapeutics in PAH. As shown in Table 11.5, several CTD-specific factors may influence the measures of response to therapy, including concomitant ILD, left ventricular diastolic dysfunction, musculoskeletal disease, and gastrointestinal disease. In an attempt to mitigate these limitations of outcome measures in CTD-PAH trials, a Delphi consensus study convening experts from multiple subspecialties involved in the care of patients with SSc and PAH recommended a set of core outcome measures be utilized in clinical trials of

SSc-PAH therapies; these measures encompassed domains such as cardiopulmonary hemodynamics, exercise testing, dyspnea, medication adherence, quality of life, and survival [209]. Recent expert opinion has suggested using TTCW as a primary outcome measure with focus on disease-specific measurement of clinical worsening (i.e., distinguishing between CTD-related and PAH-related clinical worsening) and stratifying patients by disease type and functional class at randomization [210].

Conclusions and Future Directions

Pulmonary hypertension commonly complicates CTD and is invariably associated with high morbidity and mortality. Unfortunately, despite heightened awareness for this entity in CTD patients, PH is often under-recognized in CTD. Further, while specific pulmonary vasodilator therapy has been shown to improve symptoms, quality of life, and survival in other forms of PAH, the response to therapy has been attenuated in patients with CTD-associated disease in general. However, currently employed markers of disease severity and outcome measures are inadequate for CTD-related PH and thus, identification and validation of measures relevant to CTD-associated disease is imperative. Additionally, therapies targeting pathways specific to CTD are currently under investigation and may provide directed therapy for this devastating complication of CTD.

Table 11.5 Disease-specific considerations in CTD-associated PH

Domain	Tool	Application to CTD-PAH
Hemodynamics	RHC, Echo	Group II and III disease confound assessment
Exercise testing	6MWD	Musculoskeletal disease/deconditioning
Dyspnea	Borg dyspnea	Non-PAH causes for dyspnea (ILD, anemia, etc.)
Adherence with therapy	Adverse events	Concomitant medications for CTD may interact
Pharmacodynamics	Bioavailability	Different due to GI motility, malabsorption
Quality of life	SF-36/CAMPHOR	Extra-pulmonary involvement affects QOL
Global state	Survival	Poorer survival overall compared to IPAH

Adapted with permission from Denton CP, Avouac J, Behrens F, Furst DE, Foeldvari I, Humbert M, et al. Systemic sclerosis-associated pulmonary hypertension: why disease-specific composite endpoints are needed. Arthritis Res Ther 2011;13(3):114

References

1. Chin KM, Kim NH, Rubin LJ. The right ventricle in pulmonary hypertension. Coron Artery Dis. 2005;16(1):13–8.
2. Simonneau G, Gatzoulis MA, Adatia I, Celermajer D, Denton C, Ghofrani A, et al. Updated clinical classification of pulmonary hypertension. J Am Coll Cardiol. 2013;62(25 Suppl):D34–41.
3. Mathai SC, Hassoun PM. Pulmonary arterial hypertension in connective tissue diseases. Heart Fail Clin. 2012;8(3):413–25.
4. Barnett CF, De MT. Pulmonary hypertension associated with left-sided heart disease. Heart Fail Clin. 2012;8(3):447–59.
5. Georgiopoulou VV, Kalogeropoulos AP, Borlaug BA, Gheorghiade M, Butler J. Left ventricular dysfunction with pulmonary hypertension: part 1: epidemiology, pathophysiology, and definitions. Circ Heart Fail. 2013;6(2):344–54.
6. Hatano S, Strasser T. Primary pulmonary hypertension. Report on a WHO meeting. Geneva: World Health Organization; 1975.
7. Ghofrani HA, Distler O, Gerhardt F, Gorenflo M, Grunig E, Haefeli WE, et al. Treatment of pulmonary arterial hypertension (PAH): updated recommendations of the Cologne Consensus Conference 2011. Int J Cardiol. 2011;154 Suppl 1:S20–33.
8. Jamieson SW, Kapelanski DP, Sakakibara N, Manecke GR, Thistlethwaite PA, Kerr KM, et al. Pulmonary endarterectomy: experience and lessons learned in 1,500 cases. Ann Thorac Surg. 2003; 76(5):1457–62.
9. Mayer E, Jenkins D, Lindner J, D'Armini A, Kloek J, Meyns B, et al. Surgical management and outcome of patients with chronic thromboembolic pulmonary hypertension: results from an international prospective registry. J Thorac Cardiovasc Surg. 2011; 141(3):702–10.
10. Rich S, Rabinovitch M. Diagnosis and treatment of secondary (non-category 1) pulmonary hypertension. Circulation. 2008;118(21):2190–9.
11. Launay D, Mouthon L, Hachulla E, Pagnoux C, de Groote P, Remy-Jardin M, et al. Prevalence and characteristics of moderate to severe pulmonary hypertension in systemic sclerosis with and without interstitial lung disease. J Rheumatol. 2007;34(5): 1005–11.
12. Mathai SC, Hummers LK, Champion HC, Wigley FM, Zaiman A, Hassoun PM, et al. Survival in pulmonary hypertension associated with the scleroderma spectrum of diseases: impact of interstitial lung disease. Arthritis Rheum. 2009;60(2): 569–77.
13. de Groote P, Gressin V, Hachulla E, Carpentier P, Guillevin L, Kahan A, et al. Evaluation of cardiac abnormalities by Doppler echocardiography in a large nationwide multicentric cohort of patients with systemic sclerosis. Ann Rheum Dis. 2008;67(1): 31–6.
14. Launay D, Hachulla E, Hatron PY, Jais X, Simonneau G, Humbert M. Pulmonary arterial hypertension: a rare complication of primary Sjogren syndrome: report of 9 new cases and review of the literature. Medicine (Baltimore). 2007;86(5):299–315.
15. Gunnarsson R, Andreassen AK, Molberg O, Lexberg AS, Time K, Dhainaut AS, et al. Prevalence of pulmonary hypertension in an unselected, mixed connective tissue disease cohort: results of a nationwide, Norwegian cross-sectional multicentre study and review of current literature. Rheumatology (Oxford). 2013;52(7):1208–13.
16. Chow SL, Chandran V, Fazelzad R, Johnson SR. Prognostic factors for survival in systemic lupus erythematosus associated pulmonary hypertension. Lupus. 2012;21(4):353–64.
17. Chung L, Liu J, Parsons L, Hassoun PM, McGoon M, Badesch DB, et al. Characterization of connective tissue disease-associated pulmonary arterial hypertension from REVEAL: identifying systemic sclerosis as a unique phenotype. Chest. 2010; 138(6):1383–94.
18. Minai OA. Pulmonary hypertension in polymyositis-dermatomyositis: clinical and hemodynamic characteristics and response to vasoactive therapy. Lupus. 2009;18(11):1006–10.
19. Chung SM, Lee CK, Lee EY, Yoo B, Lee SD, Moon HB. Clinical aspects of pulmonary hypertension in patients with systemic lupus erythematosus and in patients with idiopathic pulmonary arterial hypertension. Clin Rheumatol. 2006;25(6): 866–72.
20. Hatron PY, Tillie-Leblond I, Launay D, Hachulla E, Fauchais AL, Wallaert B. Pulmonary manifestations of Sjogren's syndrome. Presse Med. 2011;40(1 Pt 2):e49–64.
21. Szodoray P, Hajas A, Kardos L, Dezso B, Soos G, Zold E, et al. Distinct phenotypes in mixed connective tissue disease: subgroups and survival. Lupus. 2012;21(13):1412–22.
22. Lin DF, Yan SM, Zhao Y, Zhang W, Li MT, Zeng XF, et al. Clinical and prognostic characteristics of 573 cases of primary Sjogren's syndrome. Chin Med J (Engl). 2010;123(22):3252–7.
23. Le PJ, Launay D, Mathai SC, Hassoun PM, Humbert M. Scleroderma lung disease. Clin Rev Allergy Immunol. 2011;40(2):104–16.
24. Voelkel NF, Mizuno S, Bogaard HJ. The role of hypoxia in pulmonary vascular diseases: a perspective. Am J Physiol Lung Cell Mol Physiol. 2013;304(7):L457–65.
25. Voelkel NF, Gomez-Arroyo J, Abbate A, Bogaard HJ, Nicolls MR. Pathobiology of pulmonary arterial hypertension and right ventricular failure. Eur Respir J. 2012;40(6):1555–65.
26. Rabinovitch M. Pathobiology of pulmonary hypertension. Annu Rev Pathol. 2007;2:369–99.

27. Farkas L, Gauldie J, Voelkel NF, Kolb M. Pulmonary hypertension and idiopathic pulmonary fibrosis: a tale of angiogenesis, apoptosis, and growth factors. Am J Respir Cell Mol Biol. 2011;45(1):1–15.

28. Stewart S, Rassl D. Advances in the understanding and classification of pulmonary hypertension. Histopathology. 2009;54(1):104–16.

29. Newman JH, Wheeler L, Lane KB, Loyd E, Gaddipati R, Phillips III JA, et al. Mutation in the gene for bone morphogenetic protein receptor II as a cause of primary pulmonary hypertension in a large kindred. N Engl J Med. 2001;345(5):319–24.

30. Trembath RC, Thomson JR, Machado RD, Morgan NV, Atkinson C, Winship I, et al. Clinical and molecular genetic features of pulmonary hypertension in patients with hereditary hemorrhagic telangiectasia. N Engl J Med. 2001;345(5):325–34.

31. Nasim MT, Ogo T, Ahmed M, Randall R, Chowdhury HM, Snape KM, et al. Molecular genetic characterization of SMAD signaling molecules in pulmonary arterial hypertension. Hum Mutat. 2011;32(12): 1385–9.

32. Machado RD, Pauciulo MW, Thomson JR, Lane KB, Morgan NV, Wheeler L, et al. BMPR2 haploinsufficiency as the inherited molecular mechanism for primary pulmonary hypertension. Am J Hum Genet. 2001;68(1):92–102.

33. Morse J, Barst R, Horn E, Cuervo N, Deng Z, Knowles J. Pulmonary hypertension in scleroderma spectrum of disease: lack of bone morphogenetic protein receptor 2 mutations. J Rheumatol. 2002; 29(11):2379–81.

34. Tew MB, Arnett FC, Reveille JD, Tan FK. Mutations of bone morphogenetic protein receptor type II are not found in patients with pulmonary hypertension and underlying connective tissue diseases. Arthritis Rheum. 2002;46(10):2829–30.

35. Wipff J, Kahan A, Hachulla E, Sibilia J, Cabane J, Meyer O, et al. Association between an endoglin gene polymorphism and systemic sclerosis-related pulmonary arterial hypertension. Rheumatology (Oxford). 2007;46(4):622–5.

36. Hassoun PM, Mouthon L, Barbera JA, Eddahibi S, Flores SC, Grimminger F, et al. Inflammation, growth factors, and pulmonary vascular remodeling. J Am Coll Cardiol. 2009;54(1 Suppl):S10–9.

37. Price LC, Wort SJ, Perros F, Dorfmuller P, Huertas A, Montani D, et al. Inflammation in pulmonary arterial hypertension. Chest. 2012;141(1):210–21.

38. Tuder RM, Groves B, Badesch DB, Voelkel NF. Exuberant endothelial cell growth and elements of inflammation are present in plexiform lesions of pulmonary hypertension. Am J Pathol. 1994;144(2): 275–85.

39. Perros F, Dorfmuller P, Montani D, Hammad H, Waelput W, Girerd B, et al. Pulmonary lymphoid neogenesis in idiopathic pulmonary arterial hypertension. Am J Respir Crit Care Med. 2012;185(3): 311–21.

40. Dorfmuller P, Humbert M, Perros F, Sanchez O, Simonneau G, Muller KM, et al. Fibrous remodeling of the pulmonary venous system in pulmonary arterial hypertension associated with connective tissue diseases. Hum Pathol. 2007;38(6):893–902.

41. Steen VD. The many faces of scleroderma. Rheum Dis Clin North Am. 2008;34(1):1–15.

42. Gabrielli A, Avvedimento EV, Krieg T. Scleroderma. N Engl J Med. 2009;360(19):1989–2003.

43. Tamby MC, Humbert M, Guilpain P, Servettaz A, Dupin N, Christner JJ, et al. Antibodies to fibroblasts in idiopathic and scleroderma-associated pulmonary hypertension. Eur Respir J. 2006;28(4):799–807.

44. Nicolls MR, Taraseviciene-Stewart L, Rai PR, Badesch DB, Voelkel NF. Autoimmunity and pulmonary hypertension: a perspective. Eur Respir J. 2005; 26(6):1110–8.

45. Riemekasten G, Philippe A, Nather M, Slowinski T, Muller DN, Heidecke H, et al. Involvement of functional autoantibodies against vascular receptors in systemic sclerosis. Ann Rheum Dis. 2011;70(3): 530–6.

46. Negrini D, Passi A, De LG, Miserocchi G. Pulmonary interstitial pressure and proteoglycans during development of pulmonary edema. Am J Physiol. 1996; 270(6 Pt 2):H2000–7.

47. Sgonc R, Gruschwitz MS, Dietrich H, Recheis H, Gershwin ME, Wick G. Endothelial cell apoptosis is a primary pathogenetic event underlying skin lesions in avian and human scleroderma. J Clin Invest. 1996;98(3):785–92.

48. Ebina M, Shimizukawa M, Shibata N, Kimura Y, Suzuki T, Endo M, et al. Heterogeneous increase in CD34-positive alveolar capillaries in idiopathic pulmonary fibrosis. Am J Respir Crit Care Med. 2004;169(11):1203–8.

49. Burdick MD, Murray LA, Keane MP, Xue YY, Zisman DA, Belperio JA, et al. CXCL11 attenuates bleomycin-induced pulmonary fibrosis via inhibition of vascular remodeling. Am J Respir Crit Care Med. 2005;171(3):261–8.

50. Wang R, Ibarra-Sunga O, Verlinski L, Pick R, Uhal BD. Abrogation of bleomycin-induced epithelial apoptosis and lung fibrosis by captopril or by a caspase inhibitor. Am J Physiol Lung Cell Mol Physiol. 2000;279(1):L143–51.

51. Lewandowska K, Ciurzynski M, Gorska E, Bienias P, Irzyk K, Siwicka M, et al. Antiendothelial cells antibodies in patients with systemic sclerosis in relation to pulmonary hypertension and lung fibrosis. Adv Exp Med Biol. 2013;756:147–53.

52. LeRoy EC, Black C, Fleischmajer R, Jablonska S, Krieg T, Medsger Jr TA, et al. Scleroderma (systemic sclerosis): classification, subsets and pathogenesis. J Rheumatol. 1988;15(2):202–5.

53. Barnes J, Mayes MD. Epidemiology of systemic sclerosis: incidence, prevalence, survival, risk factors, malignancy, and environmental triggers. Curr Opin Rheumatol. 2012;24(2):165–70.

54. Ranque B, Mouthon L. Geoepidemiology of systemic sclerosis. Autoimmun Rev. 2010;9(5): A311–8.

55. Tamaki T, Mori S, Takehara K. Epidemiological study of patients with systemic sclerosis in Tokyo. Arch Dermatol Res. 1991;283(6):366–71.

56. Silman A, Jannini S, Symmons D, Bacon P. An epidemiological study of scleroderma in the West Midlands. Br J Rheumatol. 1988;27(4):286–90.

57. Allcock RJ, Forrest I, Corris PA, Crook PR, Griffiths ID. A study of the prevalence of systemic sclerosis in northeast England. Rheumatology (Oxford). 2004;43(5):596–602.

58. Mayes MD, Lacey Jr JV, Beebe-Dimmer J, Gillespie BW, Cooper B, Laing TJ, et al. Prevalence, incidence, survival, and disease characteristics of systemic sclerosis in a large US population. Arthritis Rheum. 2003;48(8):2246–55.

59. Hachulla E, Gressin V, Guillevin L, Carpentier P, Diot E, Sibilia J, et al. Early detection of pulmonary arterial hypertension in systemic sclerosis: a French nationwide prospective multicenter study. Arthritis Rheum. 2005;52(12):3792–800.

60. Mukerjee D, St GD, Coleiro B, Knight C, Denton CP, Davar J, et al. Prevalence and outcome in systemic sclerosis associated pulmonary arterial hypertension: application of a registry approach. Ann Rheum Dis. 2003;62(11):1088–93.

61. Battle RW, Davitt MA, Cooper SM, Buckley LM, Leib ES, Beglin PA, et al. Prevalence of pulmonary hypertension in limited and diffuse scleroderma. Chest. 1996;110(6):1515–9.

62. Stupi AM, Steen VD, Owens GR, Barnes EL, Rodnan GP, Medsger Jr TA. Pulmonary hypertension in the CREST syndrome variant of systemic sclerosis. Arthritis Rheum. 1986;29(4):515–24.

63. MacGregor AJ, Canavan R, Knight C, Denton CP, Davar J, Coghlan J, et al. Pulmonary hypertension in systemic sclerosis: risk factors for progression and consequences for survival. Rheumatology (Oxford). 2001;40(4):453–9.

64. Sacks DG, Okano Y, Steen VD, Curtiss E, Shapiro LS, Medsger Jr TA. Isolated pulmonary hypertension in systemic sclerosis with diffuse cutaneous involvement: association with serum anti-U3RNP antibody. J Rheumatol. 1996;23(4):639–42.

65. Murata I, Takenaka K, Yoshinoya S, Kikuchi K, Kiuchi T, Tanigawa T, et al. Clinical evaluation of pulmonary hypertension in systemic sclerosis and related disorders. A Doppler echocardiographic study of 135 Japanese patients. Chest. 1997;111(1): 36–43.

66. Fisher MR, Forfia PR, Chamera E, Housten-Harris T, Champion HC, Girgis RE, et al. Accuracy of Doppler echocardiography in the hemodynamic assessment of pulmonary hypertension. Am J Respir Crit Care Med. 2009;179(7):615–21.

67. Mathai SC, Sibley CT, Forfia PR, Mudd JO, Fisher MR, Tedford RJ, et al. Tricuspid annular plane systolic excursion is a robust outcome measure in systemic sclerosis-associated pulmonary arterial hypertension. J Rheumatol. 2011;38(11):2410–8.

68. Hinchcliff M, Fischer A, Schiopu E, Steen VD. Pulmonary hypertension assessment and recognition of outcomes in scleroderma (PHAROS): baseline characteristics and description of study population. J Rheumatol. 2011;38(10):2172–9.

69. Humbert M, Sitbon O, Chaouat A, Bertocchi M, Habib G, Gressin V, et al. Pulmonary arterial hypertension in France: results from a national registry. Am J Respir Crit Care Med. 2006;173(9): 1023–30.

70. Condliffe R, Kiely DG, Peacock AJ, Corris PA, Gibbs JS, Vrapi F, et al. Connective tissue disease-associated pulmonary arterial hypertension in the modern treatment era. Am J Respir Crit Care Med. 2009;179(2):151–7.

71. Badesch DB, Raskob GE, Elliott CG, Krichman AM, Farber HW, Frost AE, et al. Pulmonary arterial hypertension: baseline characteristics from the REVEAL registry. Chest. 2010;137(2):376–87.

72. Chung L, Domsic RT, Lingala B, Alkassab F, Bolster M, Csuka ME, et al. Survival and predictors of mortality in systemic sclerosis associated pulmonary arterial hypertension: outcomes from the PHAROS registry. Arthritis Care Res (Hoboken). 2013. [Epub ahead of print].

73. Blanco I, Mathai SC, Shafiq M, Boyce D, Kolb TM, Chami H, Hummers LK, Housten T, Chaisson N, Zaiman AL, Wigley FM, Tedford RJ, Kass DA, Damico R, Girgis RE, Hassoun PM. Severity of scleroderma-associated pulmonary arterial hypertension in African Americans. Medicine 2014. (Accepted for publication).

74. Schachna L, Wigley FM, Chang B, White B, Wise RA, Gelber AC. Age and risk of pulmonary arterial hypertension in scleroderma. Chest. 2003;124(6): 2098–104.

75. Scorza R, Caronni M, Bazzi S, Nador F, Beretta L, Antonioli R, et al. Post-menopause is the main risk factor for developing isolated pulmonary hypertension in systemic sclerosis. Ann N Y Acad Sci. 2002;966:238–46.

76. Beretta L, Caronni M, Origgi L, Ponti A, Santaniello A, Scorza R. Hormone replacement therapy may prevent the development of isolated pulmonary hypertension in patients with systemic sclerosis and limited cutaneous involvement. Scand J Rheumatol. 2006;35(6):468–71.

77. Avouac J, Airo P, Meune C, Beretta L, Dieude P, Caramaschi P, et al. Prevalence of pulmonary hypertension in systemic sclerosis in European Caucasians and metaanalysis of 5 studies. J Rheumatol. 2010; 37(11):2290–8.

78. Cox SR, Walker JG, Coleman M, Rischmueller M, Proudman S, Smith MD, et al. Isolated pulmonary hypertension in scleroderma. Intern Med J. 2005; 35(1):28–33.

79. Hachulla E, de Groote P, Gressin V, Sibilia J, Diot E, Carpentier P, et al. The three-year incidence of pulmonary arterial hypertension associated with systemic sclerosis in a multicenter nationwide longitudinal study in France. Arthritis Rheum. 2009;60(6):1831–9.

80. Ferri C, Valentini G, Cozzi F, Sebastiani M, Michelassi C, La MG, et al. Systemic sclerosis: demographic, clinical, and serologic features and survival in 1,012 Italian patients. Medicine (Baltimore). 2002;81(2):139–53.

81. Steen V, Medsger Jr TA. Predictors of isolated pulmonary hypertension in patients with systemic sclerosis and limited cutaneous involvement. Arthritis Rheum. 2003;48(2):516–22.

82. Shah AA, Wigley FM, Hummers LK. Telangiectases in scleroderma: a potential clinical marker of pulmonary arterial hypertension. J Rheumatol. 2010; 37(1):98–104.

83. Allanore Y, Borderie D, Avouac J, Zerkak D, Meune C, Hachulla E, et al. High N-terminal pro-brain natriuretic peptide levels and low diffusing capacity for carbon monoxide as independent predictors of the occurrence of precapillary pulmonary arterial hypertension in patients with systemic sclerosis. Arthritis Rheum. 2008;58(1):284–91.

84. Galie N, Hoeper MM, Humbert M, Torbicki A, Vachiery JL, Barbera JA, et al. Guidelines for the diagnosis and treatment of pulmonary hypertension. Eur Respir J. 2009;34(6):1219–63.

85. Black WC, Welch HG. Screening for disease. AJR Am J Roentgenol. 1997;168(1):3–11.

86. Humbert M, Yaici A, de Groote P, Montani D, Sitbon O, Launay D, et al. Screening for pulmonary arterial hypertension in patients with systemic sclerosis: clinical characteristics at diagnosis and long-term survival. Arthritis Rheum. 2011;63(11):3522–30.

87. Humbert M, Gerry CJ, Khanna D. Early detection and management of pulmonary arterial hypertension. Eur Respir Rev. 2012;21(126):306–12.

88. Coghlan JG, Denton CP, Grunig E, Bonderman D, Distler O, Khanna D, et al. Evidence-based detection of pulmonary arterial hypertension in systemic sclerosis: the DETECT study. Ann Rheum Dis. 2013. [Epub ahead of print].

89. Khanna D, Gladue H, Channick R, Chung L, Distler O, Furst DE, et al. Recommendations for screening and detection of connective-tissue disease associated pulmonary arterial hypertension. Arthritis Rheum. 2013;65(12):3194–201.

90. Kawut SM, Taichman DB, Archer-Chicko CL, Palevsky HI, Kimmel SE. Hemodynamics and survival in patients with pulmonary arterial hypertension related to systemic sclerosis. Chest. 2003; 123(2):344–50.

91. Fisher MR, Mathai SC, Champion HC, Girgis RE, Housten-Harris T, Hummers L, et al. Clinical differences between idiopathic and scleroderma-related pulmonary hypertension. Arthritis Rheum. 2006;54(9):3043–50.

92. Hachulla E, Carpentier P, Gressin V, Diot E, Allanore Y, Sibilia J, et al. Risk factors for death and the 3-year survival of patients with systemic sclerosis: the French ItinerAIR-Sclerodermie study. Rheumatology (Oxford). 2009;48(3):304–8.

93. Campo A, Mathai SC, Le PJ, Zaiman AL, Hummers LK, Boyce D, et al. Hemodynamic predictors of survival in scleroderma-related pulmonary arterial hypertension. Am J Respir Crit Care Med. 2010; 182(2):252–60.

94. Rubenfire M, Huffman MD, Krishnan S, Seibold JR, Schiopu E, McLaughlin VV. Survival in systemic sclerosis with pulmonary arterial hypertension has not improved in the modern era. Chest. 2013; 144(4):1282–90.

95. Mathai SC, Bueso M, Hummers LK, Boyce D, Lechtzin N, Le PJ, et al. Disproportionate elevation of N-terminal pro-brain natriuretic peptide in scleroderma-related pulmonary hypertension. Eur Respir J. 2010;35(1):95–104.

96. Overbeek MJ, Lankhaar JW, Westerhof N, Voskuyl AE, Boonstra A, Bronzwaer JG, et al. Right ventricular contractility in systemic sclerosis-associated and idiopathic pulmonary arterial hypertension. Eur Respir J. 2008;31(6):1160–6.

97. Tedford RJ, Mudd JO, Girgis RE, Mathai SC, Zaiman AL, Housten-Harris T, et al. Right ventricular dysfunction in systemic sclerosis associated pulmonary arterial hypertension. Circ Heart Fail. 2013;6(5):953–63.

98. Launay D, Humbert M, Berezne A, Cottin V, Allanore Y, Couderc LJ, et al. Clinical characteristics and survival in systemic sclerosis-related pulmonary hypertension associated with interstitial lung disease. Chest. 2011;140(4):1016–24.

99. Sharp GC, Irvin WS, Tan EM, Gould RG, Holman HR. Mixed connective tissue disease—an apparently distinct rheumatic disease syndrome associated with a specific antibody to an extractable nuclear antigen (ENA). Am J Med. 1972;52(2):148–59.

100. Okawa-Takatsuji M, Aotsuka S, Uwatoko S, Kinoshita M, Sumiya M. Increase of cytokine production by pulmonary artery endothelial cells induced by supernatants from monocytes stimulated with autoantibodies against U1-ribonucleoprotein. Clin Exp Rheumatol. 1999;17(6):705–12.

101. Bodolay E, Csipo I, Gal I, Sipka S, Gyimesi E, Szekanecz Z, et al. Anti-endothelial cell antibodies in mixed connective tissue disease: frequency and association with clinical symptoms. Clin Exp Rheumatol. 2004;22(4):409–15.

102. Smolen JS, Steiner G. Mixed connective tissue disease: to be or not to be? Arthritis Rheum. 1998; 41(5):768–77.

103. Burdt MA, Hoffman RW, Deutscher SL, Wang GS, Johnson JC, Sharp GC. Long-term outcome in mixed connective tissue disease: longitudinal clinical and serologic findings. Arthritis Rheum. 1999;42(5):899–909.

104. Lundberg I, Hedfors E. Clinical course of patients with anti-RNP antibodies. A prospective study of 32 patients. J Rheumatol. 1991;18(10):1511–9.

105. Wigley FM, Lima JA, Mayes M, McLain D, Chapin JL, Ward-Able C. The prevalence of undiagnosed pulmonary arterial hypertension in subjects with connective tissue disease at the secondary health care level of community-based rheumatologists (the UNCOVER study). Arthritis Rheum. 2005;52(7): 2125–32.

106. Sullivan WD, Hurst DJ, Harmon CE, Esther JH, Agia GA, Maltby JD, et al. A prospective evaluation emphasizing pulmonary involvement in patients with mixed connective tissue disease. Medicine (Baltimore). 1984;63(2):92–107.

107. Gunnarsson R, Aalokken TM, Molberg O, Lund MB, Mynarek GK, Lexberg AS, et al. Prevalence and severity of interstitial lung disease in mixed connective tissue disease: a nationwide, cross-sectional study. Ann Rheum Dis. 2012;71(12):1966–72.

108. Johnson SR, Granton JT. Pulmonary hypertension in systemic sclerosis and systemic lupus erythematosus. Eur Respir Rev. 2011;20(122):277–86.

109. Perez HD, Kramer N. Pulmonary hypertension in systemic lupus erythematosus: report of four cases and review of the literature. Semin Arthritis Rheum. 1981;11(1):177–81.

110. Quismorio Jr FP, Sharma O, Koss M, Boylen T, Edmiston AW, Thornton PJ, et al. Immunopathologic and clinical studies in pulmonary hypertension associated with systemic lupus erythematosus. Semin Arthritis Rheum. 1984;13(4):349–59.

111. Badui E, Garcia-Rubi D, Robles E, Jimenez J, Juan L, Deleze M, et al. Cardiovascular manifestations in systemic lupus erythematosus. Prospective study of 100 patients. Angiology. 1985;36(7):431–41.

112. Simonson JS, Schiller NB, Petri M, Hellmann DB. Pulmonary hypertension in systemic lupus erythematosus. J Rheumatol. 1989;16(7):918–25.

113. Asherson RA, Higenbottam TW, Dinh Xuan AT, Khamashta MA, Hughes GR. Pulmonary hypertension in a lupus clinic: experience with twenty-four patients. J Rheumatol. 1990;17(10):1292–8.

114. Ong ML, Veerapen K, Chambers JB, Lim MN, Manivasagar M, Wang F. Cardiac abnormalities in systemic lupus erythematosus: prevalence and relationship to disease activity. Int J Cardiol. 1992; 34(1):69–74.

115. Winslow TM, Ossipov MA, Fazio GP, Simonson JS, Redberg RF, Schiller NB. Five-year follow-up study of the prevalence and progression of pulmonary hypertension in systemic lupus erythematosus. Am Heart J. 1995;129(3):510–5.

116. Shen JY, Chen SL, Wu YX, Tao RQ, Gu YY, Bao CD, et al. Pulmonary hypertension in systemic lupus erythematosus. Rheumatol Int. 1999;18(4):147–51.

117. Johnson SR, Gladman DD, Urowitz MB, Ibanez D, Granton JT. Pulmonary hypertension in systemic lupus. Lupus. 2004;13(7):506–9.

118. Fois E, Le Guern V, Dupuy A, Humbert M, Mouthon L, Guillevin L. Noninvasive assessment of systolic pulmonary artery pressure in systemic lupus erythematosus: retrospective analysis of 93 patients. Clin Exp Rheumatol. 2010;28(6):836–41.

119. Goupille P, Fauchier L, Babuty D, Fauchier JP, Valat JP. Precapillary pulmonary hypertension dramatically improved with high doses of corticosteroids during systemic lupus erythematosus. J Rheumatol. 1994;21(10):1976–7.

120. Asherson RA, Oakley CM. Pulmonary hypertension and systemic lupus erythematosus. J Rheumatol. 1986;13(1):1–5.

121. Kim WU, Min JK, Lee SH, Park SH, Cho CS, Kim HY. Causes of death in Korean patients with systemic lupus erythematosus: a single center retrospective study. Clin Exp Rheumatol. 1999;17(5): 539–45.

122. Pope J. An update in pulmonary hypertension in systemic lupus erythematosus—do we need to know about it? Lupus. 2008;17(4):274–7.

123. Mavragani CP, Moutsopoulos HM. Sjogren's syndrome. Annu Rev Pathol. 2014;9:273–85.

124. Kokosi M, Riemer EC, Highland KB. Pulmonary involvement in Sjogren syndrome. Clin Chest Med. 2010;31(3):489–500.

125. Vassiliou VA, Moyssakis I, Boki KA, Moutsopoulos HM. Is the heart affected in primary Sjogren's syndrome? An echocardiographic study. Clin Exp Rheumatol. 2008;26(1):109–12.

126. Crowson CS, Matteson EL, Myasoedova E, Michet CJ, Ernste FC, Warrington KJ, et al. The lifetime risk of adult-onset rheumatoid arthritis and other inflammatory autoimmune rheumatic diseases. Arthritis Rheum. 2011;63(3):633–9.

127. Turesson C, McClelland RL, Christianson TJ, Matteson EL. Severe extra-articular disease manifestations are associated with an increased risk of first ever cardiovascular events in patients with rheumatoid arthritis. Ann Rheum Dis. 2007;66(1):70–5.

128. Balbir-Gurman A, Yigla M, Nahir AM, Braun-Moscovici Y. Rheumatoid pleural effusion. Semin Arthritis Rheum. 2006;35(6):368–78.

129. Marigliano B, Soriano A, Margiotta D, Vadacca M, Afeltra A. Lung involvement in connective tissue diseases: a comprehensive review and a focus on rheumatoid arthritis. Autoimmun Rev. 2013;12(11): 1076–84.

130. Dawson JK, Goodson NG, Graham DR, Lynch MP. Raised pulmonary artery pressures measured with Doppler echocardiography in rheumatoid arthritis patients. Rheumatology (Oxford). 2000;39(12): 1320–5.

131. Gonzalez-Juanatey C, Testa A, Garcia-Castelo A, Garcia-Porrua C, Llorca J, Ollier WE, et al. Echocardiographic and Doppler findings in long-term treated rheumatoid arthritis patients without clinically evident cardiovascular disease. Semin Arthritis Rheum. 2004;33(4):231–8.

132. Kay JM, Banik S. Unexplained pulmonary hypertension with pulmonary arthritis in rheumatoid disease. Br J Dis Chest. 1977;71(1):53–9.

133. Lehrman SG, Hollander RC. Severe pulmonary hypertension in a patient with rheumatoid arthritis—response to nifedipine. West J Med. 1986;145(2): 242–4.

134. Eaton AM, Serota H, Kernodle Jr GW, Uglietta JP, Crawford J, Fulkerson WJ. Pulmonary hypertension secondary to serum hyperviscosity in a patient with rheumatoid arthritis. Am J Med. 1987;82(5):1039–45.

135. Morikawa J, Kitamura K, Habuchi Y, Tsujimura Y, Minamikawa T, Takamatsu T. Pulmonary hypertension in a patient with rheumatoid arthritis. Chest. 1988;93(4):876–8.

136. Young ID, Ford SE, Ford PM. The association of pulmonary hypertension with rheumatoid arthritis. J Rheumatol. 1989;16(9):1266–9.

137. Sharma S, Vaccharajani A, Mandke J. Severe pulmonary hypertension in rheumatoid arthritis. Int J Cardiol. 1990;26(2):220–2.

138. Balagopal VP, da Costa P, Greenstone MA. Fatal pulmonary hypertension and rheumatoid vasculitis. Eur Respir J. 1995;8(2):331–3.

139. Keser G, Capar I, Aksu K, Inal V, Danaoglu Z, Savas R, et al. Pulmonary hypertension in rheumatoid arthritis. Scand J Rheumatol. 2004;33(4):244–5.

140. Castro GW, Appenzeller S, Bertolo MB, Costallat LT. Isolated pulmonary hypertension secondary to rheumatoid arthritis. Clin Rheumatol. 2006;25(6): 901–3.

141. Shariff N, Kumar A, Narang R, Malhotra A, Mukhopadhyaya S, Sharma SK. A study of pulmonary arterial hypertension in patients with rheumatoid arthritis. Int J Cardiol. 2007;115(1):75–6.

142. Udayakumar N, Venkatesan S, Rajendiran C. Pulmonary hypertension in rheumatoid arthritis–relation with the duration of the disease. Int J Cardiol. 2008;127(3):410–2.

143. Bernatsky S, Joseph L, Pineau CA, Belisle P, Boivin JF, Banerjee D, et al. Estimating the prevalence of polymyositis and dermatomyositis from administrative data: age, sex and regional differences. Ann Rheum Dis. 2009;68(7):1192–6.

144. Jacobson DL, Gange SJ, Rose NR, Graham NM. Epidemiology and estimated population burden of selected autoimmune diseases in the United States. Clin Immunol Immunopathol. 1997;84(3):223–43.

145. Mammen AL. Autoimmune myopathies: autoantibodies, phenotypes and pathogenesis. Nat Rev Neurol. 2011;7(6):343–54.

146. Vij R, Strek ME. Diagnosis and treatment of connective tissue disease-associated interstitial lung disease. Chest. 2013;143(3):814–24.

147. Adnot S. Lessons learned from cancer may help in the treatment of pulmonary hypertension. J Clin Invest. 2005;115(6):1461–3.

148. Hoeper MM, Barst RJ, Bourge RC, Feldman J, Frost AE, Galie N, et al. Imatinib mesylate as add-on therapy for pulmonary arterial hypertension: results of

the randomized IMPRES study. Circulation. 2013;127(10):1128–38.

149. Ghofrani HA, Morrell NW, Hoeper MM, Olschewski H, Peacock AJ, Barst RJ, et al. Imatinib in pulmonary arterial hypertension patients with inadequate response to established therapy. Am J Respir Crit Care Med. 2010;182(9):1171–7.

150. Ghofrani HA, Seeger W, Grimminger F. Imatinib for the treatment of pulmonary arterial hypertension. N Engl J Med. 2005;353(13):1412–3.

151. Godinas L, Guignabert C, Seferian A, Perros F, Bergot E, Sibille Y, et al. Tyrosine kinase inhibitors in pulmonary arterial hypertension: a double-edge sword? Semin Respir Crit Care Med. 2013;34(5): 714–24.

152. Girgis RE, Frost AE, Hill NS, Horn EM, Langleben D, McLaughlin VV, et al. Selective endothelin A receptor antagonism with sitaxsentan for pulmonary arterial hypertension associated with connective tissue disease. Ann Rheum Dis. 2007;66(11):1467–72.

153. Oudiz RJ, Schilz RJ, Barst RJ, Galie N, Rich S, Rubin LJ, et al. Treprostinil, a prostacyclin analogue, in pulmonary arterial hypertension associated with connective tissue disease. Chest. 2004;126(2): 420–7.

154. Denton CP, Humbert M, Rubin L, Black CM. Bosentan treatment for pulmonary arterial hypertension related to connective tissue disease: a subgroup analysis of the pivotal clinical trials and their open-label extensions. Ann Rheum Dis. 2006;65(10): 1336–40.

155. Denton CP, Pope JE, Peter HH, Gabrielli A, Boonstra A, van den Hoogen FH, et al. Long-term effects of bosentan on quality of life, survival, safety and tolerability in pulmonary arterial hypertension related to connective tissue diseases. Ann Rheum Dis. 2008; 67(9):1222–8.

156. Badesch DB, Hill NS, Burgess G, Rubin LJ, Barst RJ, Galie N, et al. Sildenafil for pulmonary arterial hypertension associated with connective tissue disease. J Rheumatol. 2007;34(12):2417–22.

157. Continuous or nocturnal oxygen therapy in hypoxemic chronic obstructive lung disease: a clinical trial. Nocturnal Oxygen Therapy Trial Group. Ann Intern Med. 1980;93(3):391–8.

158. Long term domiciliary oxygen therapy in chronic hypoxic cor pulmonale complicating chronic bronchitis and emphysema. Report of the Medical Research Council Working Party. Lancet 1981; 1(8222):681–6.

159. Mereles D, Ehlken N, Kreuscher S, Ghofrani S, Hoeper MM, Halank M, et al. Exercise and respiratory training improve exercise capacity and quality of life in patients with severe chronic pulmonary hypertension. Circulation. 2006;114(14):1482–9.

160. Grunig E, Maier F, Ehlken N, Fischer C, Lichtblau M, Blank N, et al. Exercise training in pulmonary arterial hypertension associated with connective tissue diseases. Arthritis Res Ther. 2012;14(3): R148.

161. Jais X, Launay D, Yaici A, Le PJ, Tcherakian C, Sitbon O, et al. Immunosuppressive therapy in lupus- and mixed connective tissue disease-associated pulmonary arterial hypertension: a retrospective analysis of twenty-three cases. Arthritis Rheum. 2008;58(2):521–31.

162. Sanchez O, Sitbon O, Jais X, Simonneau G, Humbert M. Immunosuppressive therapy in connective tissue diseases-associated pulmonary arterial hypertension. Chest. 2006;130(1):182–9.

163. Kato M, Kataoka H, Odani T, Fujieda Y, Otomo K, Oku K, et al. The short-term role of corticosteroid therapy for pulmonary arterial hypertension associated with connective tissue diseases: report of five cases and a literature review. Lupus. 2011;20(10): 1047–56.

164. Miyamichi-Yamamoto S, Fukumoto Y, Sugimura K, Ishii T, Satoh K, Miura Y, et al. Intensive immunosuppressive therapy improves pulmonary hemodynamics and long-term prognosis in patients with pulmonary arterial hypertension associated with connective tissue disease. Circ J. 2011;75(11): 2668–74.

165. Barst RJ, Rubin LJ, Long WA, McGoon MD, Rich S, Badesch DB, et al. A comparison of continuous intravenous epoprostenol (prostacyclin) with conventional therapy for primary pulmonary hypertension. N Engl J Med. 1996;334(5):296–301.

166. Badesch DB, Tapson VF, McGoon MD, Brundage BH, Rubin LJ, Wigley FM, et al. Continuous intravenous epoprostenol for pulmonary hypertension due to the scleroderma spectrum of disease. A randomized, controlled trial. Ann Intern Med. 2000;132(6): 425–34.

167. Farber HW, Graven KK, Kokolski G, Korn JH. Pulmonary edema during acute infusion of epoprostenol in a patient with pulmonary hypertension and limited scleroderma. J Rheumatol. 1999;26(5): 1195–6.

168. Palmer SM, Robinson LJ, Wang A, Gossage JR, Bashore T, Tapson VF. Massive pulmonary edema and death after prostacyclin infusion in a patient with pulmonary veno-occlusive disease. Chest. 1998;113(1):237–40.

169. Farber HW, Miller DP, Meltzer LA, McGoon MD. Treatment of patients with pulmonary arterial hypertension at the time of death or deterioration to functional class IV: insights from the REVEAL registry. J Heart Lung Transplant. 2013;32(11):1114–22.

170. Caravita S, Wu SC, Secchi MB, Dadone V, Bencini C, Pierini S. Long-term effects of intermittent iloprost infusion on pulmonary arterial pressure in connective tissue disease. Eur J Intern Med. 2011;22(5): 518–21.

171. Hoeper MM, Gall H, Seyfarth HJ, Halank M, Ghofrani HA, Winkler J, et al. Long-term outcome with intravenous iloprost in pulmonary arterial hypertension. Eur Respir J. 2009;34(1):132–7.

172. Olschewski H, Simonneau G, Galie N, Higenbottam T, Naeije R, Rubin LJ, et al. Inhaled iloprost for severe pulmonary hypertension. N Engl J Med. 2002;347(5):322–9.

173. McLaughlin VV, Benza RL, Rubin LJ, Channick RN, Voswinckel R, Tapson VF, et al. Addition of inhaled treprostinil to oral therapy for pulmonary arterial hypertension: a randomized controlled clinical trial. J Am Coll Cardiol. 2010; 55(18):1915–22.

174. Shao D, Park JE, Wort SJ. The role of endothelin-1 in the pathogenesis of pulmonary arterial hypertension. Pharmacol Res. 2011;63(6):504–11.

175. Shetty N, Derk CT. Endothelin receptor antagonists as disease modifiers in systemic sclerosis. Inflamm Allergy Drug Targets. 2011;10(1):19–26.

176. Girgis RE, Mathai SC, Krishnan JA, Wigley FM, Hassoun PM. Long-term outcome of bosentan treatment in idiopathic pulmonary arterial hypertension and pulmonary arterial hypertension associated with the scleroderma spectrum of diseases. J Heart Lung Transplant. 2005;24(10):1626–31.

177. Tingey T, Shu J, Smuczek J, Pope J. Meta-analysis of healing and prevention of digital ulcers in systemic sclerosis. Arthritis Care Res (Hoboken). 2013; 65(9):1460–71.

178. Galie N, Olschewski H, Oudiz RJ, Torres F, Frost A, Ghofrani HA, et al. Ambrisentan for the treatment of pulmonary arterial hypertension: results of the ambrisentan in pulmonary arterial hypertension, randomized, double-blind, placebo-controlled, multicenter, efficacy (ARIES) study 1 and 2. Circulation. 2008;117(23):3010–9.

179. Oudiz RJ, Galie N, Olschewski H, Torres F, Frost A, Ghofrani HA, et al. Long-term ambrisentan therapy for the treatment of pulmonary arterial hypertension. J Am Coll Cardiol. 2009;54(21):1971–81.

180. Iglarz M, Binkert C, Morrison K, Fischli W, Gatfield J, Treiber A, et al. Pharmacology of macitentan, an orally active tissue-targeting dual endothelin receptor antagonist. J Pharmacol Exp Ther. 2008;327(3): 736–45.

181. Pulido T, Adzerikho I, Channick RN, Delcroix M, Galie N, Ghofrani HA, et al. Macitentan and morbidity and mortality in pulmonary arterial hypertension. N Engl J Med. 2013;369(9):809–18.

182. McGoon MD, Frost AE, Oudiz RJ, Badesch DB, Galie N, Olschewski H, et al. Ambrisentan therapy in patients with pulmonary arterial hypertension who discontinued bosentan or sitaxsentan due to liver function test abnormalities. Chest. 2009;135(1):122–9.

183. Klinger JR, Abman SH, Gladwin MT. Nitric oxide deficiency and endothelial dysfunction in pulmonary arterial hypertension. Am J Respir Crit Care Med. 2013;188(6):239–46.

184. Galie N, Ghofrani HA, Torbicki A, Barst RJ, Rubin LJ, Badesch D, et al. Sildenafil citrate therapy for pulmonary arterial hypertension. N Engl J Med. 2005;353(20):2148–57.

185. Wright PJ. Comparison of phosphodiesterase type 5 (PDE5) inhibitors. Int J Clin Pract. 2006;60(8): 967–75.

186. Galie N, Brundage BH, Ghofrani HA, Oudiz RJ, Simonneau G, Safdar Z, et al. Tadalafil therapy for pulmonary arterial hypertension. Circulation. 2009;119(22):2894–903.

187. Wirostko BM, Tressler C, Hwang LJ, Burgess G, Laties AM. Ocular safety of sildenafil citrate when administered chronically for pulmonary arterial hypertension: results from phase III, randomised, double masked, placebo controlled trial and open label extension. BMJ. 2012;344:e554.

188. Ghofrani HA, Grimminger F. Soluble guanylate cyclase stimulation: an emerging option in pulmonary hypertension therapy. Eur Respir Rev. 2009;18(111):35–41.

189. Evgenov OV, Pacher P, Schmidt PM, Hasko G, Schmidt HH, Stasch JP. NO-independent stimulators and activators of soluble guanylate cyclase: discovery and therapeutic potential. Nat Rev Drug Discov. 2006;5(9):755–68.

190. Ghofrani HA, Galie N, Grimminger F, Grunig E, Humbert M, Jing ZC, et al. Riociguat for the treatment of pulmonary arterial hypertension. N Engl J Med. 2013;369(4):330–40.

191. Humbert M, Barst RJ, Robbins IM, Channick RN, Galie N, Boonstra A, et al. Combination of bosentan with epoprostenol in pulmonary arterial hypertension: BREATHE-2. Eur Respir J. 2004;24(3):353–9.

192. Mathai SC, Girgis RE, Fisher MR, Champion HC, Housten-Harris T, Zaiman A, et al. Addition of sildenafil to bosentan monotherapy in pulmonary arterial hypertension. Eur Respir J. 2007;29(3):469–75.

193. Paul GA, Gibbs JS, Boobis AR, Abbas A, Wilkins MR. Bosentan decreases the plasma concentration of sildenafil when coprescribed in pulmonary hypertension. Br J Clin Pharmacol. 2005;60(1):107–12.

194. Schermuly RT, Dony E, Ghofrani HA, Pullamsetti S, Savai R, Roth M, et al. Reversal of experimental pulmonary hypertension by PDGF inhibition. J Clin Invest. 2005;115(10):2811–21.

195. Klein M, Schermuly RT, Ellinghaus P, Milting H, Riedl B, Nikolova S, et al. Combined tyrosine and serine/threonine kinase inhibition by sorafenib prevents progression of experimental pulmonary hypertension and myocardial remodeling. Circulation. 2008;118(20):2081–90.

196. Patterson KC, Weissmann A, Ahmadi T, Farber HW. Imatinib mesylate in the treatment of refractory idiopathic pulmonary arterial hypertension. Ann Intern Med. 2006;145(2):152–3.

197. Souza R, Sitbon O, Parent F, Simonneau G, Humbert M. Long term imatinib treatment in pulmonary arterial hypertension. Thorax. 2006;61(8):736.

198. Overbeek MJ, van Nieuw Amerongen GP, Boonstra A, Smit EF, Vonk-Noordegraaf A. Possible role of imatinib in clinical pulmonary veno-occlusive disease. Eur Respir J. 2008;32(1):232–5.

199. ten Freyhaus H, Dumitrescu D, Bovenschulte H, Erdmann E, Rosenkranz S. Significant improvement

of right ventricular function by imatinib mesylate in scleroderma-associated pulmonary arterial hypertension. Clin Res Cardiol. 2009;98(4):265–7.

200. Montani D, Bergot E, Gunther S, Savale L, Bergeron A, Bourdin A, et al. Pulmonary arterial hypertension in patients treated by dasatinib. Circulation. 2012;125(17):2128–37.

201. Nagaraj C, Tang B, Balint Z, Wygrecka M, Hrzenjak A, Kwapiszewska G, et al. Src tyrosine kinase is crucial for potassium channel function in human pulmonary arteries. Eur Respir J. 2013;41(1): 85–95.

202. McMahan ZH, Wigley FM. Novel investigational agents for the treatment of scleroderma. Expert Opin Investig Drugs. 2014;23(2):183–98.

203. Le Pavec J, Girgis RE, Lechtzin N, Mathai SC, Launay D, Hummers LK, et al. Systemic sclerosis-related pulmonary hypertension associated with interstitial lung disease: impact of pulmonary arterial hypertension therapies. Arthritis Rheum. 2011;63(8):2456–64.

204. Christie JD, Edwards LB, Kucheryavaya AY, Benden C, Dobbels F, Kirk R, et al. The Registry of the International Society for Heart and Lung Transplantation: twenty-eighth adult lung and heart-lung transplant report—2011. J Heart Lung Transplant. 2011;30(10):1104–22.

205. Schachna L, Medsger Jr TA, Dauber JH, Wigley FM, Braunstein NA, White B, et al. Lung transplantation in scleroderma compared with idiopathic pulmonary fibrosis and idiopathic pulmonary arterial hypertension. Arthritis Rheum. 2006;54(12): 3954–61.

206. Saggar R, Khanna D, Furst DE, Belperio JA, Park GS, Weigt SS, et al. Systemic sclerosis and bilateral lung transplantation: a single centre experience. Eur Respir J. 2010;36(4):893–900.

207. Shitrit D, Amital A, Peled N, Raviv Y, Medalion B, Saute M, et al. Lung transplantation in patients with scleroderma: case series, review of the literature, and criteria for transplantation. Clin Transplant. 2009; 23(2):178–83.

208. Avouac J, Wipff J, Kahan A, Allanore Y. Effects of oral treatments on exercise capacity in systemic sclerosis related pulmonary arterial hypertension: a meta-analysis of randomised controlled trials. Ann Rheum Dis. 2008;67(6):808–14.

209. Distler O, Behrens F, Pittrow D, Huscher D, Denton CP, Foeldvari I, et al. Defining appropriate outcome measures in pulmonary arterial hypertension related to systemic sclerosis: a Delphi consensus study with cluster analysis. Arthritis Rheum. 2008;59(6):867–75.

210. Denton CP, Avouac J, Behrens F, Furst DE, Foeldvari I, Humbert M, et al. Systemic sclerosis-associated pulmonary hypertension: why disease-specific composite endpoints are needed. Arthritis Res Ther. 2011;13(3):114.

Respiratory Infections in the Rheumatic Disease Patient

Jonathan B. Parr, Ritu R. Gill, and Joel T. Katz

Introduction

Among the many challenges facing rheumatic patients, infection continues to play an important role in clinical outcomes. The interplay between altered host defense mechanisms and powerful immunomodulatory drugs puts rheumatic patients at risk for serious infections, which can lead to hospitalization, morbidity, or even mortality. This is especially true of respiratory infections, and clinicians must be diligent in their evaluation and management of rheumatic patients who present with symptoms suggestive of respiratory disease.

Epidemiology

Multiple studies have examined the association between rheumatic disease and risk of infection, but the evidence is strongest in patients with inflammatory arthritis. One large prospective study of patients newly diagnosed with inflammatory polyarthritis estimated their risk of infection to be at least 2.5 times higher than the general

population [1]. The risk was even higher for respiratory tract infections, with inflammatory polyarthritis patients being 3.5 times more likely (95 % CI 2.3–5.4) to develop a respiratory tract infection than the general population.

A frequently cited retrospective matched cohort study of rheumatoid arthritis (RA) patients cared for at the Mayo Clinic spanning nearly 40 years also showed increased risks of infection. After controlling for multiple risk factors, including corticosteroid use, the researchers found that RA patients were 1.7 times (95 % CI 1.4–2.0) more likely to have objectively diagnosed infection than patients without RA from the same population. They were also 1.7 times (95 % CI 1.5–2.0) more likely to develop pneumonia [2].

Unfortunately, the increased risk of infection among rheumatic patients contributes to their increased mortality rate. In a prospective study of 1,000 RA patients over 10 years, overall mortality was significantly higher in RA patients compared to controls (352 deaths among RA patients versus 221 deaths among controls). Deaths from infectious diseases, especially respiratory infections, were significantly more common in patients with RA [3].

Pathogenesis

The pathogenesis of infection in rheumatic patients is thought to depend primarily on underlying impaired host defenses and on the effects of immunomodulatory drugs. Although certain abnormalities in the immune system of rheumatic

J.B. Parr, M.D., M.P.H. • J.T. Katz, M.D., M.A. (✉)
Department of Medicine, Brigham and Women's
Hospital, 75 Francis Street, Boston, MA 02115, USA
e-mail: jonbparr@post.harvard.edu; jkatz@partners.org

R.R. Gill, M.D., M.P.H.
Department of Radiology, Brigham and Women's
Hospital, 75 Francis Street, Boston, MA 02115, USA
e-mail: rgill@partners.org

P.F. Dellaripa et al. (eds.), *Pulmonary Manifestations of Rheumatic Disease: A Comprehensive Guide*,
DOI 10.1007/978-1-4939-0770-0_12, © Springer Science+Business Media New York 2014

patients are well described, such as complement deficiency and other mechanisms in systemic lupus erythematosus (SLE) [4], much remains to be elucidated in our understanding of the pathogenesis of rheumatic diseases [5]. In addition to immune system abnormalities, structural abnormalities attributable to rheumatic disease may also predispose to infection. Chronic lung disease and rheumatoid nodules, among other risk factors, were predictors of infection in RA patients in a multivariate model [6]. Additionally, environmental factors that may contribute to the development of rheumatic diseases can also lead to an increased risk of infection. One study of twins demonstrated an increased risk of developing RA and increased RA severity among patients who smoked [7]. Tobacco use is also a known risk factor for respiratory infection.

The numerous medications used to treat rheumatic diseases can be broadly categorized as corticosteroids, disease-modifying antirheumatic drugs (DMARDs), and biologic agents. Although many of these medications have clear immunomodulatory effects, the evidence supporting an association between their use and infection is often conflicting. A recent meta-analysis of infection risk in RA patients taking glucocorticoids showed no increased risk in randomized trials [8], but observational evidence consistently supports an association between infection and corticosteroid use [6]. In one large observational study of 16,788 rheumatic patients, for example, the risk of hospitalization for pneumonia increased with prednisone use and prednisone dose [9]. Given these findings, we consider rheumatic patients taking any immunomodulatory drugs to be at increased risk of infection.

The infection risk varies by drug, however. The most commonly used DMARD, methotrexate, has antiproliferative effects on lymphocytes. Although numerous case reports have documented opportunistic infections in rheumatic patients taking low-dose methotrexate, large cohort studies have failed to demonstrate a consistently increased risk of infection in patients taking it [10]. Cyclophosphamide use was associated with the highest risk of infection among traditional DMARDs, with a relative risk of 3.26

(95 % CI 2.28–4.67) in a large case control study of RA patients treated between 1980 and 2003. In the same study, azathioprine was associated with a moderately increased relative risk of 1.52 (95 % CI 1.18–1.97), but antimalarial agents, leflunomide, sulfasalazine, cyclosporine, and others were not [11]. Among the DMARDs, this observational data confirms that clinicians must be especially wary of infection with cyclophosphamide and azathioprine. However, it is our practice to watch closely for signs of infection and to consider opportunistic infections in patients taking other DMARDs as well.

We generally regard patients taking biologic agents as being at higher risk of infection than those taking DMARDs, based on both animal models and accumulating case series of unusual infections occurring in these patients. Tumor necrosis factor-alpha (TNF-α) antagonists are the most commonly used biologic agents in rheumatic patients. TNF-α is important for granuloma formation and maintenance and has been shown to be important for protection against numerous pathogens, including *Mycobacterium tuberculosis* and others. Currently approved TNF-α antagonists include adalimumab, certolizumab, etanercept, golimumab, and infliximab. A frequently referenced meta-analysis of patients taking TNF-α antagonists showed evidence of an increased risk of serious infections requiring hospitalization. For RA patients started on TNF-α antagonists, the number needed to harm for serious infections was 59 (95 % CI, 39–125) in a 3–12-month period of treatment [12].

It is important to note, however, that there continues to be considerable debate about the risk of infection associated with TNF-α antagonists [13]. In several studies, there was no significant increased risk of serious infection requiring hospitalization between patients being treated with TNF-α antagonists and those receiving treatment with glucocorticoids [9], methotrexate [14], or other DMARDs [15, 16]. However, several studies did find increased rates of serious infection requiring hospitalization within the first 3–6 months of starting TNF-α antagonist therapy compared to patients taking DMARDs [17, 18]. Additionally, it appears that not all TNF-α antagonists are alike.

In particular, infliximab has been associated with a greater risk of infection than etanercept [19, 20]. The evidence for increased infectious complications in patients taking rituximab, a different class of biologic agent that depletes B cells, is also mixed [21, 22]. Numerous case reports, however, have described hepatitis B virus (HBV) reactivation in patients taking rituximab [23]. For practical purposes, we recommend that any patient taking biologic agent be considered to be at increased risk of infection, particularly for fungal and mycobacterial infections.

Screening and Prophylaxis for Infections

Given concerns about increased infection risks, clinicians should carefully screen patients prior to initiating immunomodulatory drugs. The American College of Rheumatology recommends screening for HBV and hepatitis C virus (HCV) in high-risk patients prior to starting leflunomide and methotrexate [24]. Additionally, all patients should be screened for latent tuberculosis infection (LTBI), HBV, and HCV prior to initiation of TNF-α antagonists [25].

Screening for LTBI can be accomplished using either traditional tuberculin skin testing (TST) or newer interferon-γ release assays (IGRAs) such as QuantiFERON®-TB Gold (Cellestis Ltd, Victoria, Australia) [26]. IGRAs are generally preferred for patients who have previously received bacillus Calmette–Guérin (BCG) vaccination or who are unlikely to return for TST reading. Patients with positive LTBI screening results should be evaluated for clinical signs of active disease and have a chest X-ray to evaluate for active tuberculosis disease (TB). If the chest X-ray is unrevealing, they should receive treatment for LTBI with 9 months of daily isoniazid or with the recently approved 12-week regimen of weekly isoniazid and rifapentine [27, 28]. Ideally, LTBI treatment should be completed prior to initiating treatment with TNF-α antagonists, but many clinicians initiate TNF-α antagonists after several months of LTBI treatment.

Additionally, clinicians should ask about activities conferring higher risk for opportunistic infections prior to initiating biologics. Specifically, activities that increase the risk of *Histoplasma* exposure should be elucidated, including spelunking, cleaning poultry houses, demolition, and others. If any of these high-risk activities are reported, a chest X-ray is appropriate for screening. If the chest X-ray shows evidence of histoplasmosis or there is clinical evidence to support a diagnosis of histoplasmosis during the 2 years preceding biologic therapy, we recommend treating patients with prophylactic itraconazole for at least 3 months prior to and at least 1 year after initiating biologics [29]. If practicing in a region endemic for coccidioidomycosis (Arizona, New Mexico, central and southern California, or southern Texas), clinicians should obtain anti-coccidioidal antibody serologies and a chest X-ray prior to starting biologics. If either the serologies or chest X-ray shows evidence of coccidioidomycosis or if the patient has a past history of coccidioidomycosis (now resolved), we recommend treating patients taking biologics with prophylactic fluconazole for at least 6–12 months. It is important to note, however, that there is considerable debate about how best to manage patients on biologics with asymptomatic coccidioidomycosis, but a suggested management algorithm was recently published [30].

In addition to the prophylactic measures described previously, vaccination is an important intervention for patients receiving treatment for rheumatic disease (Table 12.1). Influenza vaccine is recommended for patients receiving hydroxychloroquine or minocycline. Both influenza and pneumococcal vaccines are recommended for patients receiving sulfasalazine. Influenza, pneumococcal, and hepatitis B vaccines are recommended for patients receiving leflunomide, methotrexate, or biologic agents. Live vaccines (including herpes zoster and measles, mumps, and rubella vaccines) should be avoided in patients receiving biologic agents. Of note, recent recommendations from the American College of Rheumatology recommend that patients should receive the herpes zoster vaccine before beginning biologic agents [31]. While there is not

Table 12.1 Recommendations for vaccinations in patients with RA starting or currently taking DMARDs or biologic agents

	Pneumococcal[a]	Influenza[b]	Hepatitis B[c]	Live attenuated vaccinations
Before initiating therapy				
DMARD monotherapy[d]	X	X	X	X
Combination DMARDs	X	X	X	X
All biologics[e]	X	X	X	X
While already taking therapy				
DMARD monotherapy	X	X	X	X
Combination DMARDs	X	X	X	X
All biologics	X	X	X	Not recommended

Adapted with permission from Singh JA, Furst DE, Bharat A, Curtis JR, Kavanaugh AF, Kremer JM, et al. 2012 update of the 2008 American College of Rheumatology recommendations for the use of disease-modifying antirheumatic drugs and biologic agents in the treatment of rheumatoid arthritis. Arthritis Care Res (Hoboken) 2012 May;64(5):625–639

X = recommend vaccination when indicated (based on age and risk)

[a] The Centers for Disease Control and Prevention also recommends a one-time pneumococcal revaccination after 5 years for persons with chronic conditions such as RA. For persons ages ≥65 years, one-time revaccination is recommended if they were vaccinated ≥5 years previously and were age <65 years at the time of the primary vaccination

[b] Intramuscular

[c] If hepatitis risk factors are present (e.g., intravenous drug abuse, multiple sex partners in the previous 6 months, health-care personnel)

[d] DMARDs include hydroxychloroquine, leflunomide, methotrexate, minocycline, and sulfasalazine

[e] Biologics include TNF-α antagonists (adalimumab, certolizumab pegol, etanercept, golimumab, and infliximab) and other agents (abatacept, rituximab, and tocilizumab)

definitive data to guide this practice, we recommend that it be administered at least 30 days before beginning biologic therapy. For select patients already taking biologic agents, it may be reasonable to hold the biologic agent for a period of time, administer the herpes zoster vaccine, and then reinitiate biologic therapy 30 days later.

Additionally, patients receiving moderate- and high-dose glucocorticoids should receive prophylaxis for *Pneumocystis* pneumonia (PCP). While consensus guidelines are lacking, we recommend PCP prophylaxis with trimethoprim–sulfamethoxazole (at least one double-strength tablet three times weekly) to patients who are taking glucocorticoids equivalent to at least 20 mg of prednisone for at least 1 month or to those taking glucocorticoids in combination with another immunosuppressive drug such as a TNF-α antagonist. Patients who are taking both methotrexate and trimethoprim–sulfamethoxazole (TMP-SMX) are at increased risk of methotrexate toxicity, but methotrexate is generally well tolerated in patients receiving prophylactic doses (rather than twice daily treatment doses) of TMP-SMX. There is some concern that patients with SLE may be more likely to have allergic reactions to sulfonamide-containing antibiotics. This concern has prompted some clinicians to use atovaquone rather than TMP-SMX for PCP prophylaxis in SLE patients [32], but it remains our practice to use TMP-SMX in SLE patients without a known TMP-SMX allergy.

Clinical Syndromes

Pulmonary infections account for an important portion of infections in rheumatic patients, and they are a major driver of hospitalization, morbidity, and mortality. In one study, 21–25 % of all infections in different cohorts of SLE patients were pulmonary infections [33]. Numerous pulmonary infections have been reported in rheumatic patients, but we will focus on two broad syndromes: pneumonia—the most commonly encountered pulmonary infection—and TB, which is an important consideration in patients taking TNF-α antagonists.

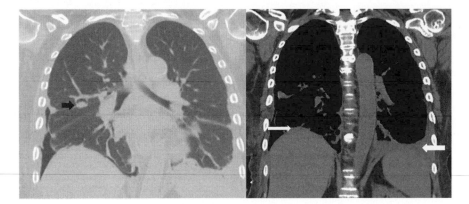

Fig. 12.1 Bilateral empyemas in a 57-year-old woman with RA being treated with methotrexate. Coronal computed tomography (CT) images (*left*: lung windows; *right*: soft tissue windows) demonstrated bilateral empyemas (*white arrows*) and multiple cavitary lung nodules consistent with rheumatoid nodules (*black arrow*). Diagnostic thoracentesis and microbial cultures confirmed bilateral *Staphylococcus aureus* pyogenic empyemas

Pneumonia

All rheumatic patients deserve special attention when they present with symptoms suggestive of pneumonia, especially those taking biologic agents. Typical signs and symptoms of pneumonia may be absent or attenuated, and imaging studies may be falsely negative. Patients with suspected pneumonia should be evaluated and treated for common bacterial pathogens, including *Streptococcus pneumoniae*, *Mycoplasma pneumoniae*, *Haemophilus influenzae*, *Chlamydia pneumoniae*, and *Legionella* spp. In 2011, the US Food and Drug Administration (FDA) added a black box warning to TNF-α antagonists for *Legionella* pneumonia. Between 1999 and 2010, 80 cases of *Legionella* pneumonia and four deaths in patients taking TNF-α antagonists were reported to the FDA's adverse events reporting system (AERS) [34].

For rheumatic patients with community-acquired pneumonia, we generally initiate treatment with either a respiratory fluoroquinolone (e.g., levofloxacin or moxifloxacin) or a beta-lactam in addition to an advanced-generation macrolide (e.g., azithromycin). For hospitalized rheumatic patients with healthcare-associated or hospital-acquired pneumonia, initial antibiotic coverage should be broadened to include nosocomial pathogens including methicillin-resistant *Staphylococcus aureus* (MRSA) and *Pseudomonas aeruginosa* (Fig. 12.1). Typical regimens include a combination of three antibiotics as follows: (1) piperacillin–tazobactam, an antipseudomonal cephalosporin (e.g., ceftazidime or cefepime), or an antipseudomonal carbapenem (e.g., imipenem or meropenem), (2) vancomycin, and (3) an antipseudomonal fluoroquinolone (e.g., levofloxacin or ciprofloxacin) or an aminoglycoside. Complete antibiotic recommendations are available from the Infectious Diseases Society of America [35, 36].

Uncommon pathogens must also be considered, especially given the growing body of observational evidence linking biologic agent use with bacterial, fungal, and viral pneumonias. Multiple cases of fungal pneumonia have been reported to the AERS. In response to 240 reported cases of histoplasmosis [37], the FDA added a black box warning to TNF-α antagonists for pulmonary and disseminated histoplasmosis (Figs. 12.2 and 12.3), coccidioidomycosis, and blastomycosis [38]. The risk of developing histoplasmosis appears to be higher with infliximab than etanercept [19]. In rheumatic patients with newly diagnosed histoplasmosis, antifungal therapy should be initiated promptly—usually with itraconazole or amphotericin B in consultation with an infectious diseases specialist. We also recommend stopping TNF-α antagonists in these patients if

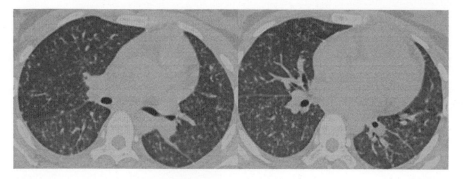

Fig. 12.2 Disseminated histoplasmosis in a 37-year-old woman with SLE being treated with rituximab. Axial CT images showed new diffuse miliary nodules, which were felt to be consistent with reactivation of histoplasmosis. The diagnosis was made initially by urinary *Histoplasma* antigen testing and then confirmed by positive *Histoplasma* serologies

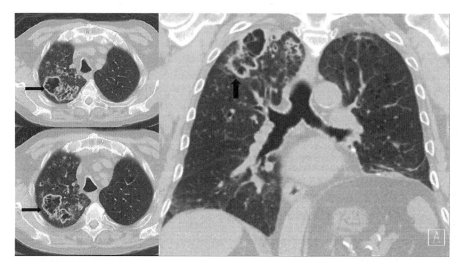

Fig. 12.3 Reactivation histoplasmosis in a 50-year-old with RA being treated with methotrexate. Axial and coronal CT images showed cavitary lesions (*bold black arrows*) with surrounding parenchymal nodular opacities in the right upper lobe. Transbronchial biopsy findings were consistent with histoplasmosis

possible, at least until the clinical infection is under control, and careful observation for signs of an immune reconstitution inflammatory syndrome (IRIS) following discontinuation of the TNF-α antagonist, which has been reported in case studies [29].

There are limited data regarding coccidioidomycosis in patients treated with biologics or DMARDs from two clinics in Arizona between 2007 and 2009. Of the 44 patients who developed coccidioidomycosis while under treatment for rheumatic disease, 29 developed pulmonary infection, 9 developed disseminated disease, and 6 developed asymptomatic positive coccidioidal serologies. In addition to beginning treatment with antifungal therapy, the majority stopped immunomodulatory therapy initially but were later able to resume it [39]. We recommend that rheumatic patients who are diagnosed with coccidioidomycosis pneumonia discontinue immunomodulatory therapy if possible and receive treatment with antifungal medication (typically fluconazole) in consultation with an infectious diseases specialist.

PCP was reported to the AERS in 84 patients taking infliximab, 49 of whom had RA, between 1998 and 2003. Many patients were also taking other immunosuppressants, including glucocorticoids. The mean time between infliximab infusion and onset of pneumonia symptoms was 21 days, and 23 patients died [40]. A case control study of 21 patients on infliximab who were diagnosed with PCP in Japan found an increased risk of PCP in patients older than 65, taking 6 mg or more of prednisolone, or with coexisting pulmonary disease [41]. Additionally, fatal PCP was reported in an RA patient treated with rituximab [42]. Based on this evidence, we recommend that PCP be considered in rheumatic patients who develop pneumonia, particularly those in whom hypoxia is a prominent clinical feature, and that treatment with TMP-SMX be initiated promptly when clinical suspicion is high. Adjunctive corticosteroids should be initiated for moderate to severe disease [43]. Bronchoscopy is superior to induced sputum for confirmation of the diagnosis. Other fungal pathogens must also be considered, as multiple cases of *Cryptococcus* and *Aspergillus* pneumonia in patients taking biologic agents have been reported [19].

Viral pneumonia has also been reported as a severe complication in patients taking TNF-α antagonists [44]. The risk of herpes simplex virus (HSV) infections may be increased in rheumatic patients in general [9], and an increased risk of HSV infection has been suggested in large observational studies of rheumatic patients taking TNF-α antagonists [45]. Reactivation of varicella zoster virus (VZV) is common in patients taking TNF-α antagonists, and severe VZV pneumonia was reported in a patient with psoriatic arthritis taking etanercept [46].

Several common clinical scenarios deserve special mention. Because rheumatic patients are more likely to develop interstitial lung disease (ILD) than the general population, clinicians are often forced to determine whether worsened respiratory symptoms represent an ILD flare or an infectious process. Similarly, patients with connective tissue disease who develop lung involvement often present with symptoms and radiographic findings that could also suggest an underlying infectious process. Because the radiographic and clinical findings associated with ILD and connective tissue disease with lung involvement are similar to those found in a variety of infections, we recommend that clinicians maintain a high index of suspicion for infection, especially for fungal infections, tuberculosis, and other uncommon pathogens. Noninvasive diagnostic studies such as β-glucan (to evaluate for PCP and fungal infections) and specific serologic or urine markers (to evaluate for histoplasmosis, coccidioidomycosis, and blastomycosis) can be extremely valuable. Induced sputum or early bronchoscopy with lavage can often differentiate infectious disease from ILD flares with minimal risk. In challenging cases, we utilize a multidisciplinary approach involving careful review of imaging studies with a radiologist, discussion with an infectious diseases specialist, and consultation with a pulmonologist.

Tuberculosis

There appears to be an increased risk of TB reactivation in patients with rheumatic disease taking TNF-α antagonists and possibly among rheumatic patients in general (Fig. 12.4). In one study of patients in Spain prior to the widespread use of TNF-α antagonists, the incidence risk ratio of pulmonary TB in patients with RA compared to the general population was 3.68 (95 % CI 2.36–5.92) [47]. In a separate prospective study conducted before widespread use of TNF-α antagonists, however, the risk of TB among RA patients was not increased compared to the general population [48].

The risk of developing TB is increased in patients taking TNF-α antagonists, presumably due to the importance of TNF-α for granuloma formation and maintenance described earlier. In a study of patients in Korea, the risk ratio of TB in RA patients not taking TNF-α antagonists was 8.9 (95 % CI 4.6–17.2) and 30.1 in those taking infliximab [49]. Reactivation of LTBI is the most common etiology among patients in the United States, but development of primary TB must also be considered—especially in patients with risk

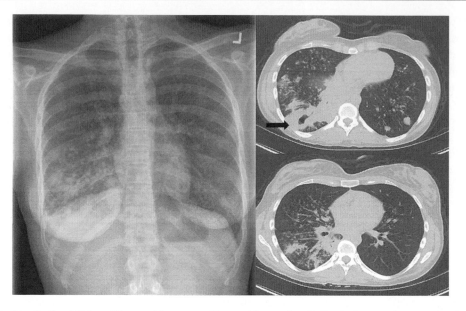

Fig. 12.4 Reactivation TB in a 29-year-old woman with RA being treated with methotrexate. Chest X-ray (postero-anterior view) and axial CT images showed multifocal bilateral parenchymal opacities with tree-in bud nodularity, evidence of cavitation in the superior segment of the right lower lobe (*bold black arrows*), and transbronchial spread of infection. Induced sputum examination and culture confirmed infection with *Mycobacterium tuberculosis*

factors for recent TB exposure. The risk of extrapulmonary TB appears to be higher in patients taking TNF-α antagonists than in members of the general population.

In a study of 112,300 patients with RA, 386 cases of TB occurred after RA treatment. The relative risk of developing TB in RA patients who received treatment with biologic agents compared to RA patients who did not receive any biologics or DMARDs was 1.5 (95 % 1.1–1.9) [50]. The incidence of TB was 2.57 (95 % 1.89–3.26) per 1,000 person-years among patients treated with TNF-α antagonists. 73 % of these patients developed pulmonary TB, and the median time to presentation of TB was 17 weeks (range 1–71 weeks) from the first prescription of infliximab and 79 weeks (range 3–168 weeks) from the first prescription of etanercept. Interestingly, the risk of developing TB was lower in patients taking corticosteroids concurrently. A recent meta-analysis also found differences between TNF-α antagonists—the risk of TB was 3–4 times higher for infliximab and adalimumab than for etanercept [51]. Similar to these findings, the median time to presentation of TB was 5.5 months for infliximab, 13.4 months for etanercept, and 18.5 months for adalimumab. Sixty-two percent of cases were extrapulmonary TB.

The diagnosis of TB can be particularly difficult in patients taking TNF-α antagonists. Immunosuppressive therapies can increase the risk of false-negative TSTs and chest X-rays, and they may predispose patients to more rapid progression of disease. For this reason, we recommend referral to an infectious diseases specialist when clinical suspicion for TB is high and the diagnosis is not easily confirmed. Further efforts to obtain a microbiologic diagnosis with culture (biopsy, bronchoscopy, and other modalities) are often undertaken, but the diagnosis must sometimes be made based on clinical data in the absence of confirmation by culture. When TB is diagnosed, multidrug therapy based on the patient's drug-susceptibility pattern and exposure history should be initiated, and TNF-α antagonists should be discontinued if possible. Notably, there have been reports of an IRIS-like reaction after stopping TNF-α antagonists in rheumatic patients with newly diagnosed TB [52].

The optimal strategy for managing the small subset of patients who must continue TNF-α antagonists while receiving TB treatment remains unclear, but a recent case report from Japan describes a patient with severe RA who was successfully treated for TB with only a brief cessation of her infliximab during the first several months of TB treatment [53]. Numerous other pathogens have been reported to cause granulomatous infection in patients taking TNF-α antagonists—including non-tuberculosis mycobacteria (NTM), *Candida, Histoplasma, Cryptococcus, Candida, Coccidioides, Blastomyces, Aspergillus,* and others [19]. As with tuberculosis, severe and rapidly progressive cases of these mycobacterial and fungal infections have been reported.

Because of the association between bronchiectasis and NTM disease, rheumatic patients with bronchiectasis require careful evaluation prior to the initiation of biologic agents. Although bronchiectasis is not an absolute contraindication to treatment with biologics, sputum culture and review of past sputum culture results should be performed prior to beginning therapy. NTM disease often requires prolonged treatment with multidrug regimens and is likely to be more difficult to treat in patients taking TNF-α antagonists. The small subset of patients with active NTM disease who must continue treatment with TNF-α antagonists should only do so if they are also receiving adequate treatment for their NTM disease [54].

Summary

Pulmonary infections are an important threat to rheumatic patients. Clinicians can reduce the risk of serious infections by ensuring that patients receive careful screening and appropriate vaccinations prior to initiating immunomodulatory therapy. The management of rheumatic patients who present with signs and symptoms of pulmonary infection should involve consideration of common and uncommon pathogens. This is especially true for patients taking biologic agents, which increase the risk of TB and other less commonly encountered infections.

Acknowledgment We wish to thank Dr. John Galgiani for his helpful advice regarding the management of coccidioidomycosis.

References

1. Franklin J, Lunt M, Bunn D, Symmons D, Silman A. Risk and predictors of infection leading to hospitalisation in a large primary-care-derived cohort of patients with inflammatory polyarthritis. Ann Rheum Dis. 2007;66(3):308–12.
2. Doran MF, Crowson CS, Pond GR, O'Fallon WM, Gabriel SE. Frequency of infection in patients with rheumatoid arthritis compared with controls: a population-based study. Arthritis Rheum. 2002;46(9):2287–93.
3. Mutru O, Laakso M, Isomaki H, Koota K. Ten year mortality and causes of death in patients with rheumatoid arthritis. Br Med J (Clin Res Ed). 1985;290(6484):1797–9.
4. Zandman-Goddard G, Shoenfeld Y. Infections and SLE. Autoimmunity. 2005;38(7):473–85.
5. McInnes IB, Schett G. The pathogenesis of rheumatoid arthritis. N Engl J Med. 2011;365(23):2205–19.
6. Doran MF, Crowson CS, Pond GR, O'Fallon WM, Gabriel SE. Predictors of infection in rheumatoid arthritis. Arthritis Rheum. 2002;46(9):2294–300.
7. Silman AJ, Newman J, MacGregor AJ. Cigarette smoking increases the risk of rheumatoid arthritis. Results from a nationwide study of disease-discordant twins. Arthritis Rheum. 1996;39(5):732–5.
8. Dixon WG, Suissa S, Hudson M. The association between systemic glucocorticoid therapy and the risk of infection in patients with rheumatoid arthritis: systematic review and meta-analyses. Arthritis Res Ther. 2011;13(4):R139.
9. Wolfe F, Caplan L, Michaud K. Treatment for rheumatoid arthritis and the risk of hospitalization for pneumonia: associations with prednisone, disease-modifying antirheumatic drugs, and anti-tumor necrosis factor therapy. Arthritis Rheum. 2006;54(2):628–34.
10. McLean-Tooke A, Aldridge C, Waugh S, Spickett GP, Kay L. Methotrexate, rheumatoid arthritis and infection risk: what is the evidence? Rheumatology (Oxford). 2009;48(8):867–71.
11. Bernatsky S, Hudson M, Suissa S. Anti-rheumatic drug use and risk of serious infections in rheumatoid arthritis. Rheumatology (Oxford). 2007;46(7):1157–60.
12. Bongartz T, Sutton AJ, Sweeting MJ, Buchan I, Matteson EL, Montori V. Anti-TNF antibody therapy in rheumatoid arthritis and the risk of serious infections and malignancies: systematic review and meta-analysis of rare harmful effects in randomized controlled trials. JAMA. 2006;295(19):2275–85.
13. Solomon DH, Lunt M, Schneeweiss S. The risk of infection associated with tumor necrosis factor alpha

antagonists: making sense of epidemiologic evidence. Arthritis Rheum. 2008;58(4):919–28.

14. Schneeweiss S, Setoguchi S, Weinblatt ME, Katz JN, Avorn J, Sax PE, et al. Anti-tumor necrosis factor alpha therapy and the risk of serious bacterial infections in elderly patients with rheumatoid arthritis. Arthritis Rheum. 2007;56(6):1754–64.

15. Listing J, Strangfeld A, Kary S, Rau R, von Hinueber U, Stoyanova-Scholz M, et al. Infections in patients with rheumatoid arthritis treated with biologic agents. Arthritis Rheum. 2005;52(11):3403–12.

16. Grijalva CG, Chen L, Delzell E, Baddley JW, Beukelman T, Winthrop KL, et al. Initiation of tumor necrosis factor-alpha antagonists and the risk of hospitalization for infection in patients with autoimmune diseases. JAMA. 2011;306(21):2331–9.

17. Dixon WG, Symmons DP, Lunt M, Watson KD, Hyrich KL, British Society for Rheumatology Biologics Register Control Centre Consortium, et al. Serious infection following anti-tumor necrosis factor alpha therapy in patients with rheumatoid arthritis: lessons from interpreting data from observational studies. Arthritis Rheum. 2007;56(9):2896–904.

18. Curtis JR, Patkar N, Xie A, Martin C, Allison JJ, Saag M, et al. Risk of serious bacterial infections among rheumatoid arthritis patients exposed to tumor necrosis factor alpha antagonists. Arthritis Rheum. 2007;56(4):1125–33.

19. Wallis RS, Broder MS, Wong JY, Hanson ME, Beenhouwer DO. Granulomatous infectious diseases associated with tumor necrosis factor antagonists. Clin Infect Dis. 2004;38(9):1261–5.

20. Koo S, Marty FM, Baden LR. Infectious complications associated with immunomodulating biologic agents. Infect Dis Clin North Am. 2010;24(2):285–306.

21. Rafailidis PI, Kakisi OK, Vardakas K, Falagas ME. Infectious complications of monoclonal antibodies used in cancer therapy: a systematic review of the evidence from randomized controlled trials. Cancer. 2007;109(11):2182–9.

22. Aksoy S, Dizdar O, Hayran M, Harputluoglu H. Infectious complications of rituximab in patients with lymphoma during maintenance therapy: a systematic review and meta-analysis. Leuk Lymphoma. 2009; 50(3):357–65.

23. Garcia-Rodriguez MJ, Canales MA, Hernandez-Maraver D, Hernandez-Navarro F. Late reactivation of resolved hepatitis B virus infection: an increasing complication post rituximab-based regimens treatment? Am J Hematol. 2008;83(8):673–5.

24. Saag KG, Teng GG, Patkar NM, Anuntiyo J, Finney C, Curtis JR, et al. American College of Rheumatology 2008 recommendations for the use of nonbiologic and biologic disease-modifying antirheumatic drugs in rheumatoid arthritis. Arthritis Rheum. 2008;59(6):762–84.

25. Furst DE, Keystone EC, Kirkham B, Kavanaugh A, Fleischmann R, Mease P, et al. Updated consensus statement on biological agents for the treatment of rheumatic diseases, 2008. Ann Rheum Dis. 2008;67 Suppl 3:iii2–25.

26. Mazurek GH, Jereb J, Vernon A, LoBue P, Goldberg S, Castro K, et al. Updated guidelines for using interferon gamma release assays to detect Mycobacterium tuberculosis infection—United States, 2010. MMWR Recomm Rep. 2010;59(RR-5):1–25.

27. Targeted tuberculin testing and treatment of latent tuberculosis infection. This official statement of the American Thoracic Society was adopted by the ATS Board of Directors, July 1999. This is a Joint Statement of the American Thoracic Society (ATS) and the Centers for Disease Control and Prevention (CDC). This statement was endorsed by the Council of the Infectious Diseases Society of America. (IDSA), September 1999, and the sections of this statement. Am J Respir Crit Care Med. 2000;161 (4 Pt 2):S221–47.

28. Centers for Disease Control and Prevention (CDC). Recommendations for use of an isoniazid-rifapentine regimen with direct observation to treat latent Mycobacterium tuberculosis infection. MMWR Morb Mortal Wkly Rep. 2011;60(48):1650–3.

29. Hage CA, Bowyer S, Tarvin SE, Helper D, Kleiman MB, Joseph WL. Recognition, diagnosis, and treatment of histoplasmosis complicating tumor necrosis factor blocker therapy. Clin Infect Dis. 2010; 50(1):85–92.

30. Galgiani JN, Ampel NM, Blair JE, Catanzaro A, Johnson RH, Stevens DA, et al. Coccidioidomycosis. Clin Infect Dis. 2005;41(9):1217–23.

31. Singh JA, Furst DE, Bharat A, Curtis JR, Kavanaugh AF, Kremer JM, et al. 2012 Update of the 2008 American College of Rheumatology recommendations for the use of disease-modifying antirheumatic drugs and biologic agents in the treatment of rheumatoid arthritis. Arthritis Care Res (Hoboken). 2012; 64(5):625–39.

32. Jeffries M, Bruner G, Glenn S, Sadanandan P, Carson CW, Harley JB, et al. Sulpha allergy in lupus patients: a clinical perspective. Lupus. 2008;17(3):202–5.

33. Petri M. Infection in systemic lupus erythematosus. Rheum Dis Clin North Am. 1998;24(2):423–56.

34. FDA Drug Safety Communication: Drug labels for the tumor necrosis factor-alpha (TNFα) blockers now include warnings about infection with Legionella and Listeria bacteria. 2011. Accessed 11 May 2012. http://www.fda.gov/Drugs/DrugSafety/ucm270849.htm

35. Mandell LA, Wunderink RG, Anzueto A, Bartlett JG, Campbell GD, Dean NC, et al. Infectious Diseases Society of America/American Thoracic Society consensus guidelines on the management of community-acquired pneumonia in adults. Clin Infect Dis. 2007;44 Suppl 2:S27–72.

36. American Thoracic Society, Infectious Diseases Society of America. Guidelines for the management of adults with hospital-acquired, ventilator-associated, and healthcare-associated pneumonia. Am J Respir Crit Care Med. 2005;171(4):388–416.

37. Lee JH, Slifman NR, Gershon SK, Edwards ET, Schwieterman WD, Siegel JN, et al. Life-threatening histoplasmosis complicating immunotherapy with tumor necrosis factor alpha antagonists infliximab and etanercept. Arthritis Rheum. 2002;46(10):2565–70.

38. Information for Healthcare Professionals: Cimzia (certolizumab pegol), Enbrel (etanercept), Humira (adalimumab), and Remicade (infliximab). 2008. Accessed 11 May 2012. http://www.fda.gov/Drugs/DrugSafety/PostmarketDrugSafetyInformationfor PatientsandProviders/ucm124185.htm

39. Taroumian S, Knowles SL, Lisse JR, Yanes J, Ampel NM, Vaz A, et al. Management of coccidioidomycosis in patients receiving biologic response modifiers or disease-modifying antirheumatic drugs. Arthritis Care Res (Hoboken). 2012; 64(12):1903–9.

40. Kaur N, Mahl TC. Pneumocystis jiroveci (carinii) pneumonia after infliximab therapy: a review of 84 cases. Dig Dis Sci. 2007;52(6):1481–4.

41. Harigai M, Koike R, Miyasaka N, Pneumocystis Pneumonia under Anti-Tumor Necrosis Factor Therapy (PAT) Study Group. Pneumocystis pneumonia associated with infliximab in Japan. N Engl J Med. 2007;357(18):1874–6.

42. Teichmann LL, Woenckhaus M, Vogel C, Salzberger B, Scholmerich J, Fleck M. Fatal Pneumocystis pneumonia following rituximab administration for rheumatoid arthritis. Rheumatology (Oxford). 2008; 47(8):1256–7.

43. Kaplan JE, Benson C, Holmes KH, Brooks JT, Pau A, Masur H, et al. Guidelines for prevention and treatment of opportunistic infections in HIV-infected adults and adolescents: recommendations from CDC, the National Institutes of Health, and the HIV Medicine Association of the Infectious Diseases Society of America. MMWR Recomm Rep. 2009;58(RR-4):1–207; quiz CE1-4.

44. Smith D, Letendre S. Viral pneumonia as a serious complication of etanercept therapy. Ann Intern Med. 2002;136(2):174.

45. Strangfeld A, Listing J, Herzer P, Liebhaber A, Rockwitz K, Richter C, et al. Risk of herpes zoster in patients with rheumatoid arthritis treated with anti-TNF-alpha agents. JAMA. 2009;301(7):737–44.

46. Manzano V, Ruiz P, Torres M, Gomez F. Severe pneumonia by aciclovir-resistant varicella-zoster virus during etanercept therapy. Rheumatology (Oxford). 2010;49(9):1791–3.

47. Carmona L, Hernandez-Garcia C, Vadillo C, Pato E, Balsa A, Gonzalez-Alvaro I, et al. Increased risk of tuberculosis in patients with rheumatoid arthritis. J Rheumatol. 2003;30(7):1436–9.

48. Wolfe F, Michaud K, Anderson J, Urbansky K. Tuberculosis infection in patients with rheumatoid arthritis and the effect of infliximab therapy. Arthritis Rheum. 2004;50(2):372–9.

49. Seong SS, Choi CB, Woo JH, Bae KW, Joung CL, Uhm WS, et al. Incidence of tuberculosis in Korean patients with rheumatoid arthritis (RA): effects of RA itself and of tumor necrosis factor blockers. J Rheumatol. 2007;34(4):706–11.

50. Brassard P, Kezouh A, Suissa S. Antirheumatic drugs and the risk of tuberculosis. Clin Infect Dis. 2006; 43(6):717–22.

51. Dixon WG, Hyrich KL, Watson KD, Lunt M, Galloway J, Ustianowski A, et al. Drug-specific risk of tuberculosis in patients with rheumatoid arthritis treated with anti-TNF therapy: results from the British Society for Rheumatology Biologics Register (BSRBR). Ann Rheum Dis. 2010;69(3):522–8.

52. Arend SM, Leyten EM, Franken WP, Huisman EM, van Dissel JT. A patient with de novo tuberculosis during anti-tumor necrosis factor-alpha therapy illustrating diagnostic pitfalls and paradoxical response to treatment. Clin Infect Dis. 2007;45(11): 1470–5.

53. Matsumoto T, Tanaka T, Kawase I. Infliximab for rheumatoid arthritis in a patient with tuberculosis. N Engl J Med. 2006;355(7):740–1.

54. Griffith DE, Aksamit T, Brown-Elliott BA, Catanzaro A, Daley C, Gordin F, et al. An official ATS/IDSA statement: diagnosis, treatment, and prevention of nontuberculous mycobacterial diseases. Am J Respir Crit Care Med. 2007;175(4):367–416.

Lung Transplantation for Connective Tissue Disease-Associated Lung Disease

13

Ryan Hadley and Kevin M. Chan

Introduction

Lung transplantation has been a viable treatment option for patients with connective tissue disease (CTD)-associated respiratory failure for several decades [1]. In 2006, CTD was put forth as an indication for lung transplant by the International Society of Heart and Lung Transplantation (ISHLT) [2]. Despite this, CTD is an infrequent indication for lung transplantation with only 488 CTD patients (1.3 % of all reported lung transplants) transplanted between 1995 and 2012 [3]. The scarce volume of CTD lung transplants is likely due to the extrapulmonary manifestations of multisystem disease precluding candidacy. In this chapter, we discuss the general background regarding lung transplantation as well as indications, contraindications, outcomes, and referral recommendations for lung transplant consideration in CTD patients.

R. Hadley, M.D. • K.M. Chan, M.D. (✉)
Division of Pulmonary and Critical Care Medicine, Department of Internal Medicine, University of Michigan Health System, 3916 Taubman Center, 1500 East Medical Center Drive, SPC 5360, Ann Arbor, MI 48109-5360, USA
e-mail: hadleyr@med.umich.edu;
kevichan@med.umich.edu

Lung Transplantation Overview

Lung transplantation dates to the early 1960s with 36 transplants performed between 1963 and 1974 [4]. Uniformly poor results were noted with only three patients living more than 1 month and the longest living 10 months. The major causes of death were respiratory failure due to rejection, infection, or bronchial disruption [5–7]. The first successful lung transplantation occurred with the advent of cyclosporine in 1981 as part of a heart-lung block for pulmonary vascular disease [8, 9]. The first successful single lung transplant (SLT) was reported in 1986 in a patient with idiopathic pulmonary fibrosis (IPF) [10]. Overall, SLT remains the predominant surgical therapy for advanced pulmonary fibrosis, although the percent of double lung transplants (DLTs) performed annually for this diagnosis has increased to 54 % in 2011 [3]. The most common indication for lung transplantation remains emphysema (34 %) followed by IPF (24 %), cystic fibrosis (17 %), alpha-1 antitrypsin-deficient emphysema (5.8 %), other forms of pulmonary fibrosis (3.7 %), and idiopathic pulmonary arterial hypertension (IPAH) (3.1 %). However, from 2001 to 2011, the percentage of recipients with emphysema decreased from 40 to 30 %, and the percentage of transplants for interstitial lung disease (ILD) increased from 17 to 29 % [3].

Much controversy continues to revolve around the optimal procedure (single vs. double lung) in patients receiving lung transplants [11–14]. The current surgical approaches and principles of postoperative

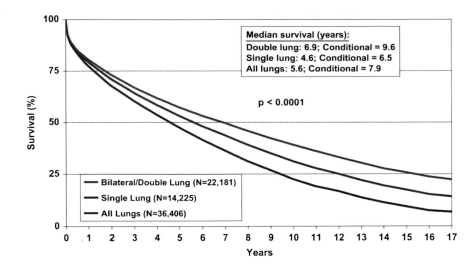

Fig. 13.1 Adult single vs. double lung transplantation survival outcomes. International Society of Lung Transplant Registry adult lung transplant recipient Kaplan–Meier survival, stratified by procedure type (transplants: January 1994–June 2011). Includes conditional median survival for the subset of recipients who were alive 1 year after transplantation (Used with permis- sion from Yusen RD, Christie JD, Edwards LB, Kucheryavaya AY, Benden C, Dipchand AI, et al. The Registry of the International Society for Heart and Lung Transplantation: Thirtieth Adult Lung and Heart-Lung Transplant Report—2013; Focus Theme: Age. The Journal of Heart and Lung Transplantation. 2013; 32(10):965–78)

management are outside the scope of this chapter [15, 16]. SLT procedures have the advantage of shorter operative times, providing organs to two rather than a single recipient, and have been shown to provide excellent outcomes to patients with emphysema and idiopathic pulmonary fibrosis [4, 13, 17–19]. Patients with suppurative lung disease such as cystic fibrosis or bronchiectasis, those with pulmonary hypertension, and patients younger than 50 years of age preferably receive a DLT. Recent data suggests improved long-term outcomes in transplant recipients treated with DLT vs. SLT (Fig. 13.1) [3, 11, 12, 14, 20]. In fact, data from 2006 to 2008 indicate bilateral lung transplantations accounted for two-thirds of all lung transplant procedures in the United States [21]. Despite these findings, this information is limited by the lack of prospective data collection, adjustment for influencing variables, and lack of randomization to ensure comparable treatment groups. As such, clear recommendations require further study.

Long-term results of lung transplantation are limited by significant complications which impair survival. Data from the Registry of the ISHLT suggests 79 % 1-year, 53 % 5-year, and 31 % 10-year survival for all recipients [3]. While emphysema patients enjoy the greatest survival advantage in the first year after lung transplantation, they have the lowest survival rate at 15 years (Fig. 13.2) [3]. Low perioperative complication rates and the advanced age of many chronic obstructive pulmonary disease (COPD) patients may contribute to this finding. Conditional median survival for those patients surviving 1 year are greatest for patients with cystic fibrosis (10.5 years) and pulmonary hypertension (10 years) compared to those with ILD (7 years) [3]. This is also likely a reflection of patient age. The most frequent causes of late death include chronic allograft rejection (obliterative bronchiolitis or bronchiolitis obliterans syndrome (BOS)), infection, and malignancy [3, 22].

Long-term data evaluating health-related quality of life (HRQL) and health status after lung transplantation is now available. Seven-year follow-up of SLT and DLT COPD patients using the St. George's Respiratory Questionnaire (SGRQ) revealed persistent improvement from pre-transplant values [23]. However, the mean absolute values of the SGRQ were greater in DLT patients, especially 4 years after transplantation [23]. In addition, while all three domains of

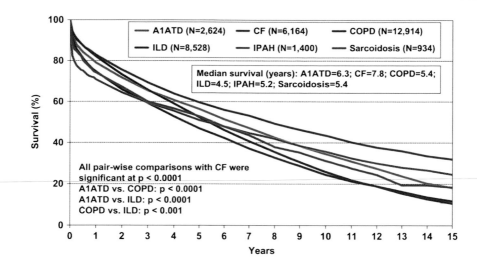

Fig. 13.2 Adult lung transplant survival stratified by recipient diagnosis. Kaplan–Meier survival by diagnosis obtained from the International Society of Heart and Lung Transplantation Registry (transplants: January 1990–June 2011). *A1ATD* α1-antitrypsin deficiency-associated chronic obstructive pulmonary disease (COPD); *COPD* non-A1ATD-associated COPD; *CF* bronchiectasis associated with cystic fibrosis (CF); *ILD* interstitial lung disease, which includes idiopathic pulmonary fibrosis (IPF);

and *IPAH* idiopathic pulmonary arterial hypertension (Used with permission from Yusen RD, Christie JD, Edwards LB, Kucheryavaya AY, Benden C, Dipchand AI, et al. The Registry of the International Society for Heart and Lung Transplantation: Thirtieth Adult Lung and Heart-Lung Transplant Report—2013; Focus Theme: Age. The Journal of Heart and Lung Transplantation. 2013;32(10):965–78)

the SGRQ improved in DLT recipients, the respiratory symptom domain lacked significant change in SLT patients. Improved long-term HRQL after DLT compared to SLT for COPD was implied [23, 24]. Rodrigue et al. administered both the SF-36 and the Transplant Specific Frequency Questionnaire (TSFQ) to lung transplant recipients [25]. After a mean follow-up of 2 years, significant improvement in 7 of 8 subscales of the SF-36 was noted but remained below that of the general population [25]. Three- to five-year posttransplant survivors reported more frequent affective, neurocognitive, and physical appearance issues. Similar findings have been described [26] in a group of 10-year survivors and are likely due to the chronic use of immunosuppressive medications, transplant comorbidities, and the development of BOS in long-term survivors.

Organ Allocation

At the time of transplant, lung allocation is based on geographic location of the donor, blood type, donor-recipient size matching, the presence of

human leukocyte antigen (HLA) antibodies directed against the donor allograft, surgical evaluation of the allograft, and the lung allocation score (LAS) [27].

In May 2005, the LAS was implemented in the United States for potential recipients greater than 12 years of age to create an allocation system that focuses on the use of objective data for the allocation of lungs based on medical urgency [27]. The LAS is based on a formula derived from risk factors associated with mortality while on the wait list and after transplantation, to determine a "transplant benefit" formula. The normalized LAS ranges from 0 to 100 with a higher score associated with a greater severity of illness. A lung review board was also implemented to provide an exception to patients when the listing center feels the LAS does not adequately reflect the severity of patient illness [28]. Four groups were devised for use in the LAS based on physiologic and statistical similarities. These include group A (obstructive lung disease), group B (pulmonary arterial hypertension, PAH), group C (cystic fibrosis), and group D (pulmonary fibrosis) [27]. Patients with CTD fall into group

B if their primary cause for respiratory failure is PAH or group D if they have ILD. These groupings are the best approximation of CTD-related disease behavior with the understanding that the number of variables for study in this patient group was too small to accurately predict outcomes [27]. A new revision of the LAS based on more recent data has been approved for implementation by the UNOS board of directors [29].

Indications for Lung Transplantation in CTD

The primary cause of death in patients with progressive systemic sclerosis (SSc) is end-stage lung disease related to PAH and/or ILD (nonspecific interstitial pneumonitis (NSIP) and/or usual interstitial pneumonitis (UIP)) [30]. Pulmonary arterial hypertension, ILD, obliterative bronchiolitis, or lymphocytic interstitial pneumonitis may also develop in patients with other CTDs including mixed connective tissue disease (MCTD), polymyositis/dermatomyositis (PM/DM), systemic lupus erythematosus (SLE), Sjögren syndrome, anti-synthetase syndrome, or rheumatoid arthritis (RA). Despite appropriate immunosuppressive management, pulmonary disease progression resulting in respiratory failure will occur in 9–12 % of patients leading to lung transplant consideration to improve patient prognosis [30–32]. Given the significant morbidity and mortality associated with lung transplantation, careful patient selection is crucial to optimize outcome [2]. A summary of potential selection criteria is presented in Table 13.1.

General Selection Criteria

Candidates for lung transplantation should have end-stage pulmonary disease that is nonresponsive to maximal medical management, have no other serious major organ system dysfunction or active systemic disease, have no active extrapulmonary infection, have the ability to ambulate and participate in pulmonary rehabilitation, have strong social support systems, have no evidence of malignancy for at least 2–5 years, have no substance addiction (including tobacco use) for at least 6 months, and have no untreatable psychiatric condition that would compromise compliance or the ability to "cope" with high-stress situations [2]. These criteria are usually designated as "absolute" contraindications, whereas several "relative" contraindications are transplant center dependent (Table 13.1).

Older recipients have a significantly worse survival [3]. The most recent update by the Pulmonary Scientific Council of the ISHLT suggests a potential upper limit for recipient age of 65 years; however, the number of recipients at or over this age limit in the United States has increased to 19 % in 2008, likely a reflection of the increasing number of recipients with fibrotic lung disease [2, 21]. A body mass index (BMI) of <17 or >30 kg/m^2 has been associated with greater 90-day mortality [33, 34]. Kanasky et al. described a mortality rate three times higher in lung recipients with a BMI >30 kg/m^2 [35]. Therefore, these criteria may be considered contraindications to transplantation. Severe osteoporosis should also be considered prior to transplant listing as it is common in patients with end-stage lung disease [36]. Accelerated bone loss as well as atraumatic fractures are associated with lung transplantation [37, 38] which may lead to long-term complications. Mechanical ventilation; prolonged extracorporeal life support; colonization with antibiotic resistant bacteria, fungi, or atypical mycobacteria; and other medical conditions including previous coronary artery bypass grafting or diabetes mellitus are additional relative contraindications for lung transplant listing [2]. Severe gastroesophageal reflux (GER) or esophageal dysmotility is also a relative contraindication to the transplant procedure and is not uncommon in patients with CTD; however, aggressive medical management or surgical correction before or after the transplant procedure has been utilized to promote good medium-term outcomes [39, 40].

While these guidelines apply to all patients considered for lung transplant referral, disease-specific criteria exist for patients with IPF and IPAH [2] (Table 13.1). Since definitive criteria for lung transplant referral has not been published for patients with CTD, IPF and IPAH criteria are extrapolated to this patient group.

Table 13.1 General and disease-specific guidelines for lung transplant referral

Guidelines for lung transplant referral	
General selection criteria	Disease-specific considerations
• **Indications**	• **Fibrotic lung disease**
– Respiratory failure refractory to maximal medical treatment	– UIP histopathology
• Absolute contraindications	– Honeycombing on HRCT
– Inability to comply with complex medical regimen	– FVC <70 % or DLCO <40 %
– Ongoing substance addiction (within 6 months) including tobacco or prescription drugs	– 15 % decrease in DLCO over 6 months
– Malignancy within 2–5 years (other than squamous and basal skin tumors or BAC)	– 10 % or greater decrease in FVC over 6 months
– Untreatable, severe organ dysfunction (e.g., kidney, liver, heart)	– Decrease in pulse oximetry below 88 % over 6-MWT
– HIV or chronic, active hepatitis B or C	– PAH or cor pulmonale in addition to ILD
– Abnormal thoracic anatomy (as determined by transplant surgeon)	– Hospitalization for respiratory failure
– Untreatable psychiatric disease	• **Pulmonary arterial hypertension**
– Bed bound or profound debility	– Any SSc-associated PAH
– Absent psychosocial support system	– NYHA class III or IV functional class despite therapy
• **Relative contraindications**	– CI <2 L/min/m²
– Severe esophageal/stomach dysmotility or GER	– Right atrial pressure >15 mmHg
– Age >65	– Rapidly progressive disease
– Poor functional status	– Low (<350 m) or worsening 6-MWT
– Severe coronary artery disease	– Signs of RV failure
– Severe osteoporosis	– ILD in addition to PAH
– Body mass index >30 or <17	• **Connective tissue disease relative contraindications**
– Colonization with resistant infectious organisms	– Active extrapulmonary CTD not thought to respond to typical posttransplant immunosuppression
– Steroid dose >20 mg of prednisone or equivalent	– SSc severe skin disease of the thorax
– Critical or unstable condition (including mechanical ventilation or ECLS)	– Digital ulceration or necrosis

BAC bronchioloalveolar carcinoma, *HIV* human immunodeficiency virus, *CTD* connective tissue disease, *SSc* systemic sclerosis, *GER* gastroesophageal reflux, *ECLS* extracorporeal life support, *UIP* usual interstitial pneumonia, *SSc* systemic sclerosis, *ILD* interstitial lung disease, *DLCO* diffusion capacity for carbon monoxide (CO), *FVC* forced vital capacity, *6-MWT* 6 min walk test, *PAH* pulmonary arterial hypertension, *NYHA* New York Heart Association, *CI* cardiac index, *RV* right ventricle, *FEV1* forced expiratory volume within 1 s, *HRCT* high-resolution computed tomography. Data from references [2, 87]

CTD-Specific Referral Considerations

Although any CTD can disable the pulmonary system to the point of needing a lung transplant, SSc is the most common indication for CTD-related lung transplantation in the United States, accounting for 75 % of all CTD procedures between January 1, 2006, and August 31, 2012 (Table 13.2) [41].

Pulmonary arterial hypertension is the principal indication for lung transplantation in CTD (50 %) [41]. Despite the advent of vasoactive agents targeting the pulmonary vessels, PAH related to CTD has a worse prognosis than IPAH with a 5-year survival of 42 % in the modern treatment era [42, 43]. This poor outcome may be driven by the predominance of SSc-related PAH in combined studies [42]. When considered

Table 13.2 Connective tissue disease-related lung transplantation in the United States 2006–2012

Diagnosis	Number	Percentage
SSc-PAH	109	50
SSc-ILD	55	25
MCTD	28	13
Sjögren	8	4
RA	16	7
Total	216	100

Number of connective tissue disease-related lung transplants performed in the United States between 1/1/2006 and 8/31/2012 as reported to the Organ Procurement Transplantation Network (OPTN). Based on OPTN [41] data as of November 30th, 2012. Data subject to change based on future data submission or correction

SSc-PAH systemic sclerosis pulmonary arterial hypertension, *SSc-ILD* systemic sclerosis-related interstitial lung disease, *MCTD* mixed connective tissue disease, *RA* rheumatoid arthritis

separately, the survival rates for patients with PAH due to SLE, RA, PM/DM, or MCTD trended toward better survival when compared to patients with SSc-related PAH (3-year survival 63–100 % vs. 47 % for SSc) [44]. Additional studies specifically evaluating PAH in SSc support a poor prognosis for these patients implicating a 3-year survival of 49–71 % [42–48] compared to 71–88 % in patients with IPAH [43, 45]. Pulmonary artery hypertension, when it coexists with ILD in SSc, has a particularly bleak prognosis, with a 3-year survival of only 28–47 % [44, 47, 48].

Patients with CTD disease-related PAH should be referred for transplant evaluation when there is persistence of New York Heart Association Functional Class III or IV symptoms despite adequate medical management, persistence of overt right heart failure (cardiac index <2.0 L/min/m², right atrial pressure >15 mmHg), a low or declining 6 min walk distance (<350 m), or concomitant ILD [2, 49–51] (Table 13.1).

In general, CTD-associated ILD is felt to have a more favorable prognosis than IPF [52, 53] though this is not a universal finding [54, 55]. Recent studies have questioned if this postulate applies to all CTDs and pathologic subtypes, specifically UIP histopathology associated with rheumatoid arthritis (RA) [56]. A retrospective analysis of RA patients with definite UIP diag-

nosed by high-resolution computed tomography (HRCT) [56] or on lung biopsy [57] had survival rates comparable to IPF. Using the abysmal prognosis of IPF as a comparator, early referral of RA patients for transplantation when UIP is diagnosed histopathologically or by HRCT should be considered. This prognosis based on the UIP subset may not extend to other CTD subtypes [52, 58].

SSc-related ILD is relatively recalcitrant to treatment, with a recent randomized trial of cyclophosphamide showing a significant but minimal effect on the rate of decline in pulmonary mechanics without having a significant impact on gas exchange [59]. Disease severity at presentation and a decline in carbon monoxide diffusing capacity (DLCO) have a substantial impact on outcome [58]. However, not all SSc patients with ILD will progress at the same rate, so serial pulmonary function testing for those with mild to moderate disease is recommended [60, 61].

Extrapolating from data supporting poor outcomes in patients with IPF as well as the CTD prognostic information discussed previously, CTD patients with a FVC <70 % and DLCO <40 % at presentation, desaturation below 88 % during 6 min walk testing, a decline in FVC of >10 % or DLCO >15 % over a 6-month period, suspected UIP histopathology, and concomitant pulmonary hypertension, should be considered for early lung transplant referral [2, 62, 63] (Table 13.1).

Other Considerations for Lung Transplantation in CTD

Medications

Multiple pharmacologic agents are administered after transplantation to prevent allograft rejection and provide prophylaxis against opportunistic infections. Coincidentally, some posttransplant immunosuppressive medications are also those used to treat CTD. Typical posttransplant maintenance immunosuppression includes a calcineurin inhibitor (tacrolimus or cyclosporine A), an antimetabolite (mycophenolate mofetil or azathioprine), and low- to moderate-dose corticosteroids. Transplant candidacy is questioned when extrapulmonary manifestations of CTD are active or the systemic disease is inadequately controlled. In addition, the use of tumor necrosis factor α blockers (TNF blockers) may impede postoperative healing or further increase the risk of infectious complications. Antimetabolites such as methotrexate, cyclophosphamide, hydroxychloroquine, or leflunomide can compound bone marrow suppression or liver toxicity when added to an already complex medication regimen. Renal dysfunction, generally attributed to calcineurin inhibitors, is particularly common after transplant [3]. As such, the regular use of nonsteroidal anti-inflammatory drugs (NSAIDS) is prohibited for pain control after the procedure [64, 65].

The exclusion of patients on the basis of the need for TNF blockers is not substantiated, but higher corticosteroid doses pre-transplant are associated with worse outcomes [3, 66]. Takagishi and colleagues reported a single-center experience of posttransplant CTD exacerbations. In their study, 2 of 22 CTD patients required supplementary immunosuppression to maintain disease control prior to transplant that was not included in the standard posttransplant regimen; both were treated with etanercept, while one required leflunomide [67]. Systemic CTD symptoms were successfully controlled after surgery using transplant immunosuppression alone except for the uncomplicated readministration of etanercept for a CTD flare in one individual [67]. The authors concluded that CTD extrapulmonary disease flares are rare after transplantation in patients with good systemic symptom control prior to the procedure.

Gastrointestinal Disease

The common involvement of esophageal smooth muscle by CTD, especially in patients with SSc or DM/PM, leads to significantly impaired peristalsis and GER. Traditionally, this has been a contraindication to lung transplantation due to the dangers of gastric content aspiration into the lung allograft and the association of GER with the development of bronchiolitis obliterans or BOS, which is the primary cause of late mortality in lung transplant recipients [68, 69]. The correlation of the presence of pepsin [70] and bile acids [71, 72] in the distal airways of lung transplant recipients with acute and chronic allograft rejection, respectively, adds to the evidence that aspiration contributes to allograft injury. Single-center studies evaluating the performance of surgical fundoplication in lung transplant recipients with GER and presumed BOS show improvement in lung function [73–75] and time free of BOS following the procedure [73]. Interestingly, the association between GER and non-transplant pulmonary deterioration is increasing [74, 76]. Prospective studies of anti-reflux surgery to prevent chronic allograft dysfunction in lung transplant recipients (RESULT) and disease progression in patients with IPF are ongoing (WRAP-IPF) [77, 78].

Patients with SSc are particularly apt to develop GER. Saravino et al. [79] found that 83 % of SSc patients with pulmonary fibrosis had evidence of increased distal acid exposure, while 55 % had ineffective esophageal motility and 22 % had abnormally low esophageal pressures [79] confirming the findings of others [80, 81]. Foregut histopathologic evaluation of the esophagus in autopsy studies of patients with SSc found that 94 % had evidence of distal smooth muscle atrophy [82], which is the likely mechanism for impaired peristalsis. Slow gastric transit, though less common than esophageal disease, frequently complicates SSc and likely worsens esophageal reflux by prolonging contact of the lower esophageal sphincter with gastric contents [83, 84]. Moreover, lung transplantation can worsen GER [85] or delay gastric transit due to surgical injury of the vagus nerve [72, 86].

Testing for esophageal and gastric pathology is suggested in patients at high risk prior to lung transplant listing [40, 87]. Saggar and colleagues described lung transplant outcomes of patients with SSc at a single center [87]. Preoperative testing included a symptom review for GER, dual pH probe monitoring, a barium esophagram, quantitative gastric emptying study, esophageal manometry, and/or upper endoscopy [87]. Patients with more than moderate GER, esophageal stricture or ulcer while on medical therapy, esophageal aperistalsis, achalasia, or abnormal gastric emptying (<25 % clearance at 90 min) were not eligible for transplantation [87]. Fourteen SSc transplant recipients who received DLT [87] were found to develop a higher rate of acute rejection than matched IPF controls (HR 2.91; $p = 0.007$). The authors hypothesized that the finding was due to the proclivity toward GER [87]. Despite these results, a recent report by Sottile et al. described good outcomes in SSc transplant recipients with GER or impaired esophageal motility [40]. Twenty three patients with SSc were compared to 46 non-CTD ILD controls [40]. GER was diagnosed based on pH probe and manometry monitoring in 52 % of the 14 patients tested in the SSc group and 41 % of the 25 patients tested in the non-CTD group, indicating a high rate of GER in all patients with ILD. A Nissen fundoplication procedure was performed in six SSc and five non-CTD patients posttransplant, some due to the development of overt aspiration in the SSc group [40]. An aggressive, multidisciplinary approach to management of the GER was utilized after transplantation to minimize the effects on the allograft. Outcomes were similar between the SSc and IPF control groups demonstrating that successful lung transplantation can be performed in SSc patients with significant esophageal disease [40].

In summary, all CTD disease patients referred for lung transplantation should be evaluated for esophageal dysfunction, and if present, candidacy for the procedure is dependent on the individual center's comfort in managing these complex patients. Our center has successfully transplanted several SSc patients with significant esophageal dysmotility utilizing a post-pyloric feeding tube after transplantation until a full (Nissen) or partial surgical wrap (Toupet) could be performed [88].

Renal, Cardiac, and Musculoskeletal Considerations

Renal dysfunction is common after transplantation with the majority (56 %) of lung transplant recipients developing impaired renal function 5 years after the procedure, some of whom require dialysis or renal transplantation [3]. The majority of renal disease stems from the use of calcineurin inhibitors, and in most instances, these medications cannot be substituted with other immunosuppressive agents. Therefore, significant kidney disease, defined as a creatinine clearance <50 mg/mL/min, is an absolute contraindication for isolated pulmonary transplantation [2]. Of particular concern are CTD patients who are at risk of acute and chronic kidney complications, such as patients with SLE or SSc. Scleroderma renal crisis (SRC), manifested by hypertension, decreased renal function, and microangiopathic hemolytic anemia can be lethal in SSc [89]. Outcomes for SRC have improved with the implementation of angiotensin-converting enzyme inhibitors (ACEi) [30], but 5-year survival after the development of SRC is still poor at 41 % [90]. Corticosteroids, an essential part of the posttransplant immunosuppressive cocktail, have been associated with the development of SRC [91–93] especially when used at a dose of >15 mg/day of prednisone or equivalent [92]. Only one case of SRC developing after lung transplantation has been described [87, 94], but it has been seen in other solid organ transplants [95]. The routine use of an ACEi in SSc patients to prevent SRC after solid organ transplantation has been suggested [87].

Patients with pulmonary hypertension and/or severe right and left ventricular dysfunction may need to be considered for a heart-lung transplant. However, the degree of isolated right ventricular dysfunction tolerated in CTD patients with PH for isolated lung transplant is institution dependent [96]. A screening echocardiogram is also a useful test for pericardial disease, which may be seen in the CTD patients that present for transplant consideration [97]. Significant, untreatable valve, conduction system, or coronary artery pathology related or unrelated to CTD must raise the consideration for heart-lung rather than lung transplantation [2].

Substantial thoracic anatomy irregularities such as severe scoliosis or kyphosis may not allow for appropriate allograft placement and function, so candidacy is at the discretion of the thoracic surgeon [2]. Myositis or respiratory muscle weakness in those at risk should be evaluated to prevent inadequate bellows function posttransplant.

SSc patients should not have skin disease of the thorax severe enough to complicate surgery or cause restrictive physiology [87]. Patients with Raynaud's phenomenon should be free of digital ulceration or necrosis as it will be a nidus for infection with immunosuppression [87].

Outcomes of Connective Tissue Disease Patients After Lung Transplant

Outcome data for CTD posttransplant has been confined to small case series and case reports. Owing to the critical mass of patients needed to publish a case series, the preponderance of data is derived from lung transplantation in SSc. The SSc literature was recently collected and reviewed by Khan [94]. None of the reviewed studies had a significant, durable difference in survival of SSc patients when compared to the various comparators in the individual studies [40, 87, 94, 98–100].

The largest of the case series was compiled by Massad and coworkers comparing 47 SSc patients to over 10,000 non-SSc lung transplant recipients utilizing the United Network for Organ Sharing (UNOS) registry database. They determined that there was no statistically significant difference in the development of BOS or 3-year survival (46 % for SSc vs. 58 % for non-SSc) between groups [98].

Schachna and colleagues compared the pre-LAS era outcomes of 29 SSc lung transplant recipients at two institutions to patients with similar disease physiology, either IPF (n=70) or IPAH (n=38) [99]. SSc patients had worse posttransplant survival at 6 months; however, the survival curves converged at 2 years to roughly 64 % for all groups indicating equivalent intermediate-term survival [99].

More recently, as discussed earlier, Saggar et al. reported on the evaluation and outcome of 14 SSc DLT recipients who were deemed candidates after exclusion of significant GER [87]. Survival and freedom from BOS for the SSc group at a median of 632 days post-procedure were excellent at 79 % and 63 %, respectively, not statistically different from a matched IPF

cohort [87]. Sottile's series of 23 SSc transplant recipients also reported favorable survival and freedom from BOS at 3 and 5 years after the procedure; however, patients with significant foregut pathology were included in this group [40].

The Toronto Lung Transplant group reported their 14-year experience on pulmonary arterial hypertension referrals [101]. While wait list mortality was worse for the CTD-PAH group compared to the remaining PAH patients (34 % vs. 11 %), 10-year survival for 16 CTD-associated PAH lung transplant recipients was exceptional at 69 %, although only two patients were at risk at year 10 [101].

Takagishi is one of the few authors to describe non-SSc CTD posttransplant recipients [67]. Using data from the Organ Procurement and Transplantation Network (OPTN) between 1991 and 2009, he found 3-year survival rates posttransplant for SLE, MCTD, Sjögren's disease, RA, and PM/DM to be 66 %, 45 %, 57 %, 58 %, and 47 %, respectively [67]. When combined, all CTD transplant patients had similar survival to IPF patients (RR at 5 years 1.04, 95 % confidence interval (CI) 0.94–1.15) but worse survival than COPD patients (RR at 5 years 1.22, 95 % CI 1.11–1.35) [67].

Analysis of all lung transplants reported to the ISHLT registry between 1999 and 2011 found that CTD was an independent risk for death in the first posttransplant year with an uncorrected relative risk (RR) of 1.36 (1.04–1.76 95 % CI; N=297) when compared to patients with ILD [3]. This risk was no longer statistically significant 5 years after the procedure [102].

Based on this review of the available case series as well as ISHLT and UNOS/OPTN data, appropriately selected CTD lung transplant recipients have an incremental increased risk of short-term mortality but reasonable intermediate-term survival when compared to similar controls [40, 67, 87, 101].

Conclusion

Lung transplantation is a viable treatment modality for carefully selected CTD patients with impending respiratory failure. While short-term mortality may be increased, intermediate-term outcome is comparable to patients with similar pathophysiology. Special attention to pre-transplant medication regimens, evaluation and treatment of esophageal pathology, and disease-specific extrapulmonary manifestations are a requisite for successful lung transplant in CTD patients. Recent data also supports the successful transplantation of CTD recipients with significant gastroesophageal dysmotility, which may increase the number of patients receiving this surgical option in the near future. We suggest referral of any potential candidate (Table 13.1) in order to provide what may be the only effective treatment of their progressive, refractory lung disease.

References

1. Levine SM, Anzueto A, Peters JI, Calhoon JH, Jenkinson SG, Bryan CL. SIngle lung transplantation in patients with systemic disease. Chest. 1994; 105(3):837–41.
2. Orens JB, Estenne M, Arcasoy S, Conte JV, Corris P, Egan JJ, et al. International guidelines for the selection of lung transplant candidates: 2006 update—a consensus report from the Pulmonary Scientific Council of the International Society for Heart and Lung Transplantation. J Heart Lung Transplant. 2006;25(7):745–55.
3. Yusen RD, Christie JD, Edwards LB, Kucheryavaya AY, Benden C, Dipchand AI, et al. The Registry of the International Society for Heart and Lung Transplantation: thirtieth adult lung and heart-lung transplant report—2013; focus theme: age. J Heart Lung Transplant. 2013;32(10):965–78.
4. Dunitz J, Hertz M. Surgical therapy for COPD: lung transplantation. Semin Respir Crit Care Med. 1999; 20(4):365–73.
5. Wildevuur C, Benfield J. A review of 23 human lung transplantation by 20 surgeons. Ann Thorac Surg. 1970;9:489–515.
6. Veith F, Koerner S. Problems in the management of lung transplant recipients. Vas Surg. 1974;8: 273–82.
7. Veith F, Koerner S, Siegelman S, et al. Single lung transplantation in experimental and human emphysema. Ann Surg. 1973;178:463–76.
8. Reitz B, Wallwork J, Hunt S, et al. Heart-lung transplantation: successful therapy for patients with pulmonary vascular disease. N Engl J Med. 1982;306: 557–64.
9. Colvin-Adams M, Valapour M, Hertz M, Heubner B, Paulson K, Dhungel V, et al. Lung and heart alloca-

tion in the United States. Am J Transplant. 2012; 12(12):3213–34.
10. Group TLT. Unilateral lung transplantation for pulmonary fibrosis. N Engl J Med. 1986;314:1140–5.
11. Force SD, Kilgo P, Neujahr DC, Pelaez A, Pickens A, Fernandez FG, et al. Bilateral lung transplantation offers better long-term survival, compared with single-lung transplantation, for younger patients with idiopathic pulmonary fibrosis. Ann Thorac Surg. 2011;91(1):244–9.
12. Neurohr C, Huppmann P, Thum D, Leuschner W, von Wulffen W, Meis T, et al. Potential functional and survival benefit of double over single lung transplantation for selected patients with idiopathic pulmonary fibrosis. Transpl Int. 2010;23(9):887–96.
13. Thabut G, Christie J, Ravaud P, Castier Y, Dauriat G, Jebrak G, et al. Survival after bilateral versus single-lung transplantation for idiopathic pulmonary fibrosis. Ann Intern Med. 2009;151(11):767–74.
14. Weiss ES, Allen JG, Merlo CA, Conte JV, Shah AS. Survival after single versus bilateral lung transplantation for high-risk patients with pulmonary fibrosis. Ann Thorac Surg. 2009;88(5):1616–26.
15. Force S, Choong C, Meyers B. Lung transplantation for emphysema. Chest Surg Clin N Am. 2003; 13(4):651–67.
16. Kotloff RM, Thabut G. Lung transplantation. Am J Respir Crit Care Med. 2011;184(2):159–71.
17. Meyers B, Patterson G. Chronic obstructive pulmonary disease. 10: bullectomy, lung volume reduction surgery, and transplantation for patients with chronic obstructive pulmonary disease. Thorax. 2003;58: 634–8.
18. Keating D, Levvey B, Kotsimbos T, Whitford H, Westall G, Williams T, et al. Lung transplantation in pulmonary fibrosis: challenging early outcomes counterbalanced by surprisingly good outcomes beyond 15 years. Transplant Proc. 2009;41(1): 289–91.
19. Meyer DM, Edwards LB, Torres F, Jessen ME, Novick RJ. Impact of recipient age and procedure type on survival after lung transplantation for pulmonary fibrosis. Ann Thorac Surg. 2005;79(3): 950–7; discussion 7–8.
20. Mason DP, Brizzio ME, Alster JM, McNeill AM, Murthy SC, Budev MM, et al. Lung transplantation for idiopathic pulmonary fibrosis. Ann Thorac Surg. 2007;84(4):1121–8.
21. Yusen RD, Shearon TH, Qian Y, Kotloff R, Barr ML, Sweet S, et al. Lung transplantation in the United States, 1999–2008. Am J Transplant. 2010;10(4p2): 1047–68.
22. Studer S, Levy R, McNeil K, Orens J. Lung transplant outcomes; a review of survival, graft function, physiology, health-related quality of life and cost-effectiveness. Eur Respir J. 2004;24:674–85.
23. Gerbase MW, Spiliopoulos A, Rochat T, Archinard M, Nicod LP. Health-related quality of life following single or bilateral lung transplantation: a 7-year

comparison to functional outcome. Chest. 2005; 128(3):1371–8.

24. Snyder LD, Palmer SM. Quality, quantity, or both?: life after lung transplantation. Chest. 2005;128(3): 1086–7.

25. Rodrigue JR, Baz MA, Kanasky JWF, MacNaughton KL. Does lung transplantation improve health-related quality of life? The University of Florida Experience. J Heart Lung Transplant. 2005; 24(6):755–63.

26. Rutherford RM, Fisher AJ, Hilton C, Forty J, Hasan A, Gould FK, et al. Functional status and quality of life in patients surviving 10 years after lung transplantation. Am J Transplant. 2005;5(5):1099–104.

27. Egan TM, Murray S, Bustami RT, Shearon TH, McCullough KP, Edwards LB, et al. Development of the new lung allocation system in the United States. Am J Transplant. 2006;6(5 Pt 2):1212–27.

28. Chan KM. Idiopathic pulmonary arterial hypertension and equity of donor lung allocation in the era of the lung allocation score: are we there yet? Am J Respir Crit Care Med. 2009;180(5):385–7.

29. UNOS/OPTN. Summary of actions taken at OPTN/ UNOS Board of Directors Meeting (November 12-13, 2012) and OPTN/UNOS Executive Committee Meetings (August 28, 2012; October 19, 2012; and November 12, 2012). 2012. p. 17.

30. Steen VD, Medsger TA. Changes in causes of death in systemic sclerosis, 1972–2002. Ann Rheum Dis. 2007;66(7):940–4.

31. Antin-Ozerkis D, Rubinowitz A, Evans J, Homer RJ, Matthay RA. Interstitial lung disease in the connective tissue diseases. Clin Chest Med. 2012;33(1): 123–49.

32. Mouthon L, Bérezné A, Guillevin L, Valeyre D. Therapeutic options for systemic sclerosis related interstitial lung diseases. Respir Med. 2010;104 Suppl 1:S59–69.

33. Madill J, Gutierrez C, Grossman J, Allard J, Chan C, Hutcheon M, et al. Nutritional assessment of the lung transplant patient: body mass index as a predictor of 90-day mortality following transplantation. J Heart Lung Transplant. 2001;20:288–96.

34. Culver DA, Mazzone PJ, Khandwala F, Blazey HC, DeCamp MM, Chapman JT. Discordant utility of ideal body weight and body mass index as predictors of mortality in lung transplant recipients. J Heart Lung Transplant. 2005;24(2):137–44.

35. Kanasky Jr WF, Anton SD, Rodrigue JR, Perri MG, Szwed T, Baz MA. Impact of body weight on long-term survival after lung transplantation. Chest. 2002; 121(2):401–6.

36. Tschopp O, Boehler A, Speich R, Weder W, Seifert B, Russi EW, et al. Osteoporosis before lung transplantation: association with low body mass index, but not with underlying disease. Am J Transplant. 2002;2(2):167–72.

37. Shane E, Papadopoulos A, Staron RB, Addesso V, Donovan D, McGregor C, et al. Bone loss and fracture after lung transplantation. Transplantation. 1999;68(2):220–7.

38. Spira A, Gutierrez C, Chaparro C, Hutcheon MA, Chan CKN. Osteoporosis and lung transplantation: a prospective study. Chest. 2000;117(2):476–81.

39. Gasper WJ, Sweet MP, Golden JA, Hoopes C, Leard LE, Kleinhenz ME, et al. Lung transplantation in patients with connective tissue disorders and esophageal dysmotility. Dis Esophagus. 2008;21(7):650–5.

40. Sottile PD, Iturbe D, Katsumoto TR, Connolly MK, Collard HR, Leard LA, et al. Outcomes in systemic sclerosis-related lung disease after lung transplantation. Transplantation. 2013;95(7):975–80.

41. (OPTN) OPTN. Based on Organ Procurement and Transplantation Network (OPTN) data as of November 30th, 2012. Transplants reported between 1/1/2006-8/31/2012. Data subject to change based on future data submission or correction. 2013.

42. Ruiz-Cano MJ, Escribano P, Alonso R, Delgado J, Carreira P, Velazquez T, et al. Comparison of baseline characteristics and survival between patients with idiopathic and connective tissue disease–related pulmonary arterial hypertension. J Heart Lung Transplant. 2009;28(6):621–7.

43. Rubenfire M, Huffman MD, Krishnan S, Seibold JR, Schiopu E, McLaughlin VV. Survival in systemic sclerosis with pulmonary arterial hypertension has not improved in the modern era. Chest. 2013; 144(4):1282–90.

44. Condliffe R, Kiely DG, Peacock AJ, Corris PA, Gibbs JS, Vrapi F, et al. Connective tissue disease-associated pulmonary arterial hypertension in the modern treatment era. Am J Respir Crit Care Med. 2009;179(2):151–7.

45. Fisher MR, Mathai SC, Champion HC, Girgis RE, Housten-Harris T, Hummers L, et al. Clinical differences between idiopathic and scleroderma-related pulmonary hypertension. Arthritis Rheum. 2006; 54(9):3043–50.

46. Campo A, Mathai SC, Le Pavec J, Zaiman AL, Hummers LK, Boyce D, et al. Hemodynamic predictors of survival in scleroderma-related pulmonary arterial hypertension. Am J Respir Crit Care Med. 2010;182(2):252–60.

47. Mathai SC, Hummers LK, Champion HC, Wigley FM, Zaiman A, Hassoun PM, et al. Survival in pulmonary hypertension associated with the scleroderma spectrum of diseases: impact of interstitial lung disease. Arthritis Rheum. 2009;60(2):569–77.

48. Launay D, Humbert M, Berezne A, Cottin V, Allanore Y, Couderc LJ, et al. Clinical characteristics and survival in systemic sclerosis-related pulmonary hypertension associated with interstitial lung disease. Chest. 2011;140(4):1016–24.

49. D'Alonzo GE, Barst RJ, Ayres SM, Bergofsky EH, Brundage BH, Detre KM, et al. Survival in patients with primary pulmonary hypertension. Results from a national prospective registry. Ann Intern Med. 1991;115(5):343–9.

50. McLaughlin VV, Shillington A, Rich S. Survival in primary pulmonary hypertension: the impact of epoprostenol therapy. Circulation. 2002;106(12): 1477–82.

51. Sitbon O, Humbert M, Nunes H, Parent F, Garcia G, Herve P, et al. Long-term intravenous epoprostenol infusion in primary pulmonary hypertension: prognostic factors and survival. J Am Coll Cardiol. 2002;40(4):780–8.

52. Park JH, Kim DS, Park IN, Jang SJ, Kitaichi M, Nicholson AG, et al. Prognosis of fibrotic interstitial pneumonia: idiopathic versus collagen vascular disease-related subtypes. Am J Respir Crit Care Med. 2007;175(7):705–11.

53. Song JW, Do K-H, Kim M-Y, Jang SJ, Colby TV, Kim DS. Pathologic and radiologic differences between idiopathic and collagen vascular disease-related usual interstitial pneumonia. Chest. 2009; 136(1):23–30.

54. Hubbard R, Venn A. The impact of coexisting connective tissue disease on survival in patients with fibrosing alveolitis. Rheumatology (Oxford). 2002; 41(6):676–9.

55. Kocheril SV, Appleton BE, Somers EC, Kazerooni EA, Flaherty KR, Martinez FJ, et al. Comparison of disease progression and mortality of connective tissue disease-related interstitial lung disease and idiopathic interstitial pneumonia. Arthritis Rheum. 2005;53(4):549–57.

56. Kim EJ, Elicker BM, Maldonado F, Webb WR, Ryu JH, Van Uden JH, et al. Usual interstitial pneumonia in rheumatoid arthritis-associated interstitial lung disease. Eur Respir J. 2010;35(6):1322–8.

57. Solomon JJ, Ryu JH, Tazelaar HD, Myers JL, Tuder R, Cool CD, et al. Fibrosing interstitial pneumonia predicts survival in patients with rheumatoid arthritis-associated interstitial lung disease (RA-ILD). Respir Med. 2013;107(8):1247–52.

58. Bouros D, Wells AU, Nicholson AG, Colby TV, Polychronopoulos V, Pantelidis P, et al. Histopathologic subsets of fibrosing alveolitis in patients with systemic sclerosis and their relationship to outcome. Am J Respir Crit Care Med. 2002;165(12):1581–6.

59. Tashkin DP, Elashoff R, Clements PJ, Goldin J, Roth MD, Furst DE, et al. Cyclophosphamide versus placebo in scleroderma lung disease. N Engl J Med. 2006;354(25):2655–66.

60. Steen VD, Conte C, Owens GR, Medsger Jr TA. Severe restrictive lung disease in systemic sclerosis. Arthritis Rheum. 1994;37(9):1283–9.

61. Plastiras SC, Karadimitrakis SP, Ziakas PD, Vlachoyiannopoulos PG, Moutsopoulos HM, Tzelepis GE. Scleroderma lung: Initial forced vital capacity as predictor of pulmonary function decline. Arthritis Care Res. 2006;55(4):598–602.

62. Lama VN, Flaherty KR, Toews GB, Colby TV, Travis WD, Long Q, et al. Prognostic value of desaturation during a 6-minute walk test in idiopathic interstitial pneumonia. Am J Respir Crit Care Med. 2003;168(9):1084–90.

63. Flaherty KR, Andrei A-C, Murray S, Fraley C, Colby TV, Travis WD, et al. Idiopathic pulmonary fibrosis: prognostic value of changes in physiology and six-minute-walk test. Am J Respir Crit Care Med. 2006;174(7):803–9.

64. Sheiner PA, Mor E, Chodoff L, Glabman S, Emre S, Schwartz ME, et al. Acute renal failure associated with the use of ibuprofen in two liver transplant recipients on FK506. Transplantation. 1994;57(7): 1132–3.

65. Soubhia RM, Mendes GE, Mendonca FZ, Baptista MA, Cipullo JP, Burdmann EA. Tacrolimus and non-steroidal anti-inflammatory drugs: an association to be avoided. Am J Nephrol. 2005;25(4):327–34.

66. McAnally KJ, Valentine VG, LaPlace SG, McFadden PM, Seoane L, Taylor DE. Effect of pre-transplantation prednisone on survival after lung transplantation. J Heart Lung Transplant. 2006;25(1): 67–74.

67. Takagishi T, Ostrowski R, Alex C, Rychlik K, Pelletiere K, Tehrani R. Survival and extrapulmonary course of connective tissue disease after lung transplantation. J Clin Rheumatol. 2012;18(6):283–9.

68. Palmer SM, Miralles AP, Howell DN, Brazer SR, Tapson VF, Davis RD. Gastroesophageal reflux as a reversible cause of allograft dysfunction after lung transplantation. Chest. 2000;118(4):1214–7.

69. Rinaldi M, Martinelli L, Volpato G, Pederzolli C, Silvestri M, Pederzolli N, et al. Gastro-esophageal reflux as cause of obliterative bronchiolitis: a case report. Transplant Proc. 1995;27(3):2006–7.

70. Stovold R, Forrest IA, Corris PA, Murphy DM, Smith JA, Decalmer S, et al. Pepsin, a biomarker of gastric aspiration in lung allografts: a putative association with rejection. Am J Respir Crit Care Med. 2007;175(12):1298–303.

71. D'Ovidio F, Singer LG, Hadjiliadis D, Pierre A, Waddell TK, de Perrot M, et al. Prevalence of gastroesophageal reflux in End-stage lung disease candidates for lung transplant. Ann Thorac Surg. 2005;80(4):1254–60.

72. D'Ovidio F, Mura M, Ridsdale R, Takahashi H, Waddell TK, Hutcheon M, et al. The effect of reflux and bile acid aspiration on the lung allograft and its surfactant and innate immunity molecules SP-A and SP-D. Am J Transplant. 2006;6(8):1930–8.

73. Cantu 3rd E, Appel 3rd JZ, Hartwig MG, Woreta H, Green C, Messier R, et al. J. Maxwell Chamberlain Memorial Paper. Early fundoplication prevents chronic allograft dysfunction in patients with gastroesophageal reflux disease. Ann Thorac Surg. 2004;78(4):1142–51; discussion-51.

74. Hoppo T, Jarido V, Pennathur A, et al. Antireflux surgery preserves lung function in patients with gastroesophageal reflux disease and end-stage lung disease before and after lung transplantation. Arch Surg. 2011;146(9):1041–7.

75. Davis Jr RD, Lau CL, Eubanks S, Messier RH, Hadjiliadis D, Steele MP, et al. Improved lung allograft function after fundoplication in patients with gastroesophageal reflux disease undergoing lung transplantation. J Thorac Cardiovasc Surg. 2003;125(3):533–42.

76. Lee JS, Ryu JH, Elicker BM, Lydell CP, Jones KD, Wolters PJ, et al. Gastroesophageal reflux therapy is associated with longer survival in patients with idiopathic pulmonary fibrosis. Am J Respir Crit Care Med. 2011;184(12):1390–4.

77. ClinicalTrials.gov. Treatment of IPF with laparoscopic anti-reflux surgery (WRAP-IPF). NIH; 2013 [updated November 2013; cited 2013 11/3/2013]; NCT01982968]. http://www.clinical trials.gov/

78. ClinicalTrials.gov. RESULT (REflux Surgery in Lung Transplantation). NIH; 2013 [updated September 16, 2013; cited 2013 11/3/2013]. http://www.clinicaltrials.gov/

79. Savarino E, Bazzica M, Zentilin P, Pohl D, Parodi A, Cittadini G, et al. Gastroesophageal reflux and pulmonary fibrosis in scleroderma. Am J Respir Crit Care Med. 2009;179(5):408–13.

80. Bassotti G, Battaglia E, Debernardi V, Germani U, Quiriconi F, Dughera L, et al. Esophageal dysfunction in scleroderma: relationship with disease subsets. Arthritis Rheum. 1997;40(12): 2252–9.

81. Sweet MP, Patti MG, Hoopes C, Hays SR, Golden JA. Gastro-oesophageal reflux and aspiration in patients with advanced lung disease. Thorax. 2009;64(2):167–73.

82. Roberts CG, Hummers LK, Ravich WJ, Wigley FM, Hutchins GM. A case-control study of the pathology of oesophageal disease in systemic sclerosis (scleroderma). Gut. 2006;55(12):1697–703.

83. Savarino E, Mei F, Parodi A, Ghio M, Furnari M, Gentile A, et al. Gastrointestinal motility disorder assessment in systemic sclerosis. Rheumatology (Oxford). 2013;52(6):1095–100.

84. Marie I, Gourcerol G, Leroi AM, Menard JF, Levesque H, Ducrotte P. Delayed gastric emptying determined using the 13C-octanoic acid breath test in patients with systemic sclerosis. Arthritis Rheum. 2012;64(7):2346–55.

85. Young LR, Hadjiliadis D, Davis RD, Palmer SM. Lung transplantation exacerbates gastroesophageal reflux disease. Chest. 2003;124(5):1689–93.

86. Au J, Hawkins T, Venables C, Morritt G, Scott CD, Gascoigne AD, et al. Upper gastrointestinal dysmotility in heart-lung transplant recipients. Ann Thorac Surg. 1993;55(1):94–7.

87. Saggar R, Khanna D, Furst DE, Belperio JA, Park GS, Weigt SS, et al. Systemic sclerosis and bilateral lung transplantation: a single centre experience. Eur Respir J. 2010;36(4):893–900.

88. Qin M, Ding G, Yang H. A clinical comparison of laparoscopic nissen and toupet fundoplication for gastroesophageal reflux disease. J Laparoendosc Adv Surg Tech A. 2013;23(7):601–4.

89. Denton CP, Lapadula G, Mouthon L, Muller-Ladner U. Renal complications and scleroderma renal crisis. Rheumatology (Oxford). 2009;48 Suppl 3:iii32–5.

90. Penn H, Howie AJ, Kingdon EJ, Bunn CC, Stratton RJ, Black CM, et al. Scleroderma renal crisis: patient characteristics and long-term outcomes. QJM. 2007;100(8):485–94.

91. DeMarco PJ, Weisman MH, Seibold JR, Furst DE, Wong WK, Hurwitz EL, et al. Predictors and outcomes of scleroderma renal crisis: the high-dose versus low-dose D-penicillamine in early diffuse systemic sclerosis trial. Arthritis Rheum. 2002; 46(11):2983–9.

92. Steen VD, Medsger Jr TA. Case-control study of corticosteroids and other drugs that either precipitate or protect from the development of scleroderma renal crisis. Arthritis Rheum. 1998;41(9):1613–9.

93. Teixeira L, Mouthon L, Mahr A, Berezne A, Agard C, Mehrenberger M, et al. Mortality and risk factors of scleroderma renal crisis: a French retrospective study of 50 patients. Ann Rheum Dis. 2008;67(1):110–6.

94. Khan IY, Singer LG, de Perrot M, Granton JT, Keshavjee S, Chau C, et al. Survival after lung transplantation in systemic sclerosis. A systematic review. Respir Med. 2013;107(12):2081–7.

95. Pham PT, Pham PC, Danovitch GM, Gritsch HA, Singer J, Wallace WD, et al. Predictors and risk factors for recurrent scleroderma renal crisis in the kidney allograft: case report and review of the literature. Am J Transplant. 2005;5(10):2565–9.

96. De Cruz S, Ross D. Lung transplantation in patients with scleroderma. Curr Opin Rheumatol. 2013; 25(6):714–8.

97. Imazio M. Pericardial involvement in systemic inflammatory diseases. Heart. 2011;97(22):1882–92.

98. Massad MG, Powell CR, Kpodonu J, Tshibaka C, Hanhan Z, Snow NJ, et al. Outcomes of lung transplantation in patients with scleroderma. World J Surg. 2005;29(11):1510–5.

99. Schachna L, Medsger TA, Dauber JH, Wigley FM, Braunstein NA, White B, et al. Lung transplantation in scleroderma compared with idiopathic pulmonary fibrosis and idiopathic pulmonary arterial hypertension. Arthritis Rheum. 2006;54(12):3954–61.

100. Shitrit D, Amital A, Peled N, Raviv Y, Medalion B, Saute M, et al. Lung transplantation in patients with scleroderma: case series, review of the literature, and criteria for transplantation. Clin Transpl. 2009; 23(2):178–83.

101. de Perrot M, Granton JT, McRae K, Pierre AF, Singer LG, Waddell TK, et al. Outcome of patients with pulmonary arterial hypertension referred for lung transplantation: a 14-year single-center experience. J Thorac Cardiovasc Surg. 2012;143(4):910–8.

102. Transplantation ISfHaL. Registries Slides. 2013 [December 6, 2013]. http://www.ishlt.org/registries/ slides.asp?slides=heartLungRegistry

Current and Emerging Treatment Options in Interstitial Lung Disease

14

Toby M. Maher

Introduction

The interstitial lung diseases (ILDs) are a group of disorders characterised by inflammation or fibrosis arising in the interstitium of the lung, that is, the space bounded by the alveolar epithelium and the capillary endothelium. Several hundred individual disorders have been identified as giving rise to ILD. In some cases, such as drug-induced ILD, the pneumoconioses and hypersensitivity pneumonitis, the cause of the ILD can be identified. However, the most common group of ILDs are the idiopathic interstitial pneumonias (IIPs); a constellation of disorders with varying histological appearances, which, as their name suggests, are of unknown aetiology. Probably the next largest group of ILDs are those associated with the connective tissue diseases (CTDs). The CTD-associated ILDs share the histological features of the IIPs but arise in the context of a defined rheumatological condition. In some cases, an apparent IIP can represent the first presentation of a CTD that only manifests months to years after the onset of respiratory symptoms. As has been discussed elsewhere, individual CTDs typically associate with specific histological lesions, with the most commonly encountered

lesion being that of fibrotic non-specific interstitial pneumonia (NSIP). However, the full spectrum of histological patterns associated with the IIPs also occurs in the context of CTD-ILD.

Broadly speaking, the treatment of ILD can be considered both in the context of the associated underlying systemic disease, on the basis of the histological lesion, and most simplistically in terms of the predominant driving pathomechanism, i.e. inflammation or fibrosis. This chapter will consider general and specific treatment approaches (as far as current evidence permits) and will look to possible future therapeutic developments.

Connective Tissue Disease-Associated Interstitial Lung Disease: A Growing Problem

The last decade or two have seen dramatic improvements in standards of care, and consequently prognosis, across the range of CTDs. These changes have been driven by a number of factors principal amongst these being the development of effective clinical trial end points permitting assessment of existing immunosuppressant therapies, the emergence of biologic therapies and improvements in some organ-specific aspects of disease management, e.g. the use of angiotensin-converting enzyme inhibitors for the treatment of scleroderma-associated renal disease. Unfortunately, the management of CTD-associated ILD has lagged behind the

T.M. Maher, M.B., M.Sc., Ph.D., F.R.C.P. (✉)
Interstitial Lung Disease Unit, Royal Brompton &
Harefield Foundation NHS Trust,
Sydney Street, London SW3 6NP, UK
e-mail: t.maher@rbht.nhs.uk

P.F. Dellaripa et al. (eds.), *Pulmonary Manifestations of Rheumatic Disease: A Comprehensive Guide*,
DOI 10.1007/978-1-4939-0770-0_14, © Springer Science+Business Media New York 2014

improvements seen in other areas of CTD treatment. Thus, for individuals with CTD, respiratory disease has grown in importance. For many CTD sufferers, disease-associated ILD is now the major cause of disability, exercise limitation and loss of quality of life. In systemic sclerosis, ILD is now the single biggest cause of mortality [1]. In rheumatoid disease, the development of ILD confers a tripling in risk of death [2]. The incidence of ILD across the different CTDs is not trivial. In rheumatoid, between 6.5 and 10 % of patients develop ILD over the course of their disease [2–7]. Those who have a usual interstitial pneumonia (UIP) pattern of disease (characterised on computed tomography (CT) by bilateral, basal and sub-pleural honeycomb change) have a prognosis indistinguishable from idiopathic pulmonary fibrosis, a disease with a median survival of 2.8–4.2 years [3, 4]. In systemic sclerosis, ILD is estimated to develop in 35 % of individuals [1, 8]. A similar proportion of individuals with idiopathic inflammatory myositis (IIM) develop clinically significant ILD [9, 10].

Treating CTD-ILD: General Principles

There are a paucity of clinical trial data to guide the management of either ILD in general or, more specifically, CTD-associated ILD. The majority of ILD clinical trial activity has been undertaken in IPF and is therefore only of limited applicability to CTD-ILD. IPF is believed to be a disease that arises as a consequence of an aberrant wound healing response in genetically susceptible individuals [11]. As such, inflammation does not appear to be a major contributor to the development of fibrosis in IPF. Importantly, the recently published PANTHER-IPF study demonstrated an increase in hospitalisations and deaths in IPF patients treated with immunosuppressant therapy (high-dose prednisolone and azathioprine) when compared to placebo alone [12]. By contrast, in CTD-ILD, immune dysregulation and autoimmune-driven pulmonary injury appear to be an important precursor to the development of fibrosis. Although trial evidence is limited, there

is a general acceptance that immunosuppressant therapy in CTD-ILD modifies the course of the disease. The same appears to be true in other ILDs (e.g. hypersensitivity pneumonitis and sarcoidosis) where an initial inflammatory insult drives the downstream development of fibrosis. In CTD-ILD (and by the same token hypersensitivity pneumonitis and sarcoidosis), once the process of fibroproliferation has been triggered, the disease pathways that are activated appear to be very similar to those seen in IPF with overexpression and activation of the archetypal profibrotic mediator transforming growth factor (TGF)-β [13], fibroblast proliferation and transformation to myofibroblasts [14], increased oxidative stress and downregulation of key anti-fibrotic molecules such as prostaglandin (PG)E$_2$ [15, 16]. Furthermore, for individuals with advanced fibrosis CTD-ILD, disease behaviour becomes indistinguishable from that seen in IPF and other end-stage IIPs with the development of disease complications including acute exacerbations, respiratory failure, secondary pulmonary hypertension, pulmonary malignancy and episodic infection. With this in mind, the treatment of CTD-ILD (Fig. 14.1) can be considered in terms of treatment of the underlying disease mechanism (inflammation), the treatment of pulmonary fibrosis (for which parallels can be drawn with IPF) and the management of disease complications including end-of-life care.

Having enunciated this therapeutic approach, it is also worth considering treatment aims when it comes to the management of ILD. In general terms, inflammatory ILD (characterised histologically by a range of lesions including cellular NSIP, organising pneumonia, desquamative interstitial pneumonia and, to a lesser extent, lymphocytic interstitial pneumonia) has the potential for major reversal with restoration of normal or near-normal tissue structure and function. Fibrotic ILD (characterised by the histological lesions of UIP and fibrotic NSIP) tends, however, to be irreversible particularly once architectural distortion and microcystic honeycombing have developed. Expected treatment outcomes therefore need to be modulated in light of the underlying interstitial abnormality.

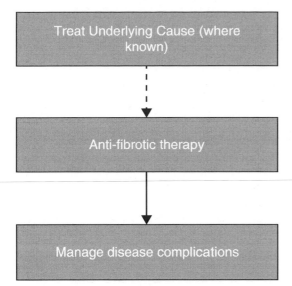

Fig. 14.1 A schematic outlining the general approach to treatment of fibrotic ILD. Where the cause of the ILD is known, e.g. connective tissue disease associated ILD, then the primary target of treatment is the underlying disease process, e.g. immuno-inflammation. However, fibrosis, once initiated, often becomes self-driving, and therapy can be separately targeted at fibroproliferative pathways. Finally, it is important not to neglect the symptomatic consequences of disease, and amelioration of symptoms should, where appropriate, be duly considered

Where inflammation predominates, it is reasonable to expect improvements in lung function and reduction in symptoms if treatment is effective. By contrast, in established fibrosis, it is unusual to see significant functional improvement with treatment; instead disease stabilisation and the prevention of progressive lung function and symptomatic decline are the key goals of therapy. Finally, whilst treatment is primarily targeted at the underlying disease mechanisms, it is important not to neglect the control of symptoms, such as cough, dyspnoea and anxiety, all of which frequently arise as a consequence of ILD.

The lack of clinical trial evidence raises a number of key unanswered questions about general treatment strategies in CTD-ILD. Whilst, for instance, it is clear that early, aggressive use of treatment in rheumatoid disease modifies disease outcomes (at least as far as joint disease is concerned), it is not clear that the same is true for CTD-ILD. This creates a dilemma for physicians

treating individuals with limited or 'early' interstitial change on thoracic CT. Although in scleroderma (where the natural history of the associated ILD is the best characterised of all the CTDs) it is known that prognosis is better in individuals with limited as compared to extensive disease, there is still an appreciable mortality risk for those with limited disease [17]. Almost all experts agreed that patients with extensive or rapidly progressive disease should be treated aggressively at the outset; however, there remains disagreement about how best to approach the management of individuals with limited disease at presentation. Carefully designed longitudinal randomised placebo-controlled trials are going to be necessary to answer this important question. Another clinical issue in CTD-ILD is the management of patients with disease activity in multiple organs. Whilst treatment decisions tend to be driven by the most life-threatening component of disease, it is not clear that a single therapeutic strategy is effective for all aspects of an individual disease. Added to this, in rheumatoid disease especially, there exists the concern that some DMARDS contribute to the development and evolution of the pulmonary complications associated with CTD [18]. It is clearly going to be a major challenge to design clinical trials to address these questions but, hopefully, such trials combined with prospective disease registries will in the future define best management of all aspects of CTD including the ILD.

Treating CTD-ILD

As has been noted, the evidence base underpinning current treatment approaches in individuals with ILD is limited. Aside from IPF, the only other disease that has seen appropriately powered randomised controlled trials is scleroderma-associated ILD. For almost all other forms of ILD, current best evidence consists of observational or open-label studies. Added to this many assumptions about the pathogenesis of ILD in individuals with CTD have been drawn from research undertaken in either IPF or else other organ systems in individuals with CTD.

For these reasons, their remains uncertainty about the key disease mechanisms that should be targeted in CTD-ILD and also by which mechanisms certain therapies that appear to be effective (e.g. rituximab) exert their therapeutic effect in the lung. Given that individual CTDs tend to be associated with different histological lesions, treatment of each condition will be considered separately, albeit acknowledging where overlap in therapeutic approaches exists. Because of the importance of progressive fibrosis in causing morbidity and mortality in those with CTD-ILD, the treatment of the fibrotic lung disease par excellence, IPF, will also be discussed. Symptom management and lung transplantation will be considered separately.

Scleroderma

Scleroderma-associated ILD is the best studied of all the CTD-ILDs, and yet there are still many unanswered questions regarding best therapy. With improvements in the treatment of renal disease and pulmonary hypertension, ILD has now become the most frequent cause of mortality in individuals with scleroderma [1]. In general, the development of ILD mirrors the changes seen in other organs and tends to occur early in the course of the disease with the greatest risk of progression being in the first 4 years after the onset of the first non-Raynaud's disease manifestation [19]. ILD is more common in diffuse systemic sclerosis and associates with the presence of the anti-Scl70 autoantibody [20]. Histologically, over 90 % of individuals with scleroderma-ILD have the lesion of NSIP with the remainder having UIP [21]. Radiologically, on HRCT, the typical appearance is of bilateral, predominantly basal sub-pleural reticulation with traction bronchiectasis. There tends to be a paucity of honeycombing but a moderate extent of ground glass attenuation [22]. Goh et al., in a landmark paper, developed an algorithm for categorising individuals according to the extent of ILD (limited or extensive) [17]. Application of this staging system (Fig. 14.2) enables prediction of individuals at high risk of ILD progression and therefore death. For this reason, most clinicians are in

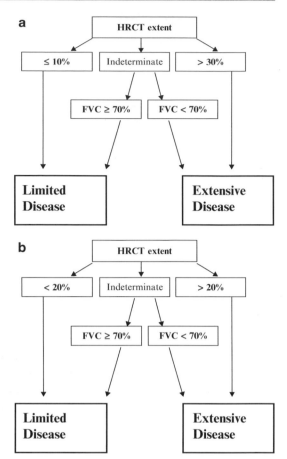

Fig. 14.2 (**a**, **b**) Flow diagram of limited/extensive staging system (**a**) with the use of formal high-resolution computed tomography (HRCT) scores, for the purposes of analysis, and (**b**) as applied in clinical practice (Used with permission from Goh NS, Desai SR, Veeraraghavan S, et al. Interstitial lung disease in systemic sclerosis: a simple staging system. Am J Respir Crit Care Med 2008;177:1248–54)

agreement that patients with extensive scleroderma-ILD merit early and aggressive immunomodulatory therapy. Opinion is more divided on how best to manage limited disease with many electing to simply observe and only commence therapy if there is evidence of disease progression on serial lung function testing.

Cyclophosphamide

The alkylating agent cyclophosphamide has been assessed as a treatment for scleroderma-ILD in two multicentre randomised, placebo-controlled trials. The first of these studies, by Tashkin et al., compared oral cyclophosphamide (at a dose of 2 mg/kg body weight per day) or matching placebo for 1 year in 158 patients with scleroderma-associated ILD [23]. The primary end point was change in FVC at 1 year. Cyclophosphamide treatment was associated with a small (2.53 %) but statistically significant ($p = 0.03$) mean improvement in FVC when compared to placebo. There were no differences in serious adverse events between placebo and cyclophosphamide although there were more episodes of leucopoenia and haematuria in the active treatment arm. In the second study by Hoyles et al., 45 patients were randomised to receive a combination of low-dose prednisolone, six monthly infusions of cyclophosphamide (at a dose of 600 mg/m^2 body surface area) and then azathioprine (150 mg daily) or placebo alone [24]. Primary outcome was change in percent-predicted FVC and single-breath diffusing capacity for carbon monoxide (DLco) at 1 year. There was a trend ($p = 0.08$) towards improved FVC in the active treatment arm. Some experts believe these studies may have been hampered by the prevalent practice patterns of the time. As has been argued by Wells, both of these studies recruited patients at a time when cyclophosphamide was already judged by most clinicians to be the standard of care for patients with progressive scleroderma-associated ILD [25]. As such, there may have been reluctance by investigators to enrol individuals with progressive disease. Instead such individuals may have been, in the most part, treated outside the study with open-label therapy. This view is borne out by the lack of disease progression observed in the placebo arms in both studies. Given that these studies were therefore conducted in individuals with relatively stable fibrotic disease, it is perhaps unsurprising that relatively little treatment effect was observed. Several open-label retrospective studies of cyclophosphamide have been reported in the literature [26–30]. Overall these favour cyclophosphamide and tend to suggest a significant improvement in FVC. In most cases, pulsed intravenous cyclophosphamide and daily oral cyclophosphamide

appear to have similar efficacy albeit that intravenous dosing appears to be better tolerated.

Longitudinal follow-up of the study by Tashkin et al. suggests that the beneficial effect of cyclophosphamide treatment wanes over time [23, 31, 32]. Optimal duration of treatment therefore remains to be defined. As in the study by Hoyles et al., many centres follow pulsed cyclophosphamide with either azathioprine or mycophenolate mofetil (MMF) [24]. The efficacy of this approach and appropriate length of treatment regimen remain to be defined [29, 33]. Ultimately, these questions require carefully designed and appropriately powered studies to provide the necessary answers for clinicians dealing with the practical issue of how best to treat scleroderma-ILD.

Rituximab

Rituximab, a chimeric (human/mouse) monoclonal antibody with a high affinity for the CD20 surface antigen expressed on pre-B and B-lymphocytes, results in rapid depletion of B-cells from the peripheral circulation for 6–9 months [34]. Evidence for the effectiveness of B-cell depletion exists in a number of immune-mediated conditions, including rheumatoid arthritis [35–37], ANCA-associated vasculitis [38, 39] and immune thrombocytopenic purpura [40]. In a small open-label, randomised proof-of-principle study of rituximab in scleroderma (given at a dose of 375 mg/m^2 weekly for 4 weeks at baseline and again at 24 weeks), Daoussis et al. reported a significant improvement in FVC, compared to baseline, at 1 year in the rituximab group. In the active treatment group, FVC increased from 68.1 ± 19.7 % predicted to 75.6 ± 19.7 % predicted ($p = 0.0018$) [41]. In the cohort receiving best standard care, there was an overall reduction in FVC over the 12 months of the study. Rituximab has been reported as an effective rescue therapy for patients with scleroderma-ILD unresponsive to treatment with corticosteroid. An ongoing clinical trial, the RECITAL study (NCT01862926), is a placebo-controlled, randomised controlled trial testing the efficacy of rituximab compared to intravenous cyclophosphamide when given as first-line therapy in progressive CTD-ILD (including scleroderma, IIM and MCTD).

Corticosteroids

In general, high doses of corticosteroids are avoided in scleroderma because of the concern over inducing renal crisis [42]. Whilst low doses of corticosteroid have often been used in clinical studies of scleroderma-ILD as an adjunct to other immunosuppressants, the need for an optimal dose and duration of corticosteroid use in scleroderma has never been defined in an RCT.

Mycophenolate

MMF is an inosine monophosphate dehydrogenase inhibitor which reduces T- and B-cell proliferation through reduction in purine synthesis. MMF has been shown to be well tolerated in systemic sclerosis with retrospective studies suggesting that the drug has favourable effects on systemic manifestations of disease. In another retrospective study [43–47], Fischer et al. looked at MMF use in 125 individuals with CTD-ILD, the largest proportion [44] of whom had scleroderma, and were able to demonstrate that MMF was associated with reduced steroid requirement and sustained improvement in FVC [48]. The scleroderma lung study (SLS) II is currently evaluating the effect of MMF compared to cyclophosphamide in scleroderma-ILD in a 2-year RCT (NCT00883129).

Imatinib

The tyrosine kinase inhibitor, imatinib, prevents protein phosphorylation through inhibition of the specific tyrosine kinase, BCR-Abl. The drug was originally developed as a specific therapy for chronic myeloid leukaemia. In vitro studies in human lung fibroblasts and in vivo studies utilising the murine bleomycin model, albeit with the use of prophylactic dosing (i.e. at the time of bleomycin administration) of imatinib, suggest that imatinib may have anti-fibrotic actions [49]. Sabnani et al. reported the use of imatinib (200 mg daily) in combination with intravenous cyclophosphamide (500 mg every 3 weeks) in five patients with scleroderma-associated ILD [50]. The combination was well tolerated, but efficacy was not determined. In a phase IIa open-label, single-arm study, Spiera et al. reported the use of imatinib (400 mg daily) for 1 year in 24 patients with diffuse cutaneous systemic sclerosis. In this group, FVC improved, on average, by 6.4 % compared to baseline over 12 months ($p = 0.008$) [51]. More recently, Khanna et al. have reported a study of imatinib 600 mg/daily in 20 patients with scleroderma-associated ILD [52]. At this dose, imatinib was poorly tolerated with common adverse effects including fatigue, oedema, diarrhoea, nausea and vomiting, generalised rash and new-onset proteinuria. Only 60 % of subjects completed the study. No beneficial effect of imatinib on FVC was observed. These mixed results preclude the routine use of imatinib in scleroderma-ILD but are sufficient to merit further randomised, placebo-controlled studies.

Cell-Based Therapy

A number of preclinical studies have identified mesenchymal- and bone marrow-derived stem cells as a potential treatment for scleroderma-ILD. Burt et al. assessed the role of autologous non-myelo-ablative haemopoietic stem cell transplantation compared with pulsed cyclophosphamide in an open-label, randomised study of 19 patients with diffuse cutaneous systemic sclerosis and pulmonary involvement [53]. All ten subjects in the stem cell arm met the primary end point of disease improvement (either a 25 % decrease in modified Rodnan skin score or 10 % increase in FVC). In the cyclophosphamide group, by stark contrast, eight of nine subjects had disease progression despite treatment. Improvement in FVC persisted at 2 years. Ongoing, open-label studies are further evaluating stem cell transplantation for scleroderma in general and specifically for the treatment of scleroderma-ILD (NCT01413100).

Bosentan

The endothelin antagonist bosentan has a well-established role in the treatment of CTD-associated pulmonary hypertension. Preclinical data suggests that endothelin antagonism is anti-fibrotic in vitro in human lung fibroblasts and in vivo in animal models of fibrosis [54]. Following on from a phase IIa study of bosentan in IPF [55], bosentan was also studied as a potential therapy for scleroderma-ILD. Seibold et al. undertook a 12-month placebo-controlled RCT of bosentan in 163 patients with scleroderma [56]. Bosentan failed to improve either 6-min walk distance or any lung function parameters and as such is ineffective as a treatment for scleroderma-ILD. Bosentan does, however, remain an important therapeutic option for scleroderma-related pulmonary hypertension.

Summary

Although scleroderma-associated ILD is the most studied and best understood of the CTD-ILDs, there remain many important questions which need answering with appropriately designed clinical studies. Nonetheless, the treatment approach now adopted by most specialist centres is to manage patients with extensive ILD with six monthly doses of intravenous cyclophosphamide together with low-dose oral prednisolone, followed by a minimum of 18 months treatment with either azathioprine or MMF together with low-dose prednisolone. Treatment refractory extensive disease is then managed with intravenous rituximab. For individuals with limited disease but evidence of progression over time, the general approach to therapy is the use of oral azathioprine (or MMF) together with low-dose prednisolone. In limited disease, cyclophosphamide is reserved for those individuals who progress despite oral immunosuppressant therapy.

Idiopathic Inflammatory Myositis

The IIMs characteristically present with a different pattern of ILD to that seen in scleroderma. In individuals with scleroderma, even in the earliest stages of the disease, the histological lesion encountered tends to be NSIP. In the IIMs, by contrast, individuals frequently present with organising pneumonia (which often has a characteristic bilateral, predominantly basal distribution with sparing of individual lobules; Fig. 14.3) and then over time progress to develop fixed fibrosis which, if biopsied, shows the lesion of NSIP. A small proportion of individuals with the IIMs present with rapid-onset ILD and often catastrophic respiratory failure. On biopsy (or autopsy), these individuals tend to have evidence of diffuse alveolar damage. Because of the relative rarity of IIMs, there has yet to be an RCT for IIM-associated ILD. As such, current treatment approaches are informed either by therapeutic

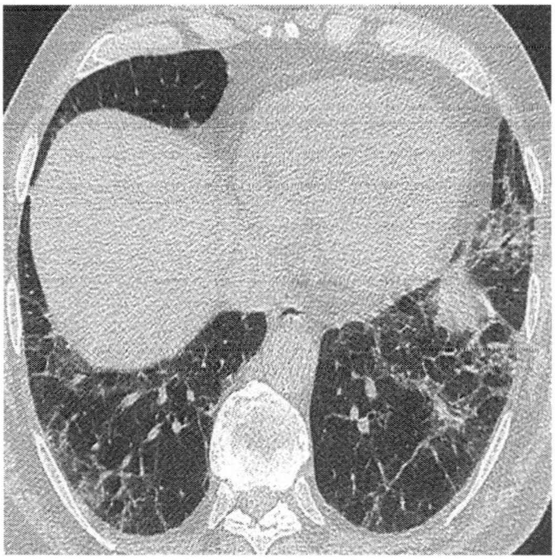

Fig. 14.3 Supine, inspiratory high-resolution CT image from a 42-year-old man with Jo-1-positive polymyositis. Image shows interstitial change with patch consolidation and lobular sparing. There is only very limited traction bronchiectasis and reticular change. The CT appearances are characteristic of the lesion of organising pneumonia with associated NSIP fibrosis that is most commonly encountered in individuals with idiopathic inflammatory myositis-associated ILD

effects seen in other CTD-ILDs or else from intervention studies targeting the systemic manifestations of the IIMs.

High-dose corticosteroids tend to be the first-line therapy for IIM-associated ILD, and in individuals for whom the predominant abnormality is organising pneumonia, these can lead to excellent treatment outcomes [57]. In individuals with mild disease, combined therapy with oral corticosteroids and either azathioprine or MMF is frequently effective. By extrapolation from scleroderma pulsed intravenous cyclophosphamide is often used as first-line therapy for individuals with extensive or rapidly progressive IIM-associated ILD [57, 58]. In individuals for whom cyclophosphamide is contraindicated or else fails to induce a therapeutic response, rituximab may be an effective alternative. In a retrospective cohort study, Keir et al. reported outcomes in nine individuals (six of whom had either polymyositis or dermatomyositis) with CTD-ILD. Overall rituximab, even though used as rescue therapy, was associated with clinically important improvements in lung function, gas exchange and radiological disease extent [59]. As with scleroderma-ILD, the efficacy of rituximab, compared to cyclophosphamide, is being tested in the RECITAL study (NCT01862926) as first-line therapy for IIM-ILD. Other oral treatment alternatives include cyclosporin and methotrexate. In a retrospective cohort study, Labirua-Iturburu et al. reported outcomes in 15 patients with anti-synthetase-associated ILD treated with a calcineurin inhibitor (either cyclosporine or tacrolimus) [60]. Calcineurin inhibitor use was associated with disease stabilisation or improvement in 87 % of patients.

In patients with treatment refractory or rapidly progressive disease, a range of therapies have been documented, in case reports or small series, as having potential efficacy. These include immunoglobulins [61], plasmapheresis [62], the T-cell-depleting agent anti-thymocyte globulin [63], the anti-complement 5 monoclonal antibody eculizumab [64], the anti-CD52 monoclonal antibody alemtuzumab [65], anti-TNFα monoclonal antibodies [66] or the IL-1 receptor antagonist anakinra [67, 68]. There is, however, insufficient evidence available to be able to select any particular therapeutic regimen over another. Clinicians should be guided by individual treatment responses when assessing the efficacy of a particular treatment.

Rheumatoid Disease

Rheumatoid-associated ILD is associated with a range of different presentations and histological lesions. A significant proportion has evidence of UIP either on biopsy or on the basis of HRCT appearances. This subgroup has a survival akin to IPF and has the poorest prognosis of any of the CTD-ILDs [2, 3, 5, 7, 69]. Other frequently encountered manifestations of RA-ILD include NSIP, smoking-related ILD, desquamative interstitial pneumonitis (DIP), lymphocytic interstitial pneumonitis (LIP) and drug-induced ILD. RA-ILD is surprisingly poorly understood. The factors predisposing to the individual presentations remain, for the most part, unknown. Similarly, there have been no RCTs in RA-ILD. Treatment guidance is based on analysis of case reports, case series, registry reviews and extrapolation from other CTD-ILDs. Potential therapies for RA-ILD that have been described in the literature include corticosteroids, azathioprine, MMF, rituximab, infliximab, cyclosporin and, more recently, the anti-interleukin (IL)-6 monoclonal antibody tocilizumab [70–73]. It is not known, however, whether many of the other disease-modifying anti-rheumatic drugs (DMARDs) are effective in slowing or preventing the progression of RA-ILD.

In general, the UIP subtype of RA-ILD is poorly responsive to immunosuppressive therapy. The recently reported PANTHER study in IPF [12], which demonstrated that combined immunosuppression with prednisolone and azathioprine in IPF is deleterious, raises the possibility that the same might be true in RA-UIP. As such, it may be best to avoid aggressive immunosuppression and extrapolate treatment approaches from IPF (as will be discussed later in this chapter). Anecdotally, other forms of ILD, particularly fibrotic NSIP, behave in a manor akin to that seen in scleroderma-ILD. On this basis, treatment regimens for non-UIP RA-ILD should probably mirror those applied in scleroderma albeit without the need to limit the peak dose of steroid used. Drug-induced lung disease represents a major challenge in RA [74]. Firstly, there are few if any features that can be used to truly differentiate drug-induced lung disease from other forms of RA-ILD. Secondly, whilst withdrawal of the offending medication is the intervention of choice, there then comes the difficulty of knowing what alternative disease-modifying agents can be used to manage the systemic manifestations of RA. From an RA-ILD, perspective corticosteroids can be considered safe, and often therapeutically effective. However, the majority of drugs that have been reported in small series to be effective for RA-ILD (e.g. infliximab and rituximab) have also been reported to cause potentially catastrophic pulmonary side effects [75]. As such the introduction of any new DMARD to an individual with existing ILD should be undertaken cautiously with regular monitoring (including lung function and serial radiographs) to ensure that there is no negative impact on the lung disease.

Other Connective Tissue Diseases

As noted earlier, the only RCTs assessing the treatment of CTD-ILD have been in scleroderma. For RA and the IIMs, there are a reasonable breadth of case series and registry data to guide potential best treatment of associated ILDs. However, for the remainder of the CTDs, there is very little information on which to formulate treatment decisions. For individuals with mixed connective tissue disease (MCTD), most centres adopt the approach of treating individuals based on whether their disease most mirrors scleroderma or IIM [76]. In short if the CT appearance is one of fibrotic NSIP then treatment reflects that used for scleroderma. On the other hand, if the appearance fits a possible histological diagnosis of fibrosing organising pneumonia, then treatment expectations and the chosen regimen should be that adopted for polymyositis or dermatomyositis.

Sjögren's syndrome is associated with chronic lymphocytic infiltration of the exocrine glands which results in mucosal dryness [77, 78]. Xerotrachea and chronic cough are frequently troublesome in Sjögren's. From the perspective of ILD, Sjögren's is most frequently associated with LIP [78]. Other associated histological lesions are UIP, NSIP and organising pneumonia [79–82]. Overall, 5-year survival in Sjögren-'related ILD is good at 84 %, and frequently the major determinant of need for treatment is symptoms [82]. Possible therapeutic strategies that have been reported in case series of individuals with Sjögren's ILD include corticosteroids, azathioprine, hydroxychloroquine, cyclophosphamide and rituximab [83, 84]. Given the very limited evidence available to guide treatment, decisions need to be made on an individual basis and should be driven by disease severity and any observed response to treatment.

Undifferentiated connective tissue disease (UCTD) is a term that has been loosely applied to a range of clinical syndromes. In the context of ILD, it has been proposed as a diagnostic label to describe individuals presenting with ILD who have features suggestive of an underlying autoimmune disorder but who fail to fulfil the diagnostic criteria for any specific CTD [85]. In a proportion of cases of NSIP, ILD can be the first manifestation of a CTD which with time declares itself more fully [86]. However, a significant minority of individuals with both NSIP and UIP have some features of CTD (e.g. Raynaud's phenomenon, positive ANA, raised inflammatory markers, etc.) but never develop a defined CTD. The relevance of such clinical features remains uncertain. Kinder et al. in a retrospective cohort study reported that features suggestive of CTD predict ILD with a better outcome [87]. Corte et al., by contrast, found no difference between outcomes for UCTD and the comparable idiopathic histological lesion [88]. Individuals with UCTD also present a therapeutic dilemma which is yet to be resolved. That is, whether they should be treated as a form of CTD with immunosuppressive therapy or whether they should be treated as idiopathic disease, e.g. IPF. Hopefully, novel deep phenotyping techniques will shine a light on this important question [89]. In the meantime, when a decision is made to treat UCTD as an autoimmune-driven phenomenon, an approach akin to that adopted in scleroderma is probably best adopted.

Anti-fibrotic Therapy: Lessons from IPF

In this chapter, thus far, the major consideration in the treatment of CTD-ILD has surrounded the management of the autoimmune-driven inflammatory component of these conditions. However, the majority of individuals with CTD-ILD develop not just inflammation but fibrosis which, in many cases, results in progressive, irreversible loss of lung function. IPF is the most common ILD and is characterised by inexorably progressive and invariably fatal fibrosis in the absence of any significant inflammation [11]. Current pathogenic paradigms emphasise the role played by aberrant wound healing responses occurring following repetitive alveolar injury in genetically

susceptible individuals. The last decade has seen a dramatic increase in clinical trial activity in IPF. Consequently, there have been many more RCTs undertaken in IPF than CTD-ILD (Table 14.1). Whilst there are clearly significant differences between CTD-ILD and IPF, there are also important synergies. As such therapies developed for IPF may be effective in preventing or slowing disease progression in, at least a proportion of, patients with fibrotic ILD occurring as a consequence of an underlying CTD.

Unlike inflammation, established fibrosis, characterised biochemically by cross-linked collagen and the deposition of other extracellular matrix proteins, is considered to be irreversible. This is especially the case when, as in the lesion of UIP, fibrosis is accompanied by destruction of the normal lacelike alveolar architecture. For this reason, the ultimate treatment goal in IPF is one of disease stabilisation. This fact has created several challenges when it comes to designing clinical trials for IPF and has resulted in a number of controversies in the field. Nonetheless, since the publication of the first true placebo-controlled

Table 14.1 Summary of late-phase IPF trials

Drug	Year	Number	Primary end point	Result
Interferon-γ	2004	330	PFS	No effect [90]
Pirfenidone	2005	107	Change in the lowest 6-MW SpO$_2$	Reduced acute exacerbations [99]
Warfarin	2005	56	Survival time	Improved survival [141]
N-acetylcysteine	2005	182	Change in VC	Reduced progression [103]
Bosentan	2008	58	Change in 6-MW distance	No effect [55]
Etanercept	2008	88	Change in FVC and DLco	No effect [142]
Interferon-γ	2009	826	Survival time	No effect [143]
Pirfenidone	2010	275	Change in VC	Reduced progression [100]
Imatinib	2010	119	Time to disease progression	No effect [144]
Sildenafil	2010	180	>20 % increase in 6-MWD	No effect [145]
Bosentan	2010	616	Time to IPF worsening	No effect [146]
Pirfenidone	2011	779	Change in % pred FVC	Reduced progression [101]
BIBF1120	2011	432	Rate of FVC decline	Trend to reduced progression [109]
Prednisolone + Azathioprine	2012	155	Change in FVC	Increased mortality [12]
Warfarin	2012	145	Progression-free survival	Increased adverse events [120]
Thalidomide	2012	24	Cough questionnaire	Reduced cough [139]
Ambrisentan	2013	492	Time to disease progression	No effect [147]
Septrin	2013	118	Change in FVC	No effect [118]

PFS progression-free survival, *6-MW(D)* 6-min walk (distance), *(F)VC* forced vital capacity, *DLco* total lung diffusion capacity for carbon monoxide

RCT in IPF in 2004, there has been an explosion in clinical trial activity [90]. This has culminated in the licencing in Europe, Canada, Japan and Asia of the first true anti-fibrotic therapy, pirfenidone [91]. This development together with ongoing trials of a range of novel therapeutic compounds has led to important changes in clinical approaches to the management of IPF. It is to be hoped that with time these advances in IPF treatment will be translated across other fibrotic ILDs including the CTD-associated ILDs.

As detailed in Table 14.1, the expansion of clinical trial activity in IPF whilst generating many negative results has also led to a rapid evolution in disease understanding, the development of clinically meaningful trial end points and identification of the fact that previously recommended treatment regimens are harmful in patients with established pulmonary fibrosis [92–94]. Furthermore, there has been a rapid expansion in pharmaceutical interest in fibrosis resulting in a large array of compounds entering early-phase clinical trials.

Pirfenidone

The major success story for IPF in the last decade has been pirfenidone. In vitro pirfenidone inhibits TGF-β-stimulated collagen synthesis, decreases synthesis by fibroblasts of extracellular matrix proteins and blocks the proliferative effects of platelet-derived growth factor (PDGF) on fibroblasts isolated from IPF lung [95–97]. In animal models of pulmonary fibrosis, pirfenidone attenuates a range of pro-fibrotic mediators whilst downregulating histological markers of cellular proliferation [96–98]. The first large-scale trial of pirfenidone was a Japanese, multicentre, randomised, placebo-controlled, phase II study of 107 subjects who received either pirfenidone 600 mg tds ($n=72$) or placebo ($n=35$) [99]. The study's Data and Safety Monitoring Board recommended early termination of study at 9 months (the planned study duration was 12 months) on ethical grounds due to an excess of acute exacerbations in the placebo arm. The primary end point, of the lowest arterial oxygen saturation measured by pulse oximetry during a 6-min walk (6 MW), was not achieved; however, there was a significant

reduction in the decline of FVC in the pirfenidone group. The trial by Azuma et al. led to the development of a 52-week, Japanese, multi-centre, double-blind, placebo-controlled, randomised phase III clinical trial in which 275 patients were randomised to either high-dose (1,800 mg/day) or low-dose (1,200 mg/day) pirfenidone or placebo [100]. Significant differences were observed in the primary end point of FVC decline between the placebo group (−0.16 L) and the high-dose group (−0.09 L) ($p=0.0416$). Progression-free survival time (with disease progression defined as more than 10 % decrease in FVC and/or death) was also significantly prolonged in the high-dose compared to the placebo group ($p<0.0280$).

The CAPACITY trials (Clinical Studies Assessing Pirfenidone in idiopathic pulmonary fibrosis) consisted of two concurrent multinational, randomised, double-blind, placebo-controlled phase III trials (004 and 006) designed to evaluate the safety and efficacy of pirfenidone in IPF patients with mild to moderate impairment in lung function [101]. In study 004, 174 patients were assigned to high-dose pirfenidone (2,403 mg/day), 87 patients to low-dose pirfenidone (1,197 mg/day), and 174 to placebo. In study 006, 171 patients were assigned high-dose pirfenidone (2,403 mg/day), and 173 patients to placebo. In study 004, the higher dose of pirfenidone met the primary end point, significantly decreasing the fall in FVC at week 72 (difference between groups of 4.4 %, $p=0.001$). By contrast, study 006 failed to meet the primary end point (FVC difference between groups of 0.6 %, $p=0.501$). However, in 006, pirfenidone did significantly reduced decline in the secondary end point of 6-MW distance (absolute difference 32 m, $p=0.0009$). The reason for the different outcomes in the two studies remains unclear. Of note, however, is the observation that whilst the rate of decline of FVC in the pirfenidone group was the same in both studies, the individuals in the 006 placebo group had a slower rate of decline compared to those in 004.

A recent Cochrane review [102], encompassing the 2 Japanese trials and CAPACITY 004 and CAPACITY 006, has shown that across the four studies pirfenidone improved progression-free survival by 30 % (HR 0.70, 95 % CI 0.56–0.88).

In light of these studies, the European Medicine Agency approved the use of pirfenidone. However, in the USA, the FDA declined to approve the medication given the failure of 006 to meet its primary end point. As a result, a phase 3 study (the ASCEND trial, NCT0136629), spanning 52 weeks, is currently underway in the USA. Pirfenidone has also been licensed for use in Japan, Canada and India.

N-Acetylcysteine

N-acetylcysteine (NAC) acts on the lung to increase intra- and extracellular levels of glutathione and exerts an antioxidant effect [103]. The bronchial and alveolar epithelium, through exposure to ambient air and a wide range of pollutants, are constantly under high levels of oxidative stress. As such evolution has equipped the lung with a number of protective mechanisms to counter the potentially deleterious consequences of reactive oxygen species and free radical exposure; these include glutathione and the supra-oxide dismutases [104, 105]. In IPF, there is evidence that these antioxidant mechanisms are impaired and that this in turn contributes to epithelial susceptibility to injury and apoptosis. Levels of the key endogenous antioxidant glutathione are four times lower in the BAL fluid of individuals with IPF when compared to healthy controls [104]. This observation led to a pilot study in which 12 weeks of treatment with NAC was shown to be sufficient to increase BAL glutathione levels [106]. This in turn led on to the development of the multicentre IFGENIA trial, and this study became the first prospective IPF trial to report a positive outcome. In total 155 patients with IPF were enrolled with 80 being assigned to treatment with NAC. Following 12 months of treatment, there was a slower rate of loss of vital capacity (VC) in the NAC-treated group with VC being 0.18 L better than that observed in the placebo-treated arm. Similarly, there was a slowing in the deterioration of DLco, by 24 % in the NAC-treated subjects [103]. The study has attracted criticism for a lack of a true placebo arm (all patients in the study, in addition to the study drug or placebo, were on prednisolone and azathioprine—the combination

of which was at the time thought to represent best treatment for IPF), a relatively high dropout rate and the fact that the results have yet to be replicated. These issues will be addressed by the ongoing PANTHER-IPF trial (NCT00650091). In the meantime, as NAC is relatively cheap and has an excellent safety profile, it is being widely used by many specialists as a treatment for many, if not all, fibrotic ILDs.

Nintedanib

Nintedanib (Boehringer Ingelheim: formally known by the development code BIBF 1120) is an orally available 6-methoxycarbonyl-substituted indolinone [107]. It acts as a multiple-receptor tyrosine kinase inhibitor which functions against three receptor families: platelet-derived growth factor (PDGF), vascular endothelial growth factor (VEGF) and fibroblast growth factor (FGF) [108]. Nintedanib was originally developed for use in cancer but has recently been tested in a phase 2b dose-ranging study in patients with IPF [109]. The TOMORROW (To Improve Pulmonary Fibrosis with BIBF1120) study, was a 12-month, 432-subject, double-blinded, randomised, dose-ranging placebo-controlled phase II trial investigating the efficacy and safety of nintedanib in IPF. The primary end point was the annual rate of FVC decline. In the highest-dose group (who took 150 mg twice daily), FVC decline was 0.06 L compared to 0.19 L in the placebo group. Hierarchical comparison of these groups (without correction for multiplicity) pointed towards a significant difference between groups ($p=0.01$). The p value corrected for the multiple group comparisons was 0.06 [109, 110]. There were also a number of clinically important and significant changes in prespecified secondary outcomes in the highest treatment dose arm compared to placebo including improved quality of life and a reduction in acute exacerbations [109, 111]. Two parallel phase three registration studies of nintedanib in IPF (NCT01335464 and NCT01335477) are currently ongoing and will report in early 2014. If these studies are positive, then nintedanib looks set to add to the armamentarium available to physicians treating individuals with IPF [107].

Future Anti-fibrotic Therapies

Based on the presumed pathogenesis of IPF as an aberrant wound healing response following repetitive alveolar injury, a wide range of potential novel therapeutic strategies are being considering (Fig. 14.4; refer to ref. [112] for a detailed review). The first of these is to try and limit or prevent alveolar injury [112]. Possible approaches to this include preventing gastro-oesophageal reflux and microaspiration [113–115], the use of antioxidants (including NOX inhibitors) with a more potent mechanism of action than NAC [116, 117] and prophylactic antimicrobials (both antibacterial and antiviral drugs having shown promising results in small pilot studies in IPF) [118, 119]. Another potential strategy is to block the coagulation cascade. Although the vitamin K antagonist warfarin, which inhibits a number of clotting cascade components, has been shown to be

deleterious in IPF [120], targeting specific factors such as FXa or the protease-activated receptors (PARs) [121, 122] may be a more effective anti-fibrotic treatment approach. Another strategy is to enhance epithelial proliferation thus stimulating restoration of epithelial integrity (a key event in the switch from fibroproliferation to scar resorption during the normal wound healing response) [15, 123]. The concern with epithelial targeted approaches is that they may increase the risk of malignancy in a disease where there is already an increased incidence of primary lung neoplasms.

The therapeutic strategy gaining the most interest in IPF is targeting of the myofibroblast. These cells are highly synthetic structural cells capable of producing large quantities of extracellular matrix. As such, they are the key effector cells in IPF and can be found in abundance within fibroblastic foci [124]. It seems likely that the main cellular target of both pirfenidone and nintedanib is the myofibroblast. A number of novel

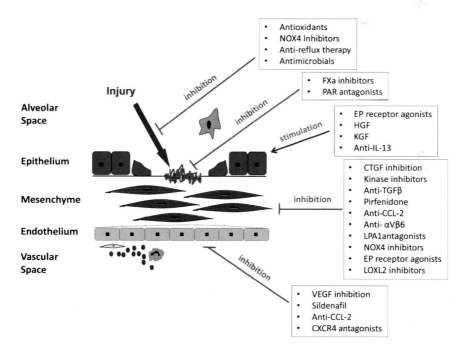

Fig. 14.4 Current understanding of the pathogenesis of IPF suggests that repetitive alveolar epithelial injury results in basement membrane denudation and activation of key pathways involved in the wound healing response. This in turn leads to fibroblast proliferation, transformation of fibroblasts to myofibroblasts, and expansion of the ECM. These effects are augmented by the influx of circulating inflammatory cells, including the putative bone marrow-derived fibroblast precursor, the fibrocyte.

Various treatments are in development targeting different aspects of IPF disease pathogenesis, through inhibition of fibrogenesis, through promotion of anti-fibrotic pathways, or through reduction of alveolar injury. *HGF* hepatocyte growth factor, *KGF* keratinocyte growth factor (Used with permission from Maher TM. Idiopathic pulmonary fibrosis: pathobiology of novel approaches to treatment. Clinics in chest medicine 2012;33:69–83) strategies have been adopted for targeting myofibroblast production of extracellular matrix proteins. These include inhibition of integrins (which play an important part in activating TGF-β), antibody-mediated blocking of connective tissue growth factor (CTGF), inhibition of lysyl oxidase homolog 2 (LOXL2) and antagonism of interleukin-13 [112]. For all of these mechanisms, there are compounds currently in early-phase clinical trials. It is to be hoped therefore that at least some of these targets will translate in to novel anti-fibrotic treatments in the next decade.

Summary

IPF clinical trials are finally bringing about advances in the treatment of this devastating disease. In Europe, the majority of specialist centres are now managing IPF patients with a combination of pirfenidone and NAC in the expectation that this should result in improved survival. The licencing of compounds with specific anti-fibrotic effects should, in time, have knock on benefits for the treatment of other diseases characterised by the development of fibrosis. It is likely that in the future and pending the necessary clinical trials drugs developed for IPF will be used to treat fibrotic CTD-associated ILD. This is especially likely to be the case for RA-ILD with UIP histology. The extensive development pipeline of anti-fibrotic compounds being tested in IPF is therefore to be welcomed by individuals with CTD-ILD and their treating physicians.

Lung Transplant

Lung transplantation is currently the only treatment for fibrotic ILD that has been shown to improve survival (Fig. 14.5) [125]. However, the benefits of treatment need to be carefully balanced against the many downsides of transplantation. These downsides include the limited availability of donor organs, the ever-present risk of both infection and rejection and the lifelong need for immunosuppressant therapy. In the UK, pulmonary fibrosis (mainly IPF) accounts for 20 % of all lung transplants [126]; however, individuals with pulmonary fibrosis have

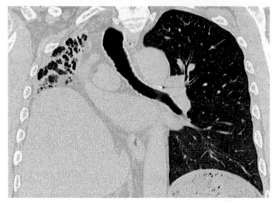

Fig. 14.5 Sagittal CT of a 56-year-old man 5 years after a left single lung transplant for idiopathic pulmonary fibrosis. The transplanted left lung has a normal appearance. The remaining right lung shows the consequences of progressive unopposed fibroproliferation with dramatic loss of volume of the right hemithorax and marked honeycomb change

the highest death rate for all diagnostic groups on the transplant waiting list [125, 126]. The 5-year survival following lung transplantation for pulmonary fibrosis is similar to other disease groups and stands at 45–50 % [127]. In a review of 47 scleroderma patients transplanted in the USA before 2005, 1- and 3-year mortalities were 67.6 and 45.9 %, respectively [128]. This was lower (albeit not statistically significantly so) than the mean outcomes for the other 10 070 patients in the US transplant register for whom survival was 75.5 and 58.8 %, respectively. Timing of referral for transplant is frequently challenging. However, criteria to address which patients and when they should be referred have been produced by the International Society for Heart and Lung Transplant (ISHLT) [129]. The ISHLT guidelines recommend that individuals with pulmonary fibrosis should be considered for transplantation if their DLCO is <40 % of predicted, if they have suffered a decrement in FVC> 10 % during the preceding 6 months or if they show a decrease in pulse oximetry <88 % saturation during a 6 MW. Active multisystem disease is a relative contraindication to lung transplant, so it is important that for individuals with CTD-ILD all aspects of their condition are considered before any decision to assess for transplant is made. Furthermore, significant other organ involvement (e.g. renal or myocardial disease in scleroderma) renders transplantation contraindicated.

Symptom Management

In a significant proportion of individuals with CTD-ILD, the disease progresses to end-stage respiratory failure and, ultimately, death. It is important therefore that consideration is given to therapeutic strategies aimed at reducing symptoms and improving quality of life. Pulmonary rehabilitation has been shown to be safe and highly effective in patients with COPD [130, 131]. In small studies of patients with pulmonary fibrosis, pulmonary rehabilitation appears to confer improvements in functional exercise capacity, dyspnoea and quality of life immediately following training [132–135]. The long-term effects of rehabilitation in pulmonary fibrosis, and specifically CTD-associated ILD, have yet to be studied. Oxygen is widely used for patients with respiratory failure due to ILD. Theoretically, at least, this may be both beneficial (in preventing the development of pulmonary hypertension) and harmful (through increasing oxidative stress and thus epithelial injury within the lung). There is, however, no trial evidence to guide the use of oxygen, either at rest, nocturnally or on exertion, in individuals with ILD of whatever cause. However, retrospective observational data demonstrate that ambulatory oxygen improves walk distance and reduces symptomatic breathlessness in individuals with exercise desaturation due to fibrotic ILD [136].

For patients with end-stage ILD, palliative use of anxiolytics, including benzodiazepines and opiates, can be very effective in alleviating the distressing symptoms of dyspnoea and the frequently associated feelings of panic which many patients experience [137]. Cough is another frequently debilitating and difficult to treat symptom of ILD. There is little evidence to support the use of any specific antitussive in ILD. In a small study of 11 patients with IPF, Horton et al. reported that thalidomide had a dramatic effect in alleviating intractable cough in IPF, suggesting a potential palliative role for this drug [138]. A larger double-blind placebo-controlled crossover trial of thalidomide for cough in IPF confirmed these findings. Although the antitussive effects of thalidomide are clinically impressive, they are offset by a number of important side effects including drowsiness, nausea and peripheral neuropathy [139]. A recent study in idiopathic cough has demonstrated that the antiepileptic drug, gabapentin, has a marked effect on cough at a dose of 1,800 mg/day. This data raises the possibility that gabapentin may also be of use in cases where there is an existing cause for the cough (i.e. ILD) [140].

Conclusions

ILD is a growing and important problem which accounts for a significant burden of morbidity and mortality in individuals with CTD. Whilst the different CTDs are associated with slightly different ILDs, in the majority of patients initial autoimmune-mediated inflammatory alveolar injury results in progressive pulmonary fibrosis. This in turn leads to impaired gas exchange which causes breathlessness, exercise limitation and, frequently, cough. For physicians treating patients with CTD-ILD, the focus of therapy is threefold and involves, first and foremost, the modulation of inflammation, secondly the inhibition of fibroproliferation and thirdly the management and control of symptoms. A wide range of immunomodulatory drugs are available for use in CTD. Unfortunately, for the most part, the effects of these drugs on the course of CTD-ILD remain unknown. The best validated therapy is that of cyclophosphamide in individuals with scleroderma-ILD. Treatment developments in IPF have made effective anti-fibrotic therapy available in the clinic with the prospect of further compounds being licensed in the near future. Whilst these drugs have yet to be trialled in CTD-ILD, it seems likely, given the overlap in pathogenic mechanisms, that they should be effective across the full spectrum of fibrosing lung disease. With the increasing availability of treatments for ILD, it is of critical importance that novel regimens are tested in well-designed and appropriately powered randomised controlled trials. In this way, the burden and suffering associated with CTD-ILD should be reduced.

Case Vignette 1: Anti-synthetase Syndrome

FG, a 38-year-old Caucasian male, presented with a 4-month history of rapidly progressive exertional dyspnoea such that he was breathless on walking 10–20 yards. He had reduced appetite and had lost 5 kg in weight. He also complained of generalised aches and pains particularly in his thighs and upper arms. He had no past medical history of note and was a lifelong non-smoker. He worked as a bank manager and had no history of significant exposures. On examination oxygen saturations were 94 % on room air and dropped to 84 % after walking up a flight of stairs. On auscultation of the chest, there were occasional fine bibasal crepitations.

Chest radiograph (Fig. 14.6a) demonstrated bilateral mid and lower zone interstitial change. An HRCT (Fig. 14.6b), undertaken at the time of the presenting chest radiograph, disclosed diffuse ground glass change, with areas of consolidation and reticulation with traction bronchiectasis. A subsequent surgical lung biopsy revealed a mixed pattern of cellular and fibrotic NSIP with a marked component of organising pneumonia (a pattern frequently seen in polymyositis). At 2 months following presentation, autoimmune profile, which had been negative, demonstrated a positive speckled ANA and positive anti-Jo-1 antibody. Serum creatine kinase was 650 U/L. A diagnosis of anti-synthetase syndrome was made.

Given the severe respiratory impairment and marked oxygen desaturation on exertion, combined treatment was commenced with three daily doses of intravenous methylprednisolone (10 mg/kg) followed by a tapering oral course of prednisolone and six monthly intravenous doses of cyclophosphamide (600 mg/m^2 body surface area). Treatment led to a dramatic and sustained improvement in respiratory symptoms. By 6 months, exercise tolerance had returned to being unlimited at a steady pace on the flat and serum creatine kinase normalised. The clinical improvement was mirrored by a marked radiographic improvement (Fig. 14.6c). Four years on from presentation, the patient remains well on maintenance therapy of azathioprine (2 mg/kg) and low-dose oral prednisolone.

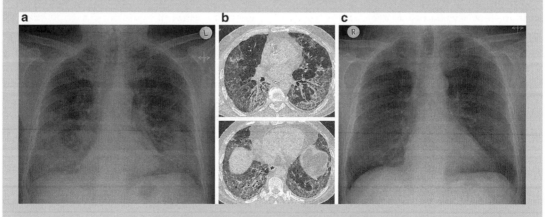

Fig. 14.6 (a–c) Plain chest radiographs and HRCT from 38-year-old man with polymyositis and associated fibrosing organising pneumonia. Radiograph on presentation (a) demonstrates bilateral lower zone interstitial change with preservation of lung volumes. High-resolution CT (b) corresponding to the presentation radiograph confirms diffuse, predominantly sub-pleural ground glass change with areas of reticulation and traction bronchiectasis admixed with consolidation. Plain chest radiograph (c) 18 months later and 12 months after completion of cyclophosphamide confirms marked improvement in previously noted interstitial change

Case Vignette 2: Diffuse Cutaneous Systemic Sclerosis

EK, a female of Middle Eastern descent, presented aged 24 years. She had a preceding 2-year history of severe Raynaud's phenomenon with digital ulceration. In the 6 months prior to presentation, she had noticed skin thickening over the hands, forearms and chest, dysphagia, 4 kg weight loss and progressively worsening exertional dyspnoea with an exercise tolerance of 30–50 yards on the flat. On clinical examination, she had microstomia, facial telangiectasia and marked skin thickening over the hands, arms and torso. Auscultation of the chest demonstrated bibasal, end-inspiratory crepitations. Autoimmune serology disclosed a positive ANA with a homogeneous pattern and a titre of 1:2560. Anti-Scl-70 antibody screen was positive. High-resolution CT of the chest (Fig. 14.7) demonstrated bilateral, basal and sub-pleural reticular change with traction bronchiectasis. Echocardiogram was normal with no evidence of pulmonary hypertension.

A diagnosis of diffuse cutaneous systemic sclerosis with associated fibrotic ILD (NSIP) was made. At the time of diagnosis the extent of ILD on CT was judged to be 25 %. Lung function demonstrated an FVC of 2.44 (67 % predicted) and TLco was 43 % predicted. On the basis that the patient fulfilled the criteria for extensive ILD treat-

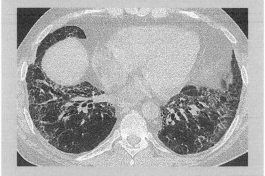

Fig. 14.7 HRCT from 24-year-old female with Scl-70-positive diffuse cutaneous systemic sclerosis. Section through the lung bases shows the characteristic appearance of scleroderma NSIP with sub-pleural reticular change, coarse ground glass and marked traction bronchiectasis

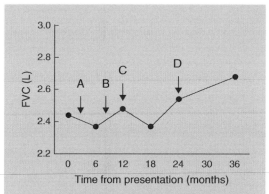

Fig. 14.8 Graph plotting change in forced vital capacity with treatment for a 26-year-old female with Scl-70-positive diffuse cutaneous systemic sclerosis. Baseline value represents date of first presentation. Treatment was commenced with intravenous cyclophosphamide and low-dose prednisolone at 2 months following presentation (A) and continued monthly for 6 months (B). Following cessation of cyclophosphamide, the patient was started on treatment with oral mycophenolate mofetil (C). Because the patient wished to become pregnant, mycophenolate was changed to azathioprine at 24 months (D)

ment was commenced with monthly doses of intravenous cyclophosphamide (600 mg/m² body surface area) and oral prednisolone (10 mg/daily). The Raynaud's was treated with losartan and a proton-pump inhibitor was commenced for symptoms of gastro-oesophageal reflux. After six doses of cyclophosphamide, treatment was changed to MMF (at a maintenance dose of 1 g twice daily), and the patient was continued on her regular dose of prednisolone.

At 24 months after presentation, EK was symptomatically much improved. She had gained 8 kg in weight with a BMI of 20.5, her exercise tolerance had become unlimited on the flat, and her skin thickening was improved with Rodnan skin score reducing from 21/51 to 11/51. By this time, the patient had married and was keen to start a family. Consequently, mycophenolate was changed to azathioprine (125 mg/daily) and losartan was stopped. Prednisolone has been continued at a dose of 7.5 mg daily. At 36 months following diagnosis, improvement has been sustained. As demonstrated in Fig. 14.8, FVC shows an upward trend and now stands at 2.68 (74 % predicted).

Case Vignette 3: Idiopathic Pulmonary Fibrosis

HT, a Caucasian male, presented aged 64 with a 3-month history of mild exertional breathlessness and troublesome dry cough. He was otherwise well with no constitutional or extra-thoracic symptoms of note. He was on no medications and had been a lifelong non-smoker. He had previously worked in dusty factory environments but had never knowingly been exposed to asbestos. Clinical examination was normal apart from fine, bibasal end-inspiratory crepitations. HRCT demonstrated bilateral lower zone reticular change with traction bronchiectasis. Surgical lung biopsy disclosed the lesion of UIP. Following multidisciplinary assessment, a diagnosis of idiopathic pulmonary fibrosis was made.

FVC at presentation was 3.03 L (66 % predicted) with a TLco 72 % predicted. Following lung biopsy, there was a stepwise deterioration in HT's exercise tolerance with a corresponding decline in his lung function. A repeat CT (Fig. 14.9) demonstrated progression of fibrosis with early honeycombing. Treatment was therefore commenced with a combination of NAC (600 mg three times daily) and pir-

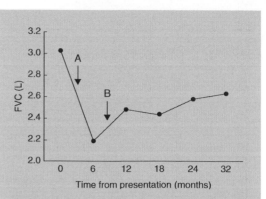

Fig. 14.10 Graph plotting change in forced vital capacity with treatment for a 64-year-old man with idiopathic pulmonary fibrosis. Baseline value represents date of first presentation. Video-assisted thoracic surgical biopsy was undertaken at 3 months. Treatment with combination *N*-acetylcysteine and pirfenidone was commenced at 9 months. The patient remains on this therapeutic regimen

fenidone (801 mg three times daily). After 2½ years of treatment, the patient remains symptomatically well with an unchanged exercise tolerance. FVC has remained stable (Fig. 14.10) and stands at 2.63 (60 % predicted), whilst TLco is 56 % predicted.

Acknowledgments Toby M. Maher is in receipt of an unrestricted academic industry grant from GSK. In the last 3 years, T.M. has received advisory board or consultancy fees from Actelion, Boehringer Ingelheim, GSK, Respironics, InterMune and Sanofi-Aventis. T.M. has received speaker's fees from UCB, Boehringer Ingelheim, InterMune and AstraZeneca. T.M.'s institution has received an unrestricted educational grant from InterMune and consultancy fees on his behalf from Novartis and Takeda.

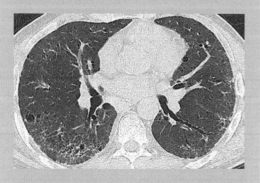

Fig. 14.9 HRCT obtained from 64-year-old man 9 months after diagnosis of idiopathic pulmonary fibrosis. The CT demonstrates the typical changes associated with the histological lesion of usual interstitial pneumonia with bilateral, basal, subpleural reticular change, early honeycombing and striking traction bronchiectasis

References

1. Tyndall AJ, Bannert B, Vonk M, et al. Causes and risk factors for death in systemic sclerosis: a study from the EULAR Scleroderma Trials and Research (EUSTAR) database. Ann Rheum Dis. 2010;69: 1809–15.

2. Olson AL, Swigris JJ, Sprunger DB, et al. Rheumatoid arthritis-interstitial lung disease-associated mortality. Am J Respir Crit Care Med. 2011;183:372–8.

3. Kim EJ, Elicker BM, Maldonado F, et al. Usual interstitial pneumonia in rheumatoid arthritis-associated interstitial lung disease. Eur Respir J. 2010;35:1322–8.

4. Kim EJ, Collard HR, King Jr TE. Rheumatoid arthritis-associated interstitial lung disease: the relevance of histopathologic and radiographic pattern. Chest. 2009;136:1397–405.

5. Koduri G, Norton S, Young A, et al. Interstitial lung disease has a poor prognosis in rheumatoid arthritis: results from an inception cohort. Rheumatology. 2010;49:1483–9.

6. Shidara K, Hoshi D, Inoue E, et al. Incidence of and risk factors for interstitial pneumonia in patients with rheumatoid arthritis in a large Japanese observational cohort, IORRA. Mod Rheumatol. 2010;20:280–6.

7. Bongartz T, Nannini C, Medina-Velasquez YF, et al. Incidence and mortality of interstitial lung disease in rheumatoid arthritis: a population-based study. Arthritis Rheum. 2010;62:1583–91.

8. Morgan C, Knight C, Lunt M, Black CM, Silman AJ. Predictors of end stage lung disease in a cohort of patients with scleroderma. Ann Rheum Dis. 2003;62:146–50.

9. Saketkoo LA, Ascherman DP, Cottin V, Christopher-Stine L, Danoff SK, Oddis CV. Interstitial lung disease in idiopathic inflammatory myopathy. Curr Rheumatol Rev. 2010;6:108–19.

10. Lega JC, Cottin V, Fabien N, Thivolet-Bejui F, Cordier JF. Interstitial lung disease associated with anti-PM/Scl or anti-aminoacyl-tRNA synthetase autoantibodies: a similar condition? J Rheumatol. 2010;37:1000–9.

11. Maher TM, Wells AU, Laurent GJ. Idiopathic pulmonary fibrosis: multiple causes and multiple mechanisms? Eur Respir J. 2007;30:835–9.

12. Idiopathic Pulmonary Fibrosis Clinical Research N, Raghu G, Anstrom KJ, King TE, Jr., Lasky JA, Martinez FJ. Prednisone, azathioprine, and N-acetylcysteine for pulmonary fibrosis. The New England journal of medicine 2012;366:1968–77.

13. Renzoni EA, Abraham DJ, Howat S, et al. Gene expression profiling reveals novel TGFbeta targets in adult lung fibroblasts. Respir Res. 2004;5:24.

14. Mutlu GM, Budinger GR, Wu M, et al. Proteasomal inhibition after injury prevents fibrosis by modulating TGF-beta(1) signalling. Thorax. 2012;67:139–46.

15. Maher TM, Evans IC, Bottoms SE, et al. Diminished prostaglandin E2 contributes to the apoptosis paradox in idiopathic pulmonary fibrosis. Am J Respir Crit Care Med. 2010;182:73–82.

16. Keerthisingam CB, Jenkins RG, Harrison NK, et al. Cyclooxygenase-2 deficiency results in a loss of the anti-proliferative response to transforming growth factor-beta in human fibrotic lung fibroblasts and promotes bleomycin-induced pulmonary fibrosis in mice. Am J Pathol. 2001;158:1411–22.

17. Goh NS, Desai SR, Veeraraghavan S, et al. Interstitial lung disease in systemic sclerosis: a simple staging system. Am J Respir Crit Care Med. 2008; 177:1248–54.

18. Navaratnam V, Ali N, Smith CJ, McKeever T, Fogarty A, Hubbard RB. Does the presence of connective tissue disease modify survival in patients with pulmonary fibrosis? Respir Med. 2011;105: 1925–30.

19. Latsi PI, Wells AU. Evaluation and management of alveolitis and interstitial lung disease in scleroderma. Curr Opin Rheumatol. 2003;15:748–55.

20. Assassi S, Sharif R, Lasky RE, et al. Predictors of interstitial lung disease in early systemic sclerosis: a prospective longitudinal study of the GENISOS cohort. Arthritis Res Ther. 2010;12:R166.

21. Bouros D, Wells AU, Nicholson AG, et al. Histopathologic subsets of fibrosing alveolitis in patients with systemic sclerosis and their relationship to outcome. Am J Respir Crit Care Med. 2002; 165:1581–6.

22. Desai SR, Veeraraghavan S, Hansell DM, et al. CT features of lung disease in patients with systemic sclerosis: comparison with idiopathic pulmonary fibrosis and nonspecific interstitial pneumonia. Radiology. 2004;232:560–7.

23. Tashkin DP, Elashoff R, Clements PJ, et al. Cyclophosphamide versus placebo in scleroderma lung disease. N Engl J Med. 2006;354:2655–66.

24. Hoyles RK, Ellis RW, Wellsbury J, et al. A multicenter, prospective, randomized, double-blind, placebo-controlled trial of corticosteroids and intravenous cyclophosphamide followed by oral azathioprine for the treatment of pulmonary fibrosis in scleroderma. Arthritis Rheum. 2006;54:3962–70.

25. Wells AU, Latsi P, McCune WJ. Daily cyclophosphamide for scleroderma: are patients with the most to gain underrepresented in this trial? Am J Respir Crit Care Med. 2007;176:952–3.

26. Domiciano DS, Bonfa E, Borges CT, et al. A long-term prospective randomized controlled study of non-specific interstitial pneumonia (NSIP) treatment in scleroderma. Clin Rheumatol. 2011;30:223–9.

27. Broad K, Pope JE. The efficacy of treatment for systemic sclerosis interstitial lung disease: results from a meta-analysis. Medical science monitor : international medical journal of experimental and clinical research 2010;16:Ra187-90.

28. Wanchu A, Suryanaryana BS, Sharma S, Sharma A, Bambery P. High-dose prednisolone and bolus cyclophosphamide in interstitial lung disease associated with systemic sclerosis: a prospective open study. Int J Rheum Dis. 2009;12:239–42.

29. Berezne A, Ranque B, Valeyre D, et al. Therapeutic strategy combining intravenous cyclophosphamide followed by oral azathioprine to treat worsening interstitial lung disease associated with systemic sclerosis: a retrospective multicenter open-label study. J Rheumatol. 2008;35:1064–72.

30. White B, Moore WC, Wigley FM, Xiao HQ, Wise RA. Cyclophosphamide is associated with pulmonary function and survival benefit in patients with scleroderma and alveolitis. Ann Intern Med. 2000; 132:947–54.

31. Theodore AC, Tseng CH, Li N, Elashoff RM, Tashkin DP. Correlation of cough with disease activity and treatment with cyclophosphamide in scleroderma interstitial lung disease: findings from the Scleroderma Lung Study. Chest. 2012;142:614–21.

32. Roth MD, Tseng CH, Clements PJ, et al. Predicting treatment outcomes and responder subsets in scleroderma-related interstitial lung disease. Arthritis Rheum. 2011;63:2797–808.

33. Dheda K, Lalloo UG, Cassim B, Mody GM. Experience with azathioprine in systemic sclerosis associated with interstitial lung disease. Clin Rheumatol. 2004;23:306–9.

34. Leandro MJ, Cambridge G, Ehrenstein MR, Edwards JC. Reconstitution of peripheral blood B cells after depletion with rituximab in patients with rheumatoid arthritis. Arthritis Rheum. 2006;54:613–20.

35. Isaacs JD, Cohen SB, Emery P, et al. Effect of baseline rheumatoid factor and anticitrullinated peptide antibody serotype on rituximab clinical response: a meta-analysis. Ann Rheum Dis. 2013;72:329–36.

36. Keystone EC, Cohen SB, Emery P, et al. Multiple courses of rituximab produce sustained clinical and radiographic efficacy and safety in patients with rheumatoid arthritis and an inadequate response to 1 or more tumor necrosis factor inhibitors: 5-year data from the REFLEX study. J Rheumatol. 2012;39: 2238–46.

37. Emery P, Fleischmann R, Filipowicz-Sosnowska A, et al. The efficacy and safety of rituximab in patients with active rheumatoid arthritis despite methotrexate treatment: results of a phase IIB randomized, double-blind, placebo-controlled, dose-ranging trial. Arthritis Rheum. 2006;54:1390–400.

38. Jones RB, Tervaert JW, Hauser T, et al. Rituximab versus cyclophosphamide in ANCA-associated renal vasculitis. N Engl J Med. 2010;363:211–20.

39. Stone JH, Merkel PA, Spiera R, et al. Rituximab versus cyclophosphamide for ANCA-associated vasculitis. N Engl J Med. 2010;363:221–32.

40. Arnold DM, Dentali F, Crowther MA, et al. Systematic review: efficacy and safety of rituximab for adults with idiopathic thrombocytopenic purpura. Ann Intern Med. 2007;146:25–33.

41. Daoussis D, Liossis SN, Tsamandas AC, et al. Effect of long-term treatment with rituximab on pulmonary function and skin fibrosis in patients with diffuse systemic sclerosis. Clin Exp Rheumatol. 2012;30: S17–22.

42. Ando K, Motojima S, Doi T, et al. Effect of glucocorticoid monotherapy on pulmonary function and survival in Japanese patients with scleroderma-related interstitial lung disease. Respir Investig. 2013;51:69–75.

43. Vanthuyne M, Blockmans D, Westhovens R, et al. A pilot study of mycophenolate mofetil combined to intravenous methylprednisolone pulses and oral low-dose glucocorticoids in severe early systemic sclerosis. Clin Exp Rheumatol. 2007;25:287–92.

44. Simeon-Aznar CP, Fonollosa-Pla V, Tolosa-Vilella C, Selva-O'Callaghan A, Solans-Laque R, Vilardell-Tarres M. Effect of mycophenolate sodium in scleroderma-related interstitial lung disease. Clin Rheumatol. 2011;30:1393–8.

45. Koutroumpas A, Ziogas A, Alexiou I, Barouta G, Sakkas LI. Mycophenolate mofetil in systemic sclerosis-associated interstitial lung disease. Clin Rheumatol. 2010;29:1167–8.

46. Gerbino AJ, Goss CH, Molitor JA. Effect of mycophenolate mofetil on pulmonary function in scleroderma-associated interstitial lung disease. Chest. 2008;133:455–60.

47. Swigris JJ, Olson AL, Fischer A, et al. Mycophenolate mofetil is safe, well tolerated, and preserves lung function in patients with connective tissue disease-related interstitial lung disease. Chest. 2006;130: 30–6.

48. Fischer A, Brown KK, Du Bois RM, et al. Mycophenolate mofetil improves lung function in connective tissue disease-associated interstitial lung disease. J Rheumatol. 2013;40:640–6.

49. Daniels CE, Wilkes MC, Edens M, et al. Imatinib mesylate inhibits the profibrogenic activity of TGF-beta and prevents bleomycin-mediated lung fibrosis. J Clin Invest. 2004;114:1308–16.

50. Sabnani I, Zucker MJ, Rosenstein ED, et al. A novel therapeutic approach to the treatment of scleroderma-associated pulmonary complications: safety and efficacy of combination therapy with imatinib and cyclophosphamide. Rheumatology. 2009;48:49–52.

51. Spiera RF, Gordon JK, Mersten JN, et al. Imatinib mesylate (Gleevec) in the treatment of diffuse cutaneous systemic sclerosis: results of a 1-year, phase IIa, single-arm, open-label clinical trial. Ann Rheum Dis. 2011;70:1003–9.

52. Khanna D, Saggar R, Mayes MD, et al. A one-year, phase I/IIa, open-label pilot trial of imatinib mesylate in the treatment of systemic sclerosis-associated active interstitial lung disease. Arthritis Rheum. 2011;63:3540–6.

53. Burt RK, Shah SJ, Dill K, et al. Autologous non-myeloablative haemopoietic stem-cell transplantation compared with pulse cyclophosphamide once per month for systemic sclerosis (ASSIST): an open-label, randomised phase 2 trial. Lancet. 2011;378: 498–506.

54. Park SH, Saleh D, Giaid A, Michel RP. Increased endothelin-1 in bleomycin-induced pulmonary fibrosis and the effect of an endothelin receptor antagonist. Am J Respir Crit Care Med. 1997;156: 600–8.

55. King Jr TE, Behr J, Brown KK, et al. BUILD-1: a randomized placebo-controlled trial of bosentan in

idiopathic pulmonary fibrosis. Am J Respir Crit Care Med. 2008;177:75–81.

56. Seibold JR, Denton CP, Furst DE, et al. Randomized, prospective, placebo-controlled trial of bosentan in interstitial lung disease secondary to systemic sclerosis. Arthritis Rheum. 2010;62:2101–8.

57. Ingegnoli F, Lubatti C, Ingegnoli A, Boracchi P, Zeni S, Meroni PL. Interstitial lung disease outcomes by high-resolution computed tomography (HRCT) in Anti-Jo1 antibody-positive polymyositis patients: a single centre study and review of the literature. Autoimmun Rev. 2012;11:335–40.

58. Mok CC, To CH, Szeto ML. Successful treatment of dermatomyositis-related rapidly progressive interstitial pneumonitis with sequential oral cyclophosphamide and azathioprine. Scand J Rheumatol. 2003;32:181–3.

59. Keir GJ, Maher TM, Hansell DM, et al. Severe interstitial lung disease in connective tissue disease: Rituximab as rescue therapy. Eur Respir J. 2012; 40(3):641–8.

60. Labirua-Iturburu A, Selva-O'Callaghan A, Martinez-Gomez X, Trallero-Araguas E, Labrador-Horrillo M, Vilardell-Tarres M. Calcineurin inhibitors in a cohort of patients with antisynthetase-associated interstitial lung disease. Clin Exp Rheumatol. 2013;31:436–9.

61. Bakewell CJ, Raghu G. Polymyositis associated with severe interstitial lung disease: remission after three doses of IV immunoglobulin. Chest. 2011;139: 441–3.

62. Bozkirli DE, Kozanoglu I, Bozkirli E, Yucel E. Antisynthetase syndrome with refractory lung involvement and myositis successfully treated with double filtration plasmapheresis. J Clin Apher. 2013; 28(6):422–5.

63. Lindberg C, Trysberg E, Tarkowski A, Oldfors A. Anti-T-lymphocyte globulin treatment in inclusion body myositis: a randomized pilot study. Neurology. 2003;61:260–2.

64. Gordon PA, Winer JB, Hoogendijk JE, Choy EH. Immunosuppressant and immunomodulatory treatment for dermatomyositis and polymyositis. The Cochrane database of systematic reviews 2012;8: Cd003643.

65. Thompson B, Corris P, Miller JA, Cooper RG, Halsey JP, Isaacs JD. Alemtuzumab (Campath-1H) for treatment of refractory polymyositis. J Rheumatol. 2008;35:2080–2.

66. Park JK, Yoo HG, Ahn DS, Jeon HS, Yoo WH. Successful treatment for conventional treatment-resistant dermatomyositis-associated interstitial lung disease with adalimumab. Rheumatol Int. 2012;32: 3587–90.

67. Zong M, Dorph C, Dastmalchi M, et al. Anakinra treatment in patients with refractory inflammatory myopathies and possible predictive response biomarkers: a mechanistic study with 12 months follow-up. Annals of the rheumatic diseases; Epub 2013 Apr 26.

68. Furlan A, Botsios C, Ruffatti A, Todesco S, Punzi L. Antisynthetase syndrome with refractory polyarthritis and fever successfully treated with the IL-1 receptor antagonist, anakinra: A case report. Joint Bone Spine. 2008;75:366–7.

69. Solomon JJ, Ryu JH, Tazelaar HD, et al. Fibrosing interstitial pneumonia predicts survival in patients with rheumatoid arthritis-associated interstitial lung disease (RA-ILD). Respir Med. 2013;107(8):1247–52.

70. Vij R, Strek ME. Diagnosis and treatment of connective tissue disease-associated interstitial lung disease. Chest. 2013;143:814–24.

71. Saketkoo LA, Espinoza LR. Rheumatoid arthritis interstitial lung disease: mycophenolate mofetil as an antifibrotic and disease-modifying antirheumatic drug. Arch Intern Med. 2008;168:1718–9.

72. Antoniou KM, Mamoulaki M, Malagari K, et al. Infliximab therapy in pulmonary fibrosis associated with collagen vascular disease. Clin Exp Rheumatol. 2007;25:23–8.

73. Mohr M, Jacobi AM. Interstitial lung disease in rheumatoid arthritis: response to IL-6R blockade. Scand J Rheumatol. 2011;40:400–1.

74. Atzeni F, Boiardi L, Salli S, Benucci M, Sarzi-Puttini P. Lung involvement and drug-induced lung disease in patients with rheumatoid arthritis. Expert Rev Clin Immunol. 2013;9:649–57.

75. Perez-Alvarez R, Perez-de-Lis M, Diaz-Lagares C, et al. Interstitial lung disease induced or exacerbated by TNF-targeted therapies: analysis of 122 cases. Semin Arthritis Rheum. 2011;41:256–64.

76. Gutsche M, Rosen GD, Swigris JJ. Connective tissue disease-associated interstitial lung disease: a review. Curr Respir Care Rep. 2012;1:224–32.

77. Fischer A, Swigris JJ, du Bois RM, et al. Minor salivary gland biopsy to detect primary Sjogren syndrome in patients with interstitial lung disease. Chest. 2009;136:1072–8.

78. Swigris JJ, Berry GJ, Raffin TA, Kuschner WG. Lymphoid interstitial pneumonia: a narrative review. Chest. 2002;122:2150–64.

79. Borie R, Schneider S, Debray MP, et al. Severe chronic bronchiolitis as the presenting feature of primary Sjogren's syndrome. Respir Med. 2011;105: 130–6.

80. Watanabe M, Naniwa T, Hara M, Arakawa T, Maeda T. Pulmonary manifestations in Sjogren's syndrome: correlation analysis between chest computed tomographic findings and clinical subsets with poor prognosis in 80 patients. J Rheumatol. 2010;37:365–73.

81. Parambil JG, Myers JL, Lindell RM, Matteson EL, Ryu JH. Interstitial lung disease in primary Sjogren syndrome. Chest. 2006;130:1489–95.

82. Ito I, Nagai S, Kitaichi M, et al. Pulmonary manifestations of primary Sjogren's syndrome: a clinical, radiologic, and pathologic study. Am J Respir Crit Care Med. 2005;171:632–8.

83. Seror R, Sordet C, Guillevin L, et al. Tolerance and efficacy of rituximab and changes in serum B cell

biomarkers in patients with systemic complications of primary Sjogren's syndrome. Ann Rheum Dis. 2007;66:351–7.

84. Kokosi M, Riemer EC, Highland KB. Pulmonary involvement in Sjogren syndrome. Clin Chest Med. 2010;31:489–500.

85. Fischer A, du Bois R. Interstitial lung disease in connective tissue disorders. Lancet. 2012;380:689–98.

86. Travis WD, Hunninghake G, King Jr TE, et al. Idiopathic nonspecific interstitial pneumonia: report of an American Thoracic Society project. Am J Respir Crit Care Med. 2008;177:1338–47.

87. Kinder BW, Collard HR, Koth L, et al. Idiopathic nonspecific interstitial pneumonia: lung manifestation of undifferentiated connective tissue disease? Am J Respir Crit Care Med. 2007;176:691–7.

88. Corte TJ, Copley SJ, Desai SR, et al. Significance of connective tissue disease features in idiopathic interstitial pneumonia. Eur Respir J. 2012;39:661–8.

89. Maher TM. Beyond the diagnosis of idiopathic pulmonary fibrosis; the growing role of systems biology and stratified medicine. Curr Opin Pulm Med. 2013;19:460–5.

90. Raghu G, Brown KK, Bradford WZ, et al. A placebo-controlled trial of interferon gamma-1b in patients with idiopathic pulmonary fibrosis. N Engl J Med. 2004;350:125–33.

91. Maher TM. Pirfenidone in idiopathic pulmonary fibrosis. Drugs Today (Barc). 2010;46:473–82.

92. Raghu G, Collard HR, Anstrom KJ, et al. Idiopathic pulmonary fibrosis: clinically meaningful primary endpoints in phase 3 clinical trials. Am J Respir Crit Care Med. 2012;185:1044–8.

93. Wells AU, Behr J, Costabel U, et al. Hot of the breath: mortality as a primary end-point in IPF treatment trials: the best is the enemy of the good. Thorax. 2012;67:938–40.

94. Vancheri C, du Bois RM. A progression-free endpoint for idiopathic pulmonary fibrosis trials: lessons from cancer. Eur Respir J. 2013;41:262–9.

95. Gurujeyalakshmi G, Hollinger MA, Giri SN. Pirfenidone inhibits PDGF isoforms in bleomycin hamster model of lung fibrosis at the translational level. Am J Physiol. 1999;276:L311–8.

96. Iyer SN, Gurujeyalakshmi G, Giri SN. Effects of pirfenidone on transforming growth factor-beta gene expression at the transcriptional level in bleomycin hamster model of lung fibrosis. J Pharmacol Exp Ther. 1999;291:367–73.

97. Iyer SN, Gurujeyalakshmi G, Giri SN. Effects of pirfenidone on procollagen gene expression at the transcriptional level in bleomycin hamster model of lung fibrosis. J Pharmacol Exp Ther. 1999;289:211–8.

98. Oku H, Shimizu T, Kawabata T, et al. Antifibrotic action of pirfenidone and prednisolone: different effects on pulmonary cytokines and growth factors in bleomycin-induced murine pulmonary fibrosis. Eur J Pharmacol. 2008;590:400–8.

99. Azuma A, Nukiwa T, Tsuboi E, et al. Double-blind, placebo-controlled trial of pirfenidone in patients with idiopathic pulmonary fibrosis. Am J Respir Crit Care Med. 2005;171:1040–7.

100. Taniguchi H, Ebina M, Kondoh Y, et al. Pirfenidone in idiopathic pulmonary fibrosis. Eur Respir J. 2010;35:821–9.

101. Noble PW, Albera C, Bradford WZ, et al. Pirfenidone in patients with idiopathic pulmonary fibrosis (CAPACITY): two randomised trials. Lancet. 2011;377:1760–9.

102. Spagnolo P, Del Giovane C, Luppi F, et al. Non-steroid agents for idiopathic pulmonary fibrosis. The Cochrane database of systematic reviews 2010:CD003134.

103. Demedts M, Behr J, Buhl R, et al. High-dose acetylcysteine in idiopathic pulmonary fibrosis. N Engl J Med. 2005;353:2229–42.

104. Cantin AM, Hubbard RC, Crystal RG. Glutathione deficiency in the epithelial lining fluid of the lower respiratory tract in idiopathic pulmonary fibrosis. Am Rev Respir Dis. 1989;139:370–2.

105. Kinnula VL, Hodgson UA, Lakari EK, et al. Extracellular superoxide dismutase has a highly specific localization in idiopathic pulmonary fibrosis/usual interstitial pneumonia. Histopathology. 2006;49:66–74.

106. Behr J, Maier K, Degenkolb B, Krombach F, Vogelmeier C. Antioxidative and clinical effects of high-dose N-acetylcysteine in fibrosing alveolitis. Adjunctive therapy to maintenance immunosuppression. Am J Respir Crit Care Med. 1997;156:1897–901.

107. Woodcock HV, Molyneaux PL, Maher TM. Reducing lung function decline in patients with idiopathic pulmonary fibrosis: potential of nintedanib. Drug Des Dev Ther. 2013;7:503–10.

108. Roth GJ, Heckel A, Colbatzky F, et al. Design, synthesis, and evaluation of indolinones as triple angio-kinase inhibitors and the discovery of a highly specific 6-methoxycarbonyl-substituted indolinone (BIBF 1120). J Med Chem. 2009;52:4466–80.

109. Richeldi L, Costabel U, Selman M, et al. Efficacy of a tyrosine kinase inhibitor in idiopathic pulmonary fibrosis. N Engl J Med. 2011;365:1079–87.

110. Richeldi L, Brown KK, Costabel U, et al. Efficacy of the tyrosine kinase inhibitor BIBF 1120 in patients with IPF: consistent pattern of primary endpoint results in sensitivity analyses of the TOMORROW trial. Am J Respir Crit Care Med. 2012;185:A3633.

111. Brown KK, Richeldi L, Costabel U, et al. Treatment of IPF with the tyrosine kinase inhibitor BIBF 1120: patient-reported outcomes in the TOMORROW trial. Am J Respir Crit Care Med. 2012;185:A3634.

112. Maher TM. Idiopathic pulmonary fibrosis: pathobiology of novel approaches to treatment. Clin Chest Med. 2012;33:69–83.

113. Raghu G, Meyer KC. Silent gastro-oesophageal reflux and microaspiration in IPF: mounting evidence for anti-reflux therapy? Eur Respir J. 2012;39:242–5.

114. Raghu G, Yang ST, Spada C, Hayes J, Pellegrini CA. Sole treatment of acid gastroesophageal reflux in idiopathic pulmonary fibrosis: a case series. Chest. 2006;129:794–800.

115. Lee JS, Ryu JH, Elicker BM, et al. Gastroesophageal reflux therapy is associated with longer survival in idiopathic pulmonary fibrosis. Am J Respir Crit Care Med. 2011;184(12):1390–4.

116. Amara N, Goven D, Prost F, Muloway R, Crestani B, Boczkowski J. NOX4/NADPH oxidase expression is increased in pulmonary fibroblasts from patients with idiopathic pulmonary fibrosis and mediates TGFbeta1-induced fibroblast differentiation into myofibroblasts. Thorax. 2010;65:733–8.

117. Laleu B, Gaggini F, Orchard M, et al. First in class, potent, and orally bioavailable NADPH oxidase isoform 4 (Nox4) inhibitors for the treatment of idiopathic pulmonary fibrosis. J Med Chem. 2010;53: 7715–30.

118. Shulgina L, Cahn AP, Chilvers ER, et al. Treating idiopathic pulmonary fibrosis with the addition of co-trimoxazole: a randomised controlled trial. Thorax. 2013;68:155–62.

119. Egan JJ, Adamali HI, Lok SS, Stewart JP, Woodcock AA. Ganciclovir antiviral therapy in advanced idiopathic pulmonary fibrosis: an open pilot study. Pulm Med. 2011;2011:240805.

120. Noth I, Anstrom KJ, Calvert SB, et al. A placebo-controlled randomized trial of warfarin in idiopathic pulmonary fibrosis. Am J Respir Crit Care Med. 2012;186:88–95.

121. Scotton CJ, Krupiczojc MA, Konigshoff M, et al. Increased local expression of coagulation factor X contributes to the fibrotic response in human and murine lung injury. J Clin Invest. 2009;119: 2550–63.

122. Chambers RC. Procoagulant signalling mechanisms in lung inflammation and fibrosis: novel opportunities for pharmacological intervention? Br J Pharmacol. 2008;153:S367–S78.

123. Mizuno S, Matsumoto K, Li MY, Nakamura T. HGF reduces advancing lung fibrosis in mice: a potential role for MMP-dependent myofibroblast apoptosis. FASEB J. 2005;19:580–2.

124. Phan SH. Biology of fibroblasts and myofibroblasts. Proc Am Thorac Soc. 2008;5:334–7.

125. Mackay LS, Anderson RL, Parry G, Lordan J, Corris PA, Fisher AJ. Pulmonary fibrosis: rate of disease progression as a trigger for referral for lung transplantation. Thorax. 2007;62:1069–73.

126. Christie JD, Edwards LB, Kucheryavaya AY, et al. The Registry of the International Society for Heart and Lung Transplantation: twenty-seventh official adult lung and heart-lung transplant report—2010. J Heart Lung Transplant. 2010;29:1104–18.

127. Schachna L, Medsger Jr TA, Dauber JH, et al. Lung transplantation in scleroderma compared with idiopathic pulmonary fibrosis and idiopathic pulmonary arterial hypertension. Arthritis Rheum. 2006;54: 3954–61.

128. Massad MG, Powell CR, Kpodonu J, et al. Outcomes of lung transplantation in patients with scleroderma. World J Surg. 2005;29:1510–5.

129. Orens JB, Estenne M, Arcasoy S, et al. International guidelines for the selection of lung transplant candidates: 2006 update—a consensus report from the Pulmonary Scientific Council of the International Society for Heart and Lung Transplantation. J Heart Lung Transpl. 2006;25:745–55.

130. Kon SS, Clark AL, Dilaver D, et al. Response of the COPD Assessment Test to pulmonary rehabilitation in unselected chronic respiratory disease. Respirology. 2013;18:974–7.

131. Polkey MI, Moxham J. Attacking the disease spiral in chronic obstructive pulmonary disease: an update. Clin Med. 2011;11:461–4.

132. Bajwah S, Ross JR, Peacock JL, et al. Interventions to improve symptoms and quality of life of patients with fibrotic interstitial lung disease: a systematic review of the literature. Thorax. 2013;68(9): 867–79.

133. Swigris JJ, Fairclough DL, Morrison M, et al. Benefits of pulmonary rehabilitation in idiopathic pulmonary fibrosis. Respir Care. 2011;56:783–9.

134. Ryerson CJ, Garvey C, Collard HR. Pulmonary rehabilitation for interstitial lung disease. Chest. 2010;138:240–1; author reply 1–2.

135. Swigris JJ, Brown KK, Make BJ, Wamboldt FS. Pulmonary rehabilitation in idiopathic pulmonary fibrosis: a call for continued investigation. Respir Med. 2008;102:1675–80.

136. Visca D, Montgomery A, de Lauretis A, et al. Ambulatory oxygen in interstitial lung disease. Eur Respir J. 2011;38:987–90.

137. Ryerson CJ, Collard HR, Pantilat SZ. Management of dyspnea in interstitial lung disease. Curr Opin Support Palliat Care. 2010;4:69–75.

138. Horton MR, Danoff SK, Lechtzin N. Thalidomide inhibits the intractable cough of idiopathic pulmonary fibrosis. Thorax. 2008;63:749.

139. Horton MR, Santopietro V, Mathew L, et al. Thalidomide for the treatment of cough in idiopathic pulmonary fibrosis: a randomized trial. Ann Intern Med. 2012;157:398–406.

140. Ryan NM, Birring SS, Gibson PG. Gabapentin for refractory chronic cough: a randomised, double-blind, placebo-controlled trial. Lancet. 2012;380: 1583–9.

141. Kubo H, Nakayama K, Yanai M, et al. Anticoagulant therapy for idiopathic pulmonary fibrosis. Chest. 2005;128:1475–82.

142. Raghu G, Brown KK, Costabel U, et al. Treatment of idiopathic pulmonary fibrosis with etanercept: an exploratory, placebo-controlled trial. Am J Respir Crit Care Med. 2008;178:948–55.

143. King Jr TE, Albera C, Bradford WZ, et al. Effect of interferon gamma-1b on survival in patients with idiopathic pulmonary fibrosis (INSPIRE): a multi-centre, randomised, placebo-controlled trial. Lancet. 2009;374:222–8.

144. Daniels CE, Lasky JA, Limper AH, Mieras K, Gabor E, Schroeder DR. Imatinib treatment for idiopathic pulmonary fibrosis: Randomized placebo-controlled trial results. Am J Respir Crit Care Med. 2010;181:604–10.

145. Zisman DA, Schwarz M, Anstrom KJ, Collard HR, Flaherty KR, Hunninghake GW. A controlled trial of sildenafil in advanced idiopathic pulmonary fibrosis. N Engl J Med. 2010;363:620–8.

146. King Jr TE, Brown KK, Raghu G, et al. BUILD-3: a randomized, controlled trial of bosentan in idiopathic pulmonary fibrosis. Am J Respir Crit Care Med. 2011;184:92–9.

147. Raghu G, Behr J, Brown KK, et al. Treatment of idiopathic pulmonary fibrosis with ambrisentan: a parallel, randomized trial. Ann Intern Med. 2013;158:641–9.

Index

Printed by Publishers' Graphics LLC
LMO140615.23.35.4